Comprehensive Healthcare Simulation

Series Editors

Adam I. Levine, Department of Anesthesiology, Mount Sinai Medical Center, New York, USA

Samuel DeMaria Jr., Department of Anesthesiology, Mount Sinai Medical Center, New York, USA

This series focuses on the use of simulation in healthcare education, one of the most exciting and significant innovations in healthcare teaching since Halsted put forth the paradigm of "see one, do one, teach one." Each volume focuses either on the use of simulation in teaching in a specific specialty or on a cross-cutting topic of broad interest, such as the development of a simulation center. The volumes stand alone and are also designed to complement Levine, DeMaria, Schwartz, and Sim, eds., THE COMPREHENSIVE TEXTBOOK OF HEALTHCARE SIMULATION by providing detailed and practical guidance beyond the scope of the larger book and presenting the most up-to-date information available. Series Editors Drs. Adam I. Levine and Samuel DeMaria Jr. are affiliated with the Icahn School of Medicine at Mount Sinai, New York, New York, USA, home to one of the foremost simulation centers in healthcare education. Dr. Levine is widely regarded as a pioneer in the use of simulation in healthcare education. Editors of individual series volumes and their contributors are all recognized leaders in simulation-based healthcare education.

Cathy M. Smith • Nemat Alsaba
Lisa Guttman Sokoloff • Debra Nestel
Editors

Comprehensive Healthcare Simulation: Geriatric Simulation

A Focus on Older Adults as Simulated Participants

Springer

Editors
Cathy M. Smith
Baycrest Academy for Research and Education
Baycrest Centre for Geriatric Care
Toronto, ON, Canada

Nemat Alsaba
Faculty of Health Sciences and Medicine
Bond University
Gold Coast, QLD, Australia

Lisa Guttman Sokoloff
Faculty of Applied Health and Community Studies
Sheridan College
Brampton, ON, Canada

Debra Nestel
School of Clinical Sciences, Faculty of Medicine
Nursing & Health Sciences, Monash University
Clayton, VIC, Australia

ISSN 2366-4479 ISSN 2366-4487 (electronic)
Comprehensive Healthcare Simulation
ISBN 978-3-031-65741-2 ISBN 978-3-031-65742-9 (eBook)
https://doi.org/10.1007/978-3-031-65742-9

This Springer imprint is published by the registered company Springer Nature Switzerland AG
The registered company address is: Gewerbestrasse 11, 6330 Cham, Switzerland

The editors dedicate this book to Ameen (Rocky) Aljaroof, Fatemah Aljaroof, Hussain Aljaroof, Mohammed Aljaroof, Om Ali Almagdad, Turki Alsaba, Maryam Alsaihati, Essie Guttman, Karen Hirshfeld, Fay Lim-Lambie, Joe Madziak, Ruth Madziak, Stan Madziak, Cooper Nestel, Pearl Nestel, Jody Sokoloff, Mark Sokoloff, Erwin Smith, Pauline Smith, Christina Van Sickle, Robyn Vinodolac, Eileen Webb, Annie Wood, Henry Wood, and Jack Wood.

Foreword by Don Melady

As a practising emergency physician and teacher for 35 years, I devote most of my academic and pedagogic projects to improving outcomes for older adults in acute care. I have long felt that education of care providers is essential, though not sufficient, to that improvement. Strangely, most of us working in acute care have received limited focussed education about the care needs of older people. In our book, *Creating a Geriatric Emergency Department* [1], John Schumacher and I argue that the three essential components of improving care for older ED patients are: people, processes, and place. It is not accidental that we place "people" first in this list. People are at the core of any effective healthcare interaction. If we want improved outcomes in healthcare for older adults, then we must have educated, well-prepared people in those interactions. Essential to that preparation is education that provides the skills, knowledge, and attitudes needed in real-life situations. Following the rise of competency-based education over the past decades, simulation has naturally become a core resource for preparing interdisciplinary clinicians for that real-life implementation. In my field, emergency medicine, simulation education overwhelmingly focusses on critical care and resuscitation, mostly of younger people. Acute care clinicians have had limited simulation resources available to prepare them for the particular challenges and needs of older patients. The authors of this book make a long-awaited and most welcome addition to the field. They provide an abundance of resources in simulation to guide the education of our people as we prepare to provide excellent care for older adults across the healthcare spectrum.

Reference

1. Melady D, Schumacher J. Creating a geriatric emergency department: a practical guide. Cambridge/New York: Cambridge University Press; 2022.

Don Melady

Schwartz-Reisman Emergency Medicine Institute,
Mount Sinai Hospital
Toronto, ON, Canada

Faculty of Medicine
University of Toronto
Toronto, ON, Canada

Foreword by Christina Johnson

The unique value of simulated participants is frequently underrated. This sits at odds with widespread recognition of the benefits of simulation in general, as offering important opportunities for health professionals to rehearse, analyse and refine their approach to challenging clinical situations without the risk of harming patients.

I have been fortunate to work with simulated participants, predominantly as the lead for interprofessional communication skills workshops, such as goals of care or breaking bad news discussions. Time and again I have witnessed the benefits as simulated participants share their insights based on lived experience. Simulated participants' authentic perspectives are uniquely illuminating as they provide health professionals with immediate reflections from those impacted by their behaviour. These are rare pearls of wisdom as healthcare consumers have so little direct involvement in the training of health professionals.

My clinical specialty is General and Geriatric Medicine, so it is no surprise that I am committed to enhancing care and collaboration with older people. The majority of people requiring health care are older. So "optimising care for older people" is everyone's business, and it makes sense to involve older people as simulated participants. This book will help everyone to advance and enhance their plans to do this. I have appreciated Professor Debra Nestel's invitations to work alongside her in professional development events. For many years, she has been at the forefront of championing the role of simulated participants and working alongside them to enhance their performance and educational benefits. This book arises from an international editorial partnership between Professor Nestel and Dr. Cathy Smith, a simulationist with extensive experience working with simulated participants (Canada); Lisa Guttman Sokoloff, Speech-Language Pathologist and former manager of a simulation centre specifically dedicated to care of older adults (Canada); and Assistant Professor Nemat Alsaba, an emergency physician, simulationist and medical educator with a passion for optimising the health care experience for older people (Australia). The book offers a wealth of useful information, covering the key considerations when working with older people as simulated participants and detailed descriptions of scenarios targeting important issues. Just a few examples include discussing the appropriate intensity of care for very sick patients with their decision-makers in Emergency, providing personal care for people living with dementia, and identifying mistreatment during a telehealth consultation, in addition to core topics such as comprehensive assessment, falls, swallowing, dementia and delirium.

This book is aimed at a broad audience. I think anyone working in health professions' education will find it full of ideas, wisdom and practical tips.

Monash Health - Monash Doctors Education
Clayton, VIC, Australia

Faculty of Medicine, Nursing and Health Sciences
Monash University Clayton
Clayton, VIC, Australia

Christina Johnson

Preface

It is well established that as the proportion of older adults in the world's population ages exponentially, training healthcare providers and teams in the care of older adults will become increasingly important. The involvement of older adult simulated participants (SPs) can support development of the expertise associated with offering high-quality person-centred care for older adults. Older adult SPs can provide authenticity in learning, promote learner engagement, and reduce the risk of ageism or bias in the portrayal of older adults.

This book is the product of an international community of leading scholars in older adult SP methodology. This is a specialised field of simulation practice. There are specific considerations in working with older adult SPs related to potential cognitive, physical, and sensory changes associated with ageing that they may experience. This book provides guidance to deepen understanding of how to work with older adult SPs in a manner that promotes their safety and effective learning outcomes.

The book reflects the deep experience, evidence-based practice, and pragmatism of scholars working with older adult simulated participants. Over 4 years, our editorial team regularly met to share our own practices, to identify the work of scholars around the world, and to hear the voices of older adult SPs themselves.

As the editors, we sincerely hope that this book will be an invaluable resource and source of inspiration to advance this field. We are deeply grateful to all our colleagues who have contributed.

Toronto, ON, Canada — Cathy M. Smith
Gold Coast, QLD, Australia — Nemat Alsaba
Clayton, VIC, Australia — Debra Nestel
Brampton, ON, Canada — Lisa Guttman Sokoloff

Acknowledgements

We express our gratitude to all the authors, simulated participants (SPs), and others who have influenced this book, generously offering their expertise and experience. We especially acknowledge the many older adult SPs with whom we have worked over many years across several institutions.

Contents

Part I

Introduction

1 A Focus on Older Adults as Simulated Participants

Cathy M. Smith, Nemat Alsaba, Debra Nestel, and Lisa Guttman Sokoloff

Key Messages

1. As the proportion of older adults in the world's population ages exponentially, training healthcare providers and teams in the care of older adults will become increasingly important.
2. The involvement of older adult simulated participants (SPs) can support development of competencies associated with the person-centred care of older adults.
3. Engaging with older adult SPs can provide authenticity, promote increased learner engagement, and reduce the risk of ageism or bias in the portrayal of older adults.
4. There are specific considerations in working with older adult SPs related to potential cognitive, physical, and sensory changes associated with ageing that they may experience.
5. This book provides guidance to deepen understanding of how to work with older adult SPs in a manner that promotes their safety and effective learning outcomes.

C. M. Smith (✉)
Baycrest Academy for Research and Education, Baycrest Centre for Geriatric Care, Toronto, ON, Canada
e-mail: CSmith4@baycrest.org

N. Alsaba
Faculty of Health Sciences and Medicine, Bond University, Gold Coast, QLD, Australia
e-mail: Nalsaba@bond.edu.au

D. Nestel
School of Clinical Sciences, Faculty of Medicine, Nursing & Health Sciences, Monash University, Clayton, VIC, Australia

Department of Surgery (Austin Precinct), University of Melbourne, Parkville, VIC, Australia
e-mail: debra.nestel@monash.edu

L. G. Sokoloff
Faculty of Applied Health and Community Studies, Sheridan College, Brampton, ON, Canada

Department of Speech Pathology, Temerty Faculty of Medicine, University of Toronto, Toronto, ON, Canada
e-mail: lisa.sokoloff@sheridancollege.ca

Introduction

As the proportion of older adults in the world's population continues to age exponentially [1], training healthcare providers and teams in the care of older adults will become increasingly important [2]. Older adults often have complex medical and psychosocial issues [3]. Simulation is recognized as being an effective educational method to train teams in caring for older adults [2]. Simulated participants (SPs) are well people trained to portray individuals such as patients and their family members [4, 5]. SP methodology is an established and effective simulation modality especially valuable when competencies relate to the development of person-centred skills that consider the whole life of a person rather than just their experience as a patient [6] or focus on how teams look after and care for older adults and their families on a daily basis [7]. Working with older adult SPs can bring authenticity to encounters, promoting strong engagement from learners [4–6]. However, there is limited information and a lack of broader understanding about working with older adult SPs and those who support them to create authentic, safe, and effective simulations [7].

This book was designed to be a core reference, a comprehensive guide to deepen understanding of how to work with older adult SPs in a safe and effective manner. The theoretical constructs are supported by practical applications and hopefully will foster innovation. Elements of evidence-informed practice related to simulation methodology are synthesized with relevant clinical evidence related to caring for older adults. Our aim is to provide a nuanced understanding of the issues but still be broad enough to support local educational practices. The book presents strategies suitable for implementation by those who are responsible for working with SPs, at all levels of experience and with varying degrees of resources to build, develop, and sustain SP programmes that include older adults. The contents build on an evidence-informed framework for engaging with older adult SPs [8] and include practical templates, guides, worksheets, case studies, examples of scenarios, tips, and key messages.

C. M. Smith et al. (eds.), *Comprehensive Healthcare Simulation: Geriatric Simulation*, Comprehensive Healthcare Simulation,
https://doi.org/10.1007/978-3-031-65742-9_1

We believe this book will be a practical resource for educators, academics, and other healthcare providers who use simulation as an educational method related to care of older adults.

Terms

Researchers, educators, clinicians, and older adult SPs from across the globe contributed to this book. As has been noted in other publications, this diversity of practice and contexts reflects differences in understanding and use of terms [9–11]. While we respect these differences, the words we use matter. To this end, we provide some definitions about specific terms to clarify the editors' preferred terms.

Geriatric or Gerontological Simulation

Simulation focused on the care of older adults is sometimes referred to as *geriatric* or *gerontological* simulation. These terms refer to the medical specialty or healthcare area rather than descriptors of an older adult, which could be perceived as derogatory.

Learner

Different terms (e.g. learner, participant, trainee, student) are used generally and in this book by various authors to refer to the people for whom the simulation experience has been designed and that relate to stages of their training or experience. For consistency and clarity, we use the term *learner.*

Older Adult

Drawing on definitions from the World Health Organization and the United Nations, we refer to older adults as being 60 years of age and over [1, 12]. We use the term *older adult* to describe this age group as it is recognized by organizations such as the American Medical Association as being a respectful way of referring to adults in this age group rather than using terms such as "elderly", "senior", "pensioners", "retired", or "the aged" which can "connote discrimination and certain negative stereotypes that may undercut research-based recommendations for better serving our needs as we age" [13, p. 1386].

Scenario

The term *scenario* refers to all the information that is required to run a simulation, that is, the complete documentation for a simulation session.

Simulated Participant

Simulated participants (SPs) are well people carefully trained to portray others (such as patients, family members, healthcare professionals, or clients) for educational, assessment, and research purposes. The acronym SP is understood to mean various things depending on the context, including "standardized patient" and "simulated patient." Drawing on international advocacy, we use SP to mean "simulated participant" [9, 14, 15], a more inclusive phrase that reflects all human role players in simulation and the person-centred presentation of older peoples' experiences in healthcare, one that can include patients, carers, family members, healthcare professionals, and others.

Simulation

A pioneer of contemporary simulation, David Gaba, defined *simulation* as "… a technique … to replace or amplify real experiences with guided experiences, often immersive in nature, that evoke or replicate substantial aspects of the real world in a fully interactive manner" [16, p. 12]. This definition aptly describes how the authenticity offered by working with an older adult SP can engage learners in a powerful manner [4–6]. The *Healthcare Simulation Dictionary*'s (2020) definition expands on the contexts in which simulation can be applied and which older adult SPs can work, noting that it is: "A technique that creates a situation or environment to allow persons to experience a representation of a real event for the purpose of practice, learning, evaluation, testing, or to gain understanding of systems or human actions " [17, p. 44].

SP Educator

We refer to *SP educators* as dedicated individuals who support older adult SPs contributions. They are known by various titles (e.g. trainer, coach, educator). They come from various backgrounds, including being specialists in SP methodology and in clinical practice. Some SP educators have full-time appointments dedicated to working with SPs while others work with SPs as one of many other tasks [9].

SP Role

An *SP role* is the information provided to the SP about the character to be portrayed, including who the SP is portraying, what they are required to do, when, and how. The SP role is usually embedded in a scenario.

Working with or Engaging with SPs

We support the language of "*working with*" or "*engaging with*" SPs as a positive and respectful way to position their valuable contributions rather than "using" SPs or describing them as "tools" which may promote unhelpful objectification [18, 19].

Considerations for Working with Older SPs

There is a strong ethical imperative when working with SPs of any age to provide a psychologically and physically safe work environment [20–22]. There are standards of practice for working with SPs that provide five underlying values (safety, quality, professionalism, accountability, collaboration) and five domains (safe work environment, case development, training SPs, programme management, professional development) [9]. However, these standards are derived from a limited evidence base and do not consider nuances related to age [23]. In 2021, three of the editors of this book (CS, NA, LS) developed a collaborative framework for working with older simulated participants [8]. This framework considers how to foster a safe physical and psychological environment for older adult SPs before, during, and after a simulation, with particular reference to physical, cognitive, and sensory changes that older adult SPs may experience. Contributors to this book were provided with this framework and were encouraged to also draw on their own practices of working with older adult SPs.

Origins of This Book

As editors, we have significant experience in healthcare simulation practice. We all have extensive experience working with SPs and with older adult SPs in several countries, including Australia, Canada, Hong Kong (China), and the United Kingdom. We came together to develop this book due to our shared curiosity around this topic and a recognition, through our previous research and experiences, that there are gaps in what is known about supporting older adult SPs. These gaps include knowledge about how to recognize, understand, and accommodate potential changes in older adult SPs or ways to run simulations with them in a safe and effective manner.

Editors

Cathy M. Smith is an educator who has worked for over 30 years in simulation-based health providers' education and assessment. She is based in Canada. Consulting with various organizations around the world, she supports learners in undergraduate, graduate, continuing education, and faculty development contexts, both in person and virtually. Her prior experience in performance has guided her approach as a simulation educator in promoting the safe and effective implementation of simulation scenarios. Her particular focus is on SPs, beginning her journey in this field as an SP. She has become increasingly involved in engaging with and learning from older adult SPs at the Baycrest Centre for Geriatric Care. Her research interests, informed by her PhD in Drama, include exploring the role of performance in simulation as well as ways of supporting older adult SPs and applying evidence-informed practices to SP methodology.

Nemat Alsaba is an emergency physician and an experienced medical educator with 25 years of clinical experience with a particular interest in geriatric emergency medicine (GEM). She also holds a simulation leadership role at Bond University as the Director of the Bond simulation programme and a Consultant at the Bond Translational Simulation Collaborative. Driving her passion for caring for older adults is guided by her mantra in educational and advocacy activities: "To care for those who once cared for us is one of our highest honors." Nemat combines her skills and passion for caring for older people to improve their care and health outcomes across the healthcare and educational system (undergraduate and postgraduate training). She has been disseminating GEM knowledge through creating workshops, resources, and educational activities nationally and internationally. She is currently based in Australia but has lived and worked in Saudi Arabia.

Lisa Guttman Sokoloff is a speech-language pathologist who has worked with older adults for over 30 years. She is based in Canada. She has also held educational leadership positions that support interprofessional education and collaboration. In these roles, she incorporates simulation with SPs into training, especially focusing on behavioural skills such as communication. Lisa recognizes the value and authenticity that older adult SPs bring to simulation experiences. Her background as a clinician supports her work with older adult SPs as she brings her knowledge of physical, sensory, and cognitive changes in normal and pathological ageing to the team. Lisa's current research focuses on educational methods, innovative educational practices (e.g. virtual reality), and simulation.

Debra Nestel is an educator and has held leadership roles in healthcare simulation, in faculty development, and in associated research which has positioned her to identify and respond to gaps in the broader field of healthcare simulation. Debra's first degree was in sociology, and she has worked for over 35 years in health profession education in Hong Kong, London, and Melbourne. She has extensive experience of working with SPs to support the development of communication and other professional skills. She has led the development of an online network for SPs (https://www.

simulatedpatientnetwork.org/) which connects and provides resources for SPs and those with whom they work. Debra's research is usually from a qualitative paradigm.

Authors

As editors, we recognize the importance of having varied perspectives and contributions. To that end, we reached out internationally, to engage authors from multiple countries and backgrounds to share information about their work with older adult SPs. Surveys were sent through relevant listservs, social media, and professional connections, asking those who work with older adult SPs to indicate interest in participating in the book. Once all the chapter authors were confirmed, we sent a survey to our 55 authors to gather demographic information to see if the goal of diversity in authorship was met. Forty authors responded, which is a response rate of 73%.

Authors reported living and working in at least eight countries—Australia, Canada, France, Switzerland, Taiwan, Turkey, the United Kingdom, and the United States. Thirty-one of the forty responding authors identify as female or cis-woman (78%) with seven (18%) identifying as male or cis-male and two (3%) preferring not to answer.

With regard to cultural and ethnic group/background, 13 were identified as American, followed by 9 European, 6 Australian, 6 Canadian, 3 British, and 3 East Asian. Other responses included South Asian (n = 2), African (n = 1), Hispanic or Latin (n = 1) and Middle Eastern (n = 1). One author preferred not to answer. As the question allowed authors to choose multiple responses, percentages are not reported.

Besides personal diversity, we also wanted to capture perspectives from different work settings, roles, and experiences in the field of simulation. Twelve authors work in university, college, or other higher education institutions (30%), followed by healthcare services (n = 8; 20%) and simulation centres (n = 2; 5%). About half of the authors noted that they worked in multiple settings: both a simulation centre and a university or college (n = 8; 20%), a healthcare setting and a university or college (n = 6; 15%), or a simulation centre and healthcare setting (n = 2; 5%). Two authors indicated that they worked in all three environments—university, college, or other higher education institution, healthcare service, and a simulation centre (5%).

Seventeen authors (42.5%) reported that they have multiple roles related to simulation. These roles include clinical educator, curriculum leader, researcher, SP, SP trainer/educator, or administrative roles.

The authors' experiences working with SPs had a fairly equal distribution across blocks of 5 years with 14 authors having worked 16–20 plus years (35%). Seven authors (17.5%) had 5 years or less experience working with SPs.

In response to the question, "What is your highest level of Education qualification?", 15 authors reported having a PhD (37.5%), 17 held a Master's degree (42.5%), and four had a Bachelor's degree (10%). Three authors (7.5%) reported "other" qualifications and identified themselves as physicians or medical specialists. The professional backgrounds of the authors included healthcare, social sciences, social work, education, drama, and liberal arts. Professional/clinical qualifications were reported by 26 (65%) authors. These qualifications were primarily in medicine, nursing, or allied health (e.g. physiotherapist, speech-language pathologist). One author preferred not to answer any questions related to education (2.5%).

Although the survey was not completed by all authors, the 73% response rate gives us confidence that the findings are likely representative of the larger group. Readers may notice that chapters are written in different styles, reflecting the different contexts of the authors, their places of work, country of work, and other factors. While we, as editors, offered a template, especially for the scenario chapters, it was also important to us that the authors had the freedom to write in a manner that best reflects their programmes and themselves.

Structure of the Book

There are **seven parts** of the book. While we have designed the content as whole, each chapter is also intended to stand alone. Readers can work through this book in any order or according to interest, but we encourage you to refer to Parts 1, 2, and 3 for foundational methodology.

Part 1 comprises two chapters that **orient** readers to the book, including this introduction (Chap. 1) and a chapter describing the work of older adult SPs (Chap. 2).

In **Part 2**, six chapters describe the **elements of simulation practice** with older adults. These chapters focus on scenario design (Chap. 3), training older adult SPs for role portrayal (Chap. 4), fostering psychological safety in learning conversations (Chap. 5), supporting older adult SPs to provide feedback to learners (Chap. 6), programme evaluation and quality improvement approaches in older adult SP programmes (Chap. 7), and research opportunities and knowledge translation related to simulation for the care of older adults (Chap. 8). All chapters offer specific considerations when working with older adults.

Part 3 addresses **implementation** and has six chapters, including building or enhancing an SP programme with and for older adults (Chap. 9), working with volunteer older adult SPs (Chap. 10), embedding simulations for the care of older adults into programmes (Chap. 11), faculty reflections on supporting older adult SPs in giving feedback (Chap. 12), innovations in older adult SP methodology (Chap. 13), and creative development opportunities for older adult SPs (Chap. 14).

In **Parts 4, 5, and 6,** older adult SP practice is illustrated with **20 scenarios** across various professions and topics and settings also designed for different levels of learners. We reached out to international simulation educators who work with older adult SPs and invited them to share relevant scenarios. The scenarios are organized into three sections related to the type of care being provided: **Part 4** Applications: Older Adult Care and Assessment; **Part 5** Applications: Older Adult Care in an Acute Setting; and **Part 6** Applications: Older Adult Care Related to Advanced Conversations.

The scenarios demonstrate the application of theoretical descriptions from Parts 1–3. You will notice variations in approaches as there are many ways to write and deliver scenarios, reflective of the diverse contexts of SP work and the care of older adults. To that end, some topics (e.g. falls) are covered in multiple scenarios based on different learners and/or perspectives. As editors, our interest was in authors articulating what they actually do rather than in modifying their work to fit a standardized approach.

Each chapter provides background details about why the scenario was developed, who the learners are, and how the scenario has been delivered. Key information necessary for running the scenario is provided, including a scenario overview, learning objectives, participants involved, adjunct materials (e.g. presimulation resources, props, wardrobe, moulage), scenario logistics (e.g. length, schedule, room setup), and instructions to the learners, that is, everything learners need to know before engaging in the scenario. The SP role is also described, highlighting what the SP needs to know, such as the history of the current situation, the health and family health history, social/lifestyle information, the person's ideas, concerns, and expectations, possible scripted lines, and specific instructions for portraying this scenario (e.g. related to affect or behaviour). Each scenario also includes considerations for working with older adult SPs before, during, and after the scenario with reference to the collaborative framework for working with older simulated participants [8] as well as other considerations the authors have discovered along the way. Finally, lessons learned are provided with references and resources. Our intent for these parts was to provide scenarios that can be used as written or modified to suit learner needs, environment, culture, programme resources, etc.

In the final section, **Part 7**, we explore **future directions and possibilities** in engaging with older adult SPs, based on the content of this book and discoveries made during this process.

We want to express our gratitude to all the authors and older adult SPs who participated in the creation of this book, generously offering their expertise and experience. Our hope is that this book advances understanding of how to work productively and enjoyably with older adult SPs in a safe and effective manner with the ultimate goal of improving the care of older adults.

References

1. World Health Organization. Ageing and health [Internet]. WHO; 2022. https://www.who.int/news-room/fact-sheets/detail/ageing-and-health.
2. Braude P, Reedy G, Dasgupta D, Dimmock V, Jaye P, Birns J. Evaluation of a simulation training programme for geriatric medicine. Age Ageing. 2015;44(4):677–82.
3. Rentsch S, Vitale CA, Zietlow K. Prioritizing geriatrics in medical education improves care for all. Med Educ Online. 2022;27(1):2105549.
4. Dugmore H, Carr S, Saunders R. Interpreting the value of feedback: older adult voices in nursing education. Nurse Educ Pract. 2020;48:102868.
5. Alsaba N, Brazil V. Medical students' recognition and response to clinical deterioration in simulated patient scenarios. MedEdPublish. 2018;7:1–8.
6. Davis K. Utilizing older adult standardized patients to enhance the education of health professional students. Age Action. 2017;32(2):1.
7. Smith CM, Alsaba N, Nestel D, Sokoloff L. Older adults as simulated participants: a scoping review. Int J Healthc Simul. 2023; https://doi.org/10.54531/bocf7225.
8. Smith CM, Sokoloff LG, Alsaba N. Collaborative framework for working with older simulated participants (SP). BMJ Simul Technol Enhanc Learn. 2021;7(2):112.
9. Lewis KL, Bohnert CA, Gammon WL, Hölzer H, Lyman L, Smith C, et al. The Association of Standardized Patient Educators (ASPE) Standards of Best Practice (SOBP). Adv Simul. 2017;2(1):10.
10. Nestel D, Roche J, Battista A. Creating a quality improvement culture in standardized/simulated patient methodology: the role of professional societies. Adv Simul. 2017;2:18.
11. Nestel D, McNaughton N, Smith C, Schlegel C, Tierney T. Values and value in simulated participant methodology: a global perspective on contemporary practices. Med Teach. 2018;40:697–702.
12. United Nations Population Fund. Ageing in the twenty-first century: a celebration and a challenge. New York: United Nations Population Fund; 2012.
13. Lundebjerg NE, Trucil DE, Hammond EC, Applegate WB. When it comes to older adults, language matters: Journal of the American Geriatrics Society adopts modified American Medical Association style. J Am Geriatr Soc. 2017;65(7):1386–8.
14. Murphy P, Nestel D. Healthcare simulation terms: promoting critical reflection. Int J Healthc Simul. 2022;1(3):45–6.
15. Bearman M, Nestel D. The future of simulated patient methodology. In: Nestel D, Bearman M, editors. Simulated patient methodology: theory, evidence and practice. Chichester: Wiley; 2015. p. 145–9.
16. Gaba DM. The future vision of simulation in health care. Qual Saf Health Care. 2004;13(Suppl 1):i2–i10.
17. Lioce L, Anderson M, Chang T, Diaz D, Downing D, Robertson J, et al. Healthcare simulation dictionary. Rockville: Agency for Healthcare Research and Quality; 2020.
18. McNaughton N, Anderson M. Standardized patients: it's all in the words. Clin Simul Nursing. 2017;13(7):293–4.
19. Nestel D, Burn CL, Pritchard SA, Glastonbury R, Tabak D. The use of simulated patients in medical education: guide supplement 42.1 viewpoint. Med Teach. 2011;33(12):1027–9.

20. Nestel D, Sanko J, McNaughton N. Simulated participant methodologies: maintaining humanism in practice. In: Nestel D, Kelly M, Jolly B, Watson M, editors. Healthcare simulation education: evidence, theory and practice. Oxford: Wiley-Blackwell; 2018. p. 45–53.
21. Clark L, Woll A, Owens TL, Shropshire D, Kiser B, Gephardt G, et al. SP safety, autonomy and healthcare simulation practice in the COVID-19 era. BMJ Simul Technol Enhanc Learn. 2021;7(5):450.
22. Gerzina HA. Ensuring a safe and supportive work environment. In: Maxworthy JC, Palaganas JC, Epps CA, Mancini ME, editors. Comprehensive healthcare simulation: implementing best practices in standardized patient methodology. 2nd ed. Philadelphia: Lippincott Williams & Wilkins; 2020. p. 25–9.
23. Gamble A, Bearman M, Nestel D. A systematic review: children & adolescents as simulated patients in health professional education. Adv Simul. 2016;1(1):1.

Describing the Work of Older Adult Simulated Participants

2

Cathy M. Smith, Nemat Alsaba, Debra Nestel, and Lisa Guttman Sokoloff

Key Messages

1. Older adult simulated participants (SPs) can contribute to healthcare providers' education in authentic, engaging, safe, and effective ways.
2. Possible changes in cognitive, sensory, and physical abilities associated with ageing should be considered when working with older adult SPs.
3. Older adult SPs participate in a variety of activities or contexts that reflect the wider SP population practices.
4. There is an ethical imperative to carefully recruit, screen, and support older adult SPs with full consideration to their psychological and physical safety.
5. Improved reporting details in articles involving older adult SPs will facilitate the identification and implementation of effective practices.

C. M. Smith (✉)
Baycrest Academy for Research and Education, Baycrest Centre for Geriatric Care, Toronto, ON, Canada
e-mail: CSmith4@baycrest.org

N. Alsaba
Faculty of Health Sciences and Medicine, Bond University, Gold Coast, QLD, Australia
e-mail: nalsaba@bond.edu.au

D. Nestel
School of Clinical Sciences, Faculty of Medicine, Nursing & Health Sciences, Monash University, Clayton, VIC, Australia

Department of Surgery (Austin Precinct), University of Melbourne, Parkville, VIC, Australia
e-mail: debra.nestel@monash.edu

L. G. Sokoloff
Faculty of Applied Health and Community Studies, Sheridan College, Brampton, ON, Canada

Department of Speech Pathology, Temerty Faculty of Medicine, University of Toronto, Toronto, ON, Canada
e-mail: lisa.sokoloff@sheridancollege.ca

Background

There has been a worldwide exponential growth of the percentage of older adults in the population. Older adults are defined by organisations such as the World Health Organization (WHO) and the United Nations (UN) as being 60 years of age or over [1, 2]. There has been a parallel progressive increase over more than 30 years of interest in and reporting on simulation for the care of older adults. To get a broad sense of the growth of interest in the topic, we conducted a Google Scholar search (Nov 18, 2023) using the terms "geriatric simulation" or "gerontological simulation." The search yielded the following results: 3400 (1990–1999), 11,300 (2000–2009), 17,600 (2010–2019), and 18,000 (2020–2023). This increase is likely related to the recognition that upskilling and training future healthcare providers and caregivers is required to improve the multidimensional medical, psychosocial, and physiological age-related changes related to older adults' care and health outcomes [3, 4].

Designing and delivering this kind of simulation encompasses specific considerations, including selecting an appropriate simulation modality. Simulated participants (SPs), a term first proposed by Bearman and Nestel [5] and later adopted by the Association of Standardized Patient Educators (ASPE) in their Standards of Best Practice (SOBP) [6], is an inclusive term for any human role-player in simulation. SPs are well people carefully trained to portray others such as patients, family members, or clients for educational, assessment, and research purposes. SPs can support development of competencies associated with the person-centred care of older adults [7]. Eklund et al. (2019) note that "… person-centered care broadens and extends the perspective of patient-centered care by considering the whole life of the patient" [8, p. 10] rather than just their experience as a patient.

C. M. Smith et al. (eds.), *Comprehensive Healthcare Simulation: Geriatric Simulation*, Comprehensive Healthcare Simulation,
https://doi.org/10.1007/978-3-031-65742-9_2

What Is Known About Working with Older Adult SPs?

There is limited reporting of details when working with older adult SPs [9]. This gap has been emphasised in previous research about SP work and the reporting of simulation in general, along with suggested frameworks for reporting [10–12]. While there have been thousands of papers published on geriatric simulation, many focus on learner outcomes, training for educators/healthcare providers/simulationists, and programme objectives [13]. If older adult SPs are involved or mentioned, there is generally minimal information provided about them (e.g. demographics) or how they are supported in their work (e.g. how they are trained) [14]. Furthermore, in some of these activities, older adults are reported as being portrayed by much younger adults [15, 16], sometimes even being made to look older [17] which may run the risk of stereotyping and promoting ageism. Our specific interest is older adult SP involvement, their training, and approaches used to study their practices.

A Scoping Review on Working with Older Adults as SPs

To address this gap, and in preparation for this book, we conducted a scoping review [9] guided by Arksey and O'Malley's five-phase approach [18] to explore and summarise what is known about working with older adults as SPs in healthcare students' and providers' education. We focused our search on articles published between 2011 and 2021, written in English, that made specific mention of the age of the older adult SPs involved as being over 60 or close to the age of the older adult in the scenario. Twelve articles were included in the review [19–30]. While we summarise some features of the article here, for full reporting, please see the open access reference cited above. The findings of the scoping review focused on five areas: (1) characteristics of articles, (2) descriptions of SPs, (3) conceptualisation of SP roles/scenarios, (4) SP preparation, and (5) scenario implementation. Most of these areas are explored in chapters in this book. Briefly, for characteristics of articles, based on the first author's place of work, all articles were from the Global North. Journals had an education, simulation, professional-specific, or education- and professional-specific focus. Learners included specific student groups, an interprofessional group, and single healthcare professions.

Benefits and Challenges Working with Older Adult SPs

The articles in the scoping review identified that involving older adult SPs may contribute to healthcare students' and providers' training in authentic, engaging, safe, and effective ways [22, 24]. Benefits to the older adult SPs included their appreciation of being able to give back through sharing their lived experiences, learning new things, feeling valued, and social engagement [20, 23, 26, 28, 30].

Possible challenges to working with older adult SPs included concerns about their ability to do the work because of physical frailty or cognitive issues [20, 22]. There was also an ethical concern raised that the roles they were being asked to play might be too close to their own current life experience and that they possibly might not be able to de-role after a simulation session [21]. Other barriers could relate to a lack of practical guidance for how to work with older adults [20]. Older adult SPs themselves identified challenges related to potential changing cognitive and physical abilities and how these might impact their ability to continue working [21, 23, 26, 28, 30].

Recommendations from the Scoping Review

Inconsistent reporting made it challenging to synthesise practices, and in the scoping review, we made three recommendations for improved reporting of older adult SPs in research articles. First, the well-being of older adult SPs was addressed in varying degrees. There are risks, for example, when older adult SPs use details from their own lives or provide feedback without having been provided with any parameters or support. This inconsistency speaks to the need for either more rigour in SP training or, at least, in reporting about training, a call echoed in another recent scoping review related to SP training for role portrayal and feedback [31]. Second, there appeared to be little diversity in the characters and situations contained in the articles; there is an opportunity to expand the possibilities of who is represented in scenarios featuring older adult SPs. Third, there was a recognition that "words matter", and in working with older adult SPs, it starts with the way they are described. The WHO, UN, and the American Medical Association [1, 2, 32] use the word *older* as a respectful way of referring to adults in this age group rather than terms such as "elderly", "senior", or "the aged" which can connote ageism and promote stereotyping. We also recommended critical reflection of other words used to describe the living spaces of older adults (e.g. nursing home, long-term care facility) while also recognising that usage will vary across countries. The American Gerontological Society offers recommendations for various terms [32].

Contexts in Which Older Adult SPs Work

Older adult SPs participate in simulation activities that reflect those reported for the wider SP population. Drawing on the scoping review, the scenarios featured in this book and the experiences of the authors of this chapter, we outline some of these contexts. Our intention is to provide an overview recognising that there are still other contexts not known to us.

The types of tasks older adult SPs are typically asked to do include role portrayal, providing verbal feedback, facilitation of sessions, debriefing learners, and filling in assessment forms. The types of roles they might portray include a patient/resident/client and/or a family member of this person (e.g. spouse, sibling, adult child, grandparent). Older adult SPs often portray a person living with dementia. In Chap. 19, Parish and colleagues present a scenario in which an older adult SP's behavioural responses are dependent on the learner's approach and communication. The scenario was designed to promote effective and compassionate communication during personal care and is designed to be used with a variety of learners.

Falls in older adults are common. Older adult SPs can be engaged in simulations related to falls prevention, falls risk assessments, and as patients who have experienced a fall. Sample scenarios of these situations are included in Parts 4, 5, and 6 of this book. Pritchard and Blackstock (Chap. 18) designed a simulation geared towards internationally trained physiotherapists to refine and develop their skills. The simulation focuses on falls assessment, prevention, and management for a patient who has had a previous fall and subsequent fracture. Similarly, Syms and colleagues (Chap. 16) developed a simulation for medical students doing training in geriatric care with a broader goal of addressing a core competency of falls and mobility. Learners participate by completing a falls risk assessment with a 76-year-old outpatient whose daughter has expressed concern about the patient's walking. In the chapter by Patel and Hullick (Chap. 24), the authors recognise that while falls are the most common reason for older adults to be admitted to the emergency department, they are also at risk for falling while in hospital and that a team approach is required to keep them safe.

Some simulations do not focus specifically on older adults but recognise the role of older adults in the care of others. Soong et al. (2011) designed a simulation for paediatric residents where a grandparent brings a child to the emergency department due to a medication overdose [29]. The simulation was developed with the recognition that over the past few decades, the number of children being raised by grandparents has increased [29, 33]. While the focus of the simulation is on a child, an important component is communication with an older adult who has a hearing loss. Part of the postactivity feedback focuses on those communication challenges and strategies. The authors make the point that training paediatricians to work with older adults will become increasingly important as more older adults care for paediatric patients.

Older adult SPs also work in assessments (formative/summative). Sarzynski et al. (2014) detail a six station Objective Structured Clinical Examination (OSCE) designed to provide formative feedback for geriatric fellows [25]. The stations feature SPs portraying patients between the ages of 68 and 92. Although each OSCE station has specific objectives, one of the overarching goals in working with the SPs is to allow for direct observation of the fellows' clinical skills in history, examination, and complex patient management.

Older adult SPs also work with learners at various stages, including undergraduates (students) and postgraduates (trainees). Some sessions are interprofessional or team based. Karnish et al. describe a simulation involving nursing, physical therapy, and diagnostic imaging students that explores the perceptions of interprofessional socialisation in acute care including patient care, interprofessional communication, teamwork, and role appreciation [22]. In this simulation, the older adults simulate a patient who fell and was admitted to the hospital for a hip fracture that required surgery. The students review patient information independently but then approach the simulated participant as a team. In the scenarios provided later in this book, learners come from the fields of medical imaging, medicine, nursing, police and emergency services, paramedics, physiotherapy, and speech-language pathology.

Sometimes older adult SPs work individually with learners; sometimes they are paired with another SP. Miehl et al. (Chap. 31) outline a simulation that features a 61-year-old woman and her husband (63 years old). She is a military veteran, living with diabetes, and is struggling to afford her medication. She has been referred for home nursing services by a social worker at the health clinic where she receives care. Two learners (prelicensure baccalaureate nursing students) meet with the patient and her husband and are offered opportunities to demonstrate rapport building and establishment of a therapeutic relationship, recognise personal feelings and bias, and adjust priorities and practise client-centred care within the community setting.

Older adult SPs also participate in hybrid simulations with moulage, task trainers, or manikins. In Chap. 33, Seifman and Nestel describe a sequential simulation in which a 70-year-old male SP initially wears a simulated mole on his right hand. The first consultation of the SP with a surgical trainee provides opportunities to develop competence in communication with the patient. The second sequence enables the trainee to confirm the diagnosis and treatment options.

Older adult SP simulations take place in classrooms, simulation labs, places within the community (e.g. long term care facility), or online (e.g. telehealth consultation). Elcin (Chap. 34) describes a simulation focused on benefits and challenges of utilising telehealth for medical consultation and recognising possible abuse in older adults.

Expanding Work

There is scope for engaging older adult SPs in simulation activities where their knowledge and expertise would be beneficial. In Chap. 3, we learn of the value of including older adult SPs in all phases of scenario design from determining learning goals, the scenario itself, the training for role portrayal, the training for feedback, and the evaluation of the learning activity. Published research and commentaries have focused on the involvement of "real" patients, including SPs, with the lived experience of the person in a scenario, in the creation of simulation scenarios to mitigate potential bias and promote respectful representations [34–36]. Involving older adult SPs can be a valuable way to enhance their involvement in an SP programme, further promote inclusion and diversity, and enrich roles related to older adults. As part of an educational team creating an online learning programme for healthcare providers working in a memory care unit that prioritises person-centred dementia care [37] and the power of storytelling [38], one of the authors of this chapter (CS) cocreated a scenario with an SP that was focused on a woman living with dementia. The SP's lived experience formed the foundation of the persona of this woman at three different stages: prior to her dementia diagnosis, in the early stages of dementia, and in the late stages of dementia. The simulations were designed using three different formats—audio clips, video clips, and text-based scenarios [39].

Older adults can also directly contribute to research programmes. Baylor et al. (2017) describe a study designed to assess the believability and authenticity of SPs portraying communication disorders for speech-language pathologists, noting that the SP must "accurately portray the fluency, word finding, comprehension or other impairment appropriate to the disorder" [19, p. 793]. The SPs involved in portraying the disorders were members of the research team. They were carefully trained and videotaped as part of the study. In their chapter on research opportunities and knowledge translation, Purdy et al. (Chap. 8) note that older adult SPs can offer fresh perspectives and make effective research partners because of their simulation and lived experiences.

Closing

In closing, this chapter has summarised findings from a scoping review of older adult SPs together with illustrations from this book to describe the practice of older adult SPs. While the practices reflect those of the wider SP population, consideration must be given to potential age-related changes of older adult SPs. The chapter finished with considerations of expanded roles for older adult SPs.

References

1. World Health Organization. Ageing and health [Internet]. WHO; 2022. https://www.who.int/news-room/fact-sheets/detail/ageing-and-health.
2. United Nations Population Fund. Ageing in the twenty-first century: a celebration and a challenge [Internet]. United Nations Population Fund; 2012. https://www.unfpa.org/sites/default/files/pub-pdf/Ageing%20report.pdf.
3. Rentsch S, Vitale CA, Zietlow K. Prioritizing geriatrics in medical education improves care for all. Med Educ Online. 2022;27(1):2105549.
4. Braude P, Reedy G, Dasgupta D, Dimmock V, Jaye P, Birns J. Evaluation of a simulation training programme for geriatric medicine. Age Ageing. 2015;44(4):677–82.
5. Bearman M, Nestel D. The future of simulated patient methodology. In: Nestel D, Bearman M, editors. Simulated patient methodology: theory, evidence and practice. Chichester: Wiley; 2015. p. 145–9.
6. Lewis KL, Bohnert CA, Gammon WL, Hölzer H, Lyman L, Smith C, et al. The Association of Standardized Patient Educators (ASPE) Standards of Best Practice (SOBP). Adv Simul. 2017;2(1):10.
7. Smith CM, Sokoloff LG, Alsaba N. Collaborative framework for working with older simulated participants (SP). BMJ Simul Technol Enhanc Learn. 2021;7(2):112.
8. Eklund JH, Holmström IK, Kumlin T, Kaminsky E, Skoglund K, Höglander J, et al. "Same same or different?" A review of reviews of person-centered and patient-centered care. Patient Educ Counseling. 2019;102(1):3–11.
9. Smith CM, Alsaba N, Nestel D, Sokoloff L. Older adults as simulated participants: a scoping review. Int J Healthc Simul. 2023; https://doi.org/10.54531/bocf7225.
10. Howley L, Szauter K, Perkowski L, Clifton M, McNaughton N. Quality of standardised patient research reports in the medical education literature: review and recommendations. Med Educ. 2008;42(4):350–8.
11. Cheng A, Kessler D, Mackinnon R, Chang TP, Nadkarni VM, Hunt EA, et al. Reporting guidelines for health care simulation research: extensions to the CONSORT and STROBE statements. Adv Simul. 2016;1(1):25.
12. Pritchard SA, Blackstock FC, Keating JL, Nestel D. The pillars of well-constructed simulated patient programs: a qualitative study with experienced educators. Med Teach. 2017;39:1159–67.
13. Siew AL, Wong JW, Chan E-Y. Effectiveness of simulated patients in geriatric education: a scoping review. Nurse Educ Today. 2021;100:104856.
14. Keane JM, Franklin NF, Vaughan B. Simulation to educate healthcare providers working within residential age care settings: a scoping review. Nurse Educ Today. 2020;85:104228.
15. Mast ME, Sawin EM, Pantaleo KA. Life of a caregiver simulation: teaching students about frail older adults and their family caregivers. J Nurs Educ. 2012;51(7):396–402.
16. Eide WM, Johansson L, Eide LS. First-year nursing students' experiences of simulation involving care of older patients. A descriptive and exploratory study. Nurse Educ Pract. 2020;45:102797.
17. Reid-Searl K, Frost J, Crownover JG, Rhodes J, Bassett J. Adapting the use of mask Ed™ simulation in nursing programmes during the COVID-19 pandemic. Clin Simul Nursing. 2022;73:1–5.
18. Arksey H, O'Malley L. Scoping studies: towards a methodological framework. Int J Soc Res Methodol. 2005;8(1):19–32.
19. Baylor C, Burns MI, Struijk J, Herron L, Mach H, Yorkston K. Assessing the believability of standardized patients trained to portray communication disorders. Am J Speech Lang Pathol. 2017;26(3):791–805.

20. Davis K. Utilizing older adult standardized patients to enhance the education of health professional students. Age Action. 2017;32(2):1.
21. Dugmore H, Carr S, Saunders R. Interpreting the value of feedback: older adult voices in nursing education. Nurse Educ Pract. 2020;48:102868.
22. Karnish K, Shustack L, Brogan L, Capitano G, Cunfer A. Interprofessional socialization through acute-care simulation. Radiol Technol. 2019;90(6):552–62.
23. Lee DA, Maxwell CA, Miller S. "This Is Me!" perceptions of older adult simulated participants in an aging and injury simulation experience. J Trauma Nurs. 2021;28(1):10–20.
24. Quail M, Brundage SB, Spitalnick J, Allen PJ, Beilby J. Student self-reported communication skills, knowledge and confidence across standardised patient, virtual and traditional clinical learning environments. BMC Med Educ. 2016;16(1):1–12.
25. Sarzynski E, Foley K, Riekse R, Laird-Fick H, Keilman L, Barnikow T, et al. An OSCE to assess trainee management of complex older adults and to teach documentation, coding, and billing. MedEdPORTAL. 2014;10:9903.
26. Schelgel C, Smith CM. "Please let me know when I do not realize it myself": a qualitative analysis of senior simulated patients' experiences. Adv Simul. 2019;4(1):18.
27. Shawler C. Palliative and end-of-life care: using a standardized patient family for gerontological nurse practitioner students. Nurs Educ Perspect. 2011;32(3):168–72.
28. Smith CM, Sokoloff LG, Gallucci CE. 'It's like a shot in the arm': evaluating the experiences of older simulated participants in structured virtual meetings during COVID-19. Int J Healthc Simul. 2021;1(1):33–40.
29. Soong A, Evans HH, Flood K. Interviewing a grandparent caregiver with age-related hearing loss. MedEdPORTAL. 2011;7:8186.
30. Thompson J, Tiplady S, Hutchinson A, Cook G, Harrington B. Older people's views and experiences of engagement in standardised patient simulation. BMJ Simul Technol Enhanc Learn. 2017;3(4):154–8.
31. Doyle AJ, Sullivan C, O'Toole M, Tjin A, Simiceva A, Collins N, et al. Training simulated participants for role portrayal and feedback practices in communication skills training: a BEME scoping review: BEME Guide No. 86. Med Teach. 2024;46:162–78.
32. Lundebjerg NE, Trucil DE, Hammond EC, Applegate WB. When it comes to older adults, language matters: Journal of the American Geriatrics Society adopts modified American Medical Association style. J Am Geriatr Soc. 2017;65(7):1386–8.
33. Saxena D, Brotherson SE. When grandparents become parents to their grandchildren: NDSU Extension Service. Fargo: North Dakota State University; 2021.
34. Snow R. Real patient participation in simulations. In: Nestel D, Bearman M, editors. Simulated patient methodology: theory, evidence and practice. Chichester: Wiley; 2015. p. 105–9.
35. Chianáin LN, Fallis R, Johnston J, McNaughton N, Gormley G. Nothing about me without me: a scoping review of how illness experiences inform simulated participants' encounters in health profession education. BMJ Simul Technol Enhanc Learn. 2021;7(6):611.
36. Picketts L, Warren MD, Bohnert C. Diversity and inclusion in simulation: addressing ethical and psychological safety concerns when working with simulated participants. BMJ Simul Technol Enhanc Learn. 2021;7(6):590–9.
37. Nolan M, Brown J, Davies S, Nolan J, Keady J. The Senses Framework: improving care for older people through a relationship-centred approach. Getting Research into Practice (GRiP) Report No 2. 2006.
38. Tafler M, Yashinsky D. Storycare [Internet]. Toronto: Baycrest; https://www.storycare.ca/.
39. Smith C, Poerschke K, Bernick L, Kramer B, Meyer R, Adams M. Ruth's story: co-creating Inclusive, Authentic and Engaging Scenarios with Simulated Participants (SPs). Poster presented at: SIM Expo; 17–18 Oct 2022; Toronto.

Part II

Elements

A Systematic Approach to Designing Scenarios Involving Older Adult Simulated Participants

3

Linda Ní Chianáin, Suzanne Gough, and Debra Nestel

Key Messages

1. Most simulations involving SPs are scenario-based. Scenarios can facilitate knowledge and skills development for application in real clinical encounters.
2. Scenario design is increasingly a team-based, codesigned, and iterative process.
3. Simulation design frameworks are useful to scenario developers to optimise learning.
4. Older adult SPs have valuable life experience, which can be leveraged to create meaningful and authentic simulations. Codesign with individuals who have *lived experience* of the focus of a scenario (e.g. disease, service user) can provide critical insights into what needs to be learned.
5. A psychologically and physically safe environment for older adults involved in scenario-based learning is a priority.

Introduction

This chapter is about scenario development that involves older adult simulated participants (SPs). We have written the chapter for anyone interested in developing scenarios for older adult care. Design considerations span every phase of simulation practice. We use the NHET-Sim framework [1] to guide our design, describing each phase—*preparing, briefing, simulating, deroling, feedback/debriefing, reflecting,* and *evaluating*. In this chapter, our main concern is the *preparing* phase since all phases need consideration from the outset. Other chapters in this book cover the other phases in more detail. As this book focuses on older adults as SPs with *older adults* referring to individuals aged over 60 years [2], we will hereafter simply refer to older SPs. We also acknowledge and recommend published guidelines for SP-based work [3] and for broader simulation practices [4, 5]. However, these guidelines have largely evolved without specific reference to older adults. One exception is a framework specifically focused on older SPs that identified pre-, during, and postsimulation practices [6]. We have embedded this work in the NHET-Sim framework (Fig. 3.1) [1].

Foundational Concepts

Scenarios offer a story-line and context in which learners are given a task. In healthcare simulation, scenarios enable learners to apply knowledge and skills in the ways they will be required in clinical practice. Scenarios explore common and rare events and everything in between to be rehearsed by learners with feedback/debriefing and reflection. Our focus is on the design of scenarios with and/or about older adults. We direct readers to resources for broader considerations of simulation design.

Scenario documents usually include all the information required to run a simulation. A helpful metaphor can be to think of the scenario document as a *recipe*. The scenario title often denotes the expected outcome. The ingredients and instructions are described with various levels of detail. Following the instructions is likely to result in something resembling the expected outcome but there are many variables that come into play. We think about scenario docu-

The original version of the chapter has been revised. A correction to this chapter can be found at https://doi.org/10.1007/978-3-031-65742-9_36

L. N. Chianáin
Centre for Medical Education, School of Medicine, Dentistry & Biomedical Sciences, Queen's University Belfast, Belfast, Northern Ireland, UK
e-mail: L.NiChianain@qub.ac.uk

S. Gough
Faculty of Health Sciences & Medicine, Bond University, Gold Coast, QLD, Australia
e-mail: sgough@bond.edu.au

D. Nestel (✉)
School of Clinical Sciences, Faculty of Medicine, Nursing & Health Sciences, Monash University, Clayton, VIC, Australia

Department of Surgery (Austin Precinct), University of Melbourne, Parkville, VIC, Australia
e-mail: dnestel@unimelb.edu.au; debra.nestel@monash.edu

C. M. Smith et al. (eds.), *Comprehensive Healthcare Simulation: Geriatric Simulation*, Comprehensive Healthcare Simulation,
https://doi.org/10.1007/978-3-031-65742-9_3

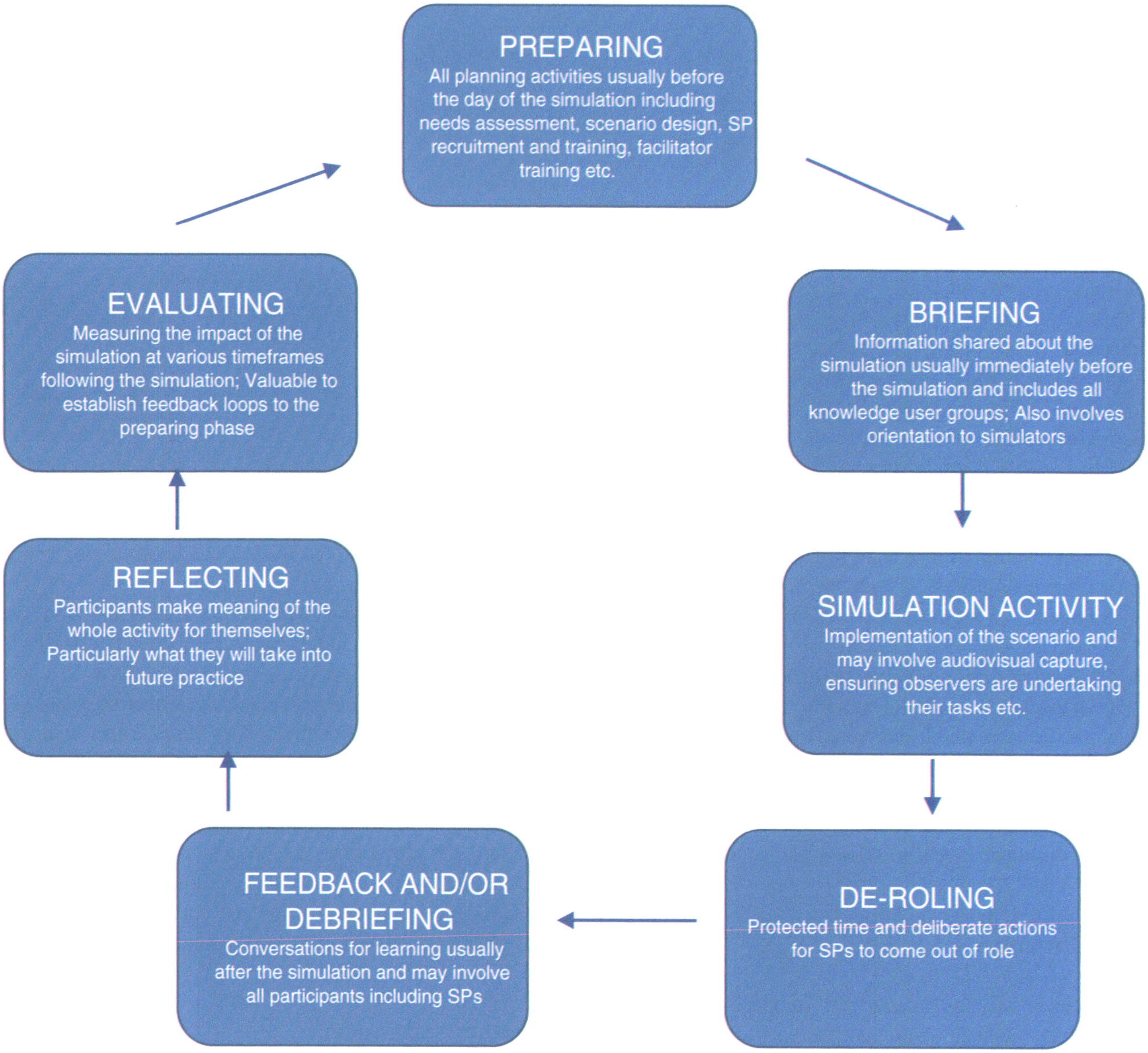

Fig. 3.1 Simulation-design framework adapted from NHET-Sim

ments containing everything you need to run the simulation and guidance on how to do it. Scenario documents come in different formats reflecting local traditions and preferences. There are several examples in Part 4 of this book. While efforts have been made to identify essential components of a scenario [7], there is little evidence to support a single approach.

Navigating Simulation Language

The language used to describe elements of scenario documents can seem complex. These may include an *SP role* or *SP script* or *SP case*. We prefer the phrase *SP role* since its focus is usually on who the SP is and what the SP is required to do and when and how. Further, SPs sometimes work in scenarios that have other simulators, such as a manikin, so it can be helpful to distinguish the information for the SP and from others involved in running the simulation. When information about SP role portrayal is referred to as an *SP script*, it can imply rigidity through the stipulation of multiple verbatim phrases. This often pushes against the naturalistic flow of communication between those involved in the simulation. While some scripting is helpful to achieve the learning objectives, we recommend keeping it to a minimum. Similarly, the phrase *SP case* seems to place a boundary around or *contain* a human experience, somehow limiting it in a way that may not feel authentic, even objectifying it. Scenario documents will also include information about the logistics of the session, guidance for learners, faculty, and administrators.

Older Adult SPs

In this section, we focus on considerations in producing a scenario document that includes older SPs. A traditional approach to scenario development has been the simulation designer (often a clinician or SP educator) who produces the scenario and then invites faculty and SPs to participate in its implementation obtaining feedback at this point. This approach has shifted to team-based development, often from the outset and is iterative in nature evolving in response to social, cultural, clinical, and other changes over time.

Older adults taking on the role of SPs will likely have extensive experience on which to draw. This may not have direct relevance to the scenario in which they will work. However, sometimes SPs will have *lived experience* of precisely the focus of the scenario (e.g. physical rehabilitation of a patient after a stroke, as a service user of an outpatient department, etc.). They may have been recruited for this direct experience, to assist in the codesign of the scenario. Whatever their experiences and degree of involvement, it is important to be sensitive to their psychological and physical safety. For example, scenarios featuring older adult abuse or life-limiting diseases may trigger emotional reactions while repetitive portrayal may be exhausting. Older SPs may have health conditions that affect their cognitive, physical, or sensory abilities. The health of any SP involved in simulation activities needs to be considered, and reasonable adjustments should be accommodated to facilitate inclusivity.

Age-related changes may affect the way older SPs process information and learn new skills. Modifying written communication (e.g. large font sizes, wider line spacing, bolded text for scripted information), use of multimedia (e.g. audio recordings and videos illustrating portrayal), provision of materials well in advance of the activity, and longer discussion times during training may assist access and support information processing.

In Box 3.1, we summarise questions older adults may have before they participate in any SP-related work. This information is helpful to know before designing scenarios to determine the content of written and spoken communications.

> Before I agree to participate, the most important information is when you want me to be there and for how long. I need to know the time commitments… There are probably some roles I would not want to do or could not do so a brief description is probably enough… [EW]

Box 3.1 Questions Older SPs May Ask Before Deciding to Participate

About the work in co-design

1. What would you like me to do? (e.g. read a document, participate in a discussion, etc.)
2. How long will you need me?
3. Who else will be there?

About the SP session

4. What is the goal of the session? (e.g. assessing communication, teaching physical examination skills, etc.)
5. Who are the learners?
6. Who else will be there?
7. What is the format of the work? (e.g. small group work, examinations such as OSCEs, etc.)
8. Will I be expected to show much emotion? [This is important for SPs to gauge their own psychological safety and their ability to play the role]
9. How long will each scenario be?
10. How many times will I play the role in one session? How many sessions will there be?
11. Do I need to give feedback? How? When? To whom?
12. Will I be required to expose any part of my body? If so, which and for what purpose?
13. Will I be required to wear any specific clothing? If so, will this be provided, or do I need to bring my own?
14. Can I use a prompt card?
15. What if I cannot hear what's being said?
16. What if I forget what I'm meant to say?
17. How will it end? Who ends it?

About preparation and training for the SP session

18. How far in advance will the scenario document be provided?
19. What training will be provided?
20. Where will it be? Who will be there?

About logistics and practicalities for co-design and SP sessions

21. Will I be paid? How much?
22. Will I be able to park close to the location? Do I pay for parking?
23. Does the building have ramp access?
24. Does the building have accessible facilities?
25. Will I be able to bring a support person?

Broad Simulation-Based Education Design Considerations

There are several resources available to assist in the design process. We have already cited standard documents from the International Nursing Association for Clinical Simulation and Learning (INACSL) and those that have been adopted by many professional societies. They cover many facets of simulation-based education including learner, faculty, and physical environment requirements. A full description of simulation design is beyond the scope of the chapter. However, we have selected specific standard documents that inform SP-based scenario design in the resources section, so we can retain our focus on older adults as SPs. We also draw attention to a framework derived from work by Kim et al. that can assist in aligning the structure, process, and intended outcomes of scenario-based learning [8]. See Box 3.2.

Box 3.2 Summary of Considerations Before the Scenario Goes Live

The following questions are derived by Kim et al. (2006) and have been adapted for scenario design.

Structure

Review relevance:

What is the level of learner?

What are goals and objectives?

What is the scenario setting?

Do the level of learner, goals and objectives and setting all align?

Review authenticity:

What sources is the scenario drawn from?

How will the learner feel regarding the authenticity of the material?

What gaps in realism are the learners required to overcome? Are they reasonable?

Process

Review engagement:

How does the learner know what to do next?

How do the learners have to interact with each other?

How do learners' actions change the outcome of the scenario?

Review the level of challenge:

What do learners have to do that they haven't already done? How will this be accounted for? How will learners know the requirements of the scenario?

How do you know that the learners will not be overwhelmed in the scenario so that they can learn?

Outcomes

Review educational design:

In general, how can the learner's performance be assessed?

In general, how does feedback occur within and after the scenario?

How does the scenario link with briefing, debriefing and reflection phases?

How does the scenario link with learners' prior knowledge?

If the scenario forms part of a curriculum, how does it fit within it?

There are several commonly cited theories that inform scenario-based learning. These include cognitive load theory [9] (ensuring a balance of intrinsic and germane with extraneous load), experiential learning theory [10] (providing learners with a concrete learning experience, feedback on that experience, distilling of key learning, and then applying that learning in a continuous cycle), situated learning [11] (giving learners the opportunity to practise in settings similar to those in which they will be expected to practise), and reflective practice [12] (individual meaning making after events with the intention of improving future practice). Again, it is beyond the scope of this chapter to cover this topic in-depth, so we provide recommendations for further reading.

NHET-Sim Phase: Preparing

The first NHET-Sim phase is *preparing*. While this effectively covers all the NHET-Sim phases, our focus is on those elements that relate mainly to older SPs and the SP role. Further, detail is shared in other chapters and in the scenarios in Part 4 of this book.

Articulating the Goal and Purpose

The goals and purpose of the learning activity need to be articulated. Be clear about what you are trying to achieve and why. Question whether the learning need you are addressing is important and whether an SP-based scenario is a meaningful way to address the need. It is easy to drift from goals and purpose so clarity from the outset is helpful.

Establishing the Design 'Team' and Knowledge User Groups

While scenarios can be written by individuals, they are now more commonly written by teams. The team may include the healthcare professionals, other subject matter experts, simulationists, and simulation operations specialists (e.g. technicians in moulage, special effects, videography, etc.). We also position SPs and individuals with lived experience of the focus of the scenario as central to the design process. Codesign opportunities may provide unique insights to further inform the goal, purpose, scenario development, and role portrayal information, and so early engagement can be beneficial [13]. See Box 3.3 for codesign examples. Think carefully about what you may need to do to be truly inclusive of older adults. You may arrange one-to-one meetings; they may need to be in person and at times that promote safe and easy travel. Ask yourself who the knowledge users are relative to the scenario. Expert guidance should be sought when the *lived experience* addressed in a scenario is distant to the simulation designers (e.g. indigeneity, sexual orientation etc.). Finally, current and past students can also offer valuable insights and can function effectively as full members of the design team. While it is impractical to include all knowledge user groups every time, bear in mind that a broad knowledge user base is likely to surface goals that may be overlooked than with a narrower base.

Box 3.3 Examples of a Co-design Process with Older Adults with 'Lived Experience'

- A hospital-based simulation team has been asked to consider developing scenarios to improve in-patient admissions. Older adults may be recruited to share their experiences of the admissions process, from initial communication to completing the admission.
- A care assistant program wants to improve experiential learning opportunities for students attending rotations in residential aged care. While students' perspectives will be important in this quality improvement activity, so will the voices of the residents and their carers, including exploration of the content of the learning experience for the students but also the ways in which the rotation impacts the residents and carers.
- Awareness training focused on older adult abuse for healthcare professionals working in the emergency department, to develop skills to identify and discuss abuse. Careful attention must be given to manage the psychological safety of older adults invited to share their lived experience of older adult abuse.
- Falls prevention simulation designed to help occupational therapists (OTs) identify risks and implement strategies to reduce/prevent falls. Inviting older adults with prior OT to observe relevant scenarios in action may offer valuable insights to the authenticity of the portrayal. Their feedback can be used to further shape the scenario.

Writing Learning Objectives

Learning objectives define what is expected to be achieved in the scenario and are usually written as behavioural or observational statements. See examples in Part 4 of this book. We share several resources to assist in the process of writing learning objectives. It is also important to note the link between learning objectives and *evaluating*. It is common to have 2–4 learning objectives in a scenario.

Learners

The learners' needs and experiences are obviously central to any educational design. Ensure you consider the learners' knowledge, prior experience, and expectations of the learning activity. See Box 3.2.

Facilitators

Similarly, think about the functions you expect of facilitators, what knowledge and experience will be optimal, and what training may be necessary to support them to work effectively. Write clear guidelines for facilitators in the scenario document (e.g. briefing notes such as allowing more time for settling the older adult SP into their physical environment, simulation activity guidance such as hand signals to call a pause and discuss in case SPs cannot easily hear you, debriefing guidance such as a large font rating or prompt forms for SPs to guide their feedback, etc.).

Templates for SP Roles

The scenario document should contain information on the SP role outlining the characteristics of the person they are portraying, their personal characteristics, and if the SP is in the role of a *patient*, then their health details and prompts and key responses should be included. Keep the SP reader in mind when you are writing the SP role. Avoid headings such as *history of presenting complaint* since this is a medicalised presentation and not usually how patients talk about their health. We have replaced this with *the patient's history of the issue, concern, or problem.* We also encourage writing with direct statements since they draw the SP immediately into the role. That is, 'You're concerned about your headaches' rather than '*Mrs. Leong is concerned about her headaches'*. See Box 3.4. SPs will also need information about logistics but that is often presented separately since it can vary across learning settings even though the SP role remains consistent.

> Sometimes too much information is confusing… I like information on my role ahead of time, but I don't want too much…. I like you to mail it me so I can read it and highlight it for myself… I prefer to give you feedback on what you've done rather than coming up with the ideas with you… [EW]

Box 3.4 Headings Commonly Found in SP Role Templates Where the Participant Is a Patient

Title of scenario
Date
Authors
Overview
Learning objectives
- After participating in this scenario, learners will be able to: … (List objectives)

Type of learning activity
- For example: Teaching in small groups with video-assisted debriefing with learner, observers and SP led by a facilitator

Description of role to be played including the patient's characteristics
- For example: You will be playing the role of Mr Alexander Wong, an 86-year-old man concerned about his loss of balance. You are co-operative and communicate easily although your voice is quiet and your movements are careful. You're really pleased to have got the appointment at short notice…

The patient's history of the issue or problem
The patient's past medical history
The patient's social information (work, lifestyle, habits, etc.)
The patient's ideas and concerns about the focus of the scenario
- For example: You think your loss of balance is related to the flu you had last month…
- For example: You are concerned because you might fall over…

The patient's expectations about what will happen in the encounter
- For example: You are expecting that you might be given some medicine or have some tests.

Opening statement
Key phrases or prompts
Considerations in playing this role
- For example: Clothing required, physical requirements, need for physical examination, moulage, etc.)

Training for Older SP Role Portrayal

Like all SPs, older SPs benefit from training for role portrayal. See Chap. 4—Training Older SPs for Role Portrayal. This includes how to portray the character as written in the SP role. The training typically includes guidance on the extent to which they can improvise or give standardised or scripted responses (e.g. opening statements and key phrases or prompts). It is important to note that *standardisation* processes can reduce authenticity. Again, see Part 4 of this book for examples.

Dry Run of the Scenario

The *preparing* phase should also include testing of the scenario to identify any issues (a dry run), so these can be rectified and refined in advance. The dry run helps to verify timings, equipment requirements, environment staging, and audiovisual testing to ensure audiovisual capture is in the right place for faculty, SPs, and learners. During this dry run, older SPs may also offer recommendations to the SP role or broader scenario document to better reflect their ideas and improve the learning activity. While you may already have addressed the questions in Box 3.2, it is a good opportunity to consider them again during the dry run.

Smith et al. (2020) refer to the 'presimulation' phase as 'know your older SPs', offering physical, cognitive, and sensory changes that may need consideration [6]. Often, we do not know who the SPs will be in our scenarios since some scenarios have a long life. It is incumbent on scenario designers to build in prompts to scenario documents to remind faculty to consider specific SP needs. For example, an older SP who is very frail may need more time and specific seating for comfort and safety; an older SP with multiple scars from previous surgery may need an adjustment to the medical history of the role they are playing to add realism to their portrayal; and so on.

NHET-Sim Phase: Briefing

The *briefing* phase can help facilitate a safe learning experience for all those involved. It can alleviate anxiety by providing information on the simulation activity [1]. Briefing can assist in ensuring that the simulation is implemented as designed. Briefing notes should form part of the scenario document as a checklist or verbatim script. The briefing occurs immediately before the scenario is implemented. Ensuring adequate time for the briefing is likely to promote learning. We think of the briefing as setting up everyone involved for success.

Briefing the Simulation Team

Briefing provides an opportunity for a shared mental model to be established by team members. All members of the simulation team usually participate, and this includes the older SP. It covers introductions (who is involved), the schedule (how the simulation activity will run from briefing to evaluation, the starting state, cues to pause and ending), learning objectives, and orientation to equipment (e.g. the SP cannot move her simulator arm for taking blood). The opportunity for questions to be asked is also important. Even at this late stage, new information may be required. Providing an opportunity for older SPs to have a final detailed run through is helpful. Take care to position yourself so they can see and hear you. Older SPs may also be introduced to learners during their briefing, but often the first time the older SP meets the learners is in role during the simulation. Briefing the older SP usually ends by taking them to the simulation space and settling them into their *starting* position for the scenario. Ensuring the scenario space is free of fall hazards, that the SP is comfortable and that they know the cue to pause the scenario should they wish.

> I like meeting the facilitator ahead of the session, so you know what they want. It doesn't always play out as the information sheets say it will, so I just leave the changes to the facilitator. Having a talk about how the session is going to work is really helpful. I usually have something to ask. It's always better that my first role is not a surprise for anyone, so a quick rehearsal makes a lot of sense. [EW]

Briefing the Learners

This includes introductions, the schedule, learning objectives, orientation to the equipment and environment, and establishing the limitations of the simulators. Exploring learners' experiences of simulation, the topic to be explored and their areas of strength and development in this area can occur during the briefing. It is also helpful to invite learners to imagine the scenario they will participate in as real—this is referred to as the *fiction contract*. The specific information of the learners' task(s) within the scenario should be shared and opportunities for questions invited. Briefing should also include information about the use of audiovisual equipment. That is, if the scenario is being recorded or live streamed, for what purpose and to whom. While it is common for briefings to be a one-way flow of information, it can be helpful to promote exchanges of ideas to set a conversational tone for debriefing and feedback.

NHET-Sim Phase: Simulation Activity

During the simulation, there may be transitional points as the scenario evolves; there may be the need to pause and discuss what is occurring in the scenario and then reset. The scenario may run its course and naturally end, or it may require cues provided to signal its end. When learner participants are observing a scenario via a live stream/a viewing area, distractions should be minimised, to avoid disrupting the flow of the scenario. Observer guides can add value to learners' experiences [14]. These observations can be integrated into the feedback/debriefing phases. Smith et al. (2020) refer to the 'during-simulation' phase as 'full support', again offering physical, cognitive, and sensory changes that may need consideration [6]. Prompting notes can be built into the role (e.g. 'I have a list of questions I want to ask you'; 'I've written down my tablets because I find them a bit confusing.').

NHET-Sim: Deroling Phase

Deroling occurs when the scenario has ended [15, 16]. This process of breaking character facilitates meaningful discussion between learners, the older SP, and others during the feedback/debriefing phase. Deroling can occur when the older SP joins the feedback/debriefing. It can be as simple as introducing the older SP to the learners, thanking them for playing the SP role and asking them how they are feeling now. It can be undertaken individually or as part of a group [15, 16]. This process can facilitate the psychological safety of all those involved in the scenario [16]. Techniques used to transition out of the role may include deep breathing, visualisation, or physical movement. Deroling is important whether or not the older SP is involved in feedback/debriefing. See Chap. 14.

NHET-Sim Phase: Feedback/Debriefing

The feedback/debriefing phase links back to the briefing phase, in which the facilitator usually leads discussion with learners, observers, SPs, and relevant others to recap what was covered [1]. There is a significant emphasis on the importance of this phase as it is associated with being explicit about learning. There are several debriefing frameworks. See recommended resources [1, 17–19]. Debriefing promotes reflection (individually and as a group), focuses on feelings and reactions, discusses the learning objectives, gathers perspectives, recognises positive performance, and explores unanticipated situations and gaps in performance. The timing of the debrief can occur immediately after the simulation, or it can be delayed [1, 17–19]. Video-assisted debriefing (VAD) can be a valuable adjunct, especially when learners cannot specifically recall what they did during the simulation. Conversely, the facilitator may wish to reaffirm positive performances, especially when learners felt they underperformed. VAD may be helpful to older SPs who can be invited to watch a specific segment of the video to prompt their reflection on what they were feeling or thinking relative to the learners' behaviours. Specifically inviting older SPs to share what they would like learners to know based on their experience of them in the simulation is invaluable. There is no specific evidence for time allocations between briefings, simulation activities, and debriefings in SP-based scenarios. However, for a 15-min scenario designed as a learning event, it would be reasonable to allocate10 min to briefing and 30 min to feedback/debriefing.

It is important that *feedback/debriefing* incorporates the SP, since SPs offer unique perspectives from within the simulation encounter. SPs can be supported to provide feedback to learners on aspects of patient-centred care and communication. Structured feedback/debriefing tools can assist the SP to focus their attention to key aspects of patient-centred care (e.g. how they felt in response to learners, whether they felt valued as a person, etc.). Training to empower SPs to provide feedback is available [20]. See Chap. 6. We acknowledge that these responsibilities of completing feedback tools and providing feedback may be daunting for the SP, not because of their age but because of the complexity of the task and the emotional weight of some of the experiences. Encouraging older SPs to record their immediate reactions can assist in later recall during debriefing.

In some instances, the older SP may not be directly involved in feedback/debriefing such as in OSCEs. They may be asked to complete rating forms, perhaps with assistance which must always be respectful of the views expressed by the older SP.

> … I like talking with the learners afterwards… You can talk about things in a different way to it being a real consult. Sometimes you're invited by the facilitator but other times you have something to say but you're not invited so it gets missed. I think it's probably important to always ask the SP is there is anything else they'd like to say. [EW]

It is also helpful to debrief SPs separately to the learners because then the purpose is about the SPs' experience of their own performance and how they may maintain or improve their own contribution to learning. In the NHET-Sim phases, we have positioned this in the *reflecting* phase (see below). The timing of the 'SP debriefing/reflection' should probably occur before the SPs leave the session. However, there may be times when they are tired and that time is short, and so it would be better to revisit on a later occasion.

NHET-Sim Phase: Reflecting

In the NHET-Sim phases, there is an overlap between the *reflecting* and *feedback/debriefing phases*. In *reflecting*, learners are urged to think about the learning they will take into their future practice and what additional learning may need to be undertaken. While this may have occurred as a group activity during debriefing, here it is intended for learners to think about the meaning of the learning for themselves. Reflection techniques can include a written, audio, or video documentation of their experience using a model to structure their reflection. For example, the Gibbs model provides structured guidance that could be used to reflect on the simulation and debriefing/feedback activities [21]. See resources.

While the *feedback/debriefing* phase is focused on the learners' development, reflection encourages SPs and faculty to develop and maintain their own performance. Write into the scenario document prompts for the SPs to reflect on their own performance—What did you do well today? Why do you think it worked? What could have improved your performance? How can you maintain or improve your performance for next time?

> I've done this work on and off for many years. I think I have got better at it, of feeling comfortable in roles … it mainly depends on the information I'm given and also the attitudes of the facilitators. Some take more time than others, giving you time to think about what we're doing and why and how we can all get better. [EW]

NHET-Sim Phase: Evaluating

The *evaluating* phase is an opportunity for learners, faculty, and older SPs to provide feedback on the whole learning experience [1, 17–19]. Return to the learning objectives to invite judgements on the extent to which they were met and from the perspectives of all those involved. While some of this information will have surfaced during the feedback/debriefing phase, then the intention was to support learners; this time the focus shifts to improving the quality of the learning experience. Each element of the learning activity can be examined—the preparation for learners, SPs, and facilitators, the learning objectives, the briefings, the observation opportunities, the feedback/debriefing, and the reflection. The evaluation can be unstructured or structured, with a rating scale or free text options, digital, or paper format. These evaluations provide valuable insights into how well the scenario went relative to meeting the learning objectives and what issues still need to be addressed. The evaluation format and method may need to be adjusted to assist older SPs to complete, whether this involves completing it with them, providing hand-written evaluations or audio collection of their evaluation comments. It will be helpful to know from SPs their experience across the whole activity to reveal what they valued and what was unhelpful, repetitive, obstructive, or unproductive.

> Some days go better than others and it can be hard to identify why but sometimes it is obvious. I can fill out forms, but I like to just tell the organisers a few key things about how the day went for me. [EW]

Smith et al. refer to the 'postsimulation' phase as 'invest and integrate' reminding us of the benefits and the adjustments to our practice we may need to make to ensure it is a truly collaborative activity [6]. Before older SPs leave, always check in to see that they are comfortable to make their way home.

Closing

This chapter provides an overview of a systematic approach to designing SP-based scenarios. Team-based and iterative scenario development can produce meaningful simulation experiences for learners. Practical examples and templates have been provided and wide-ranging resources recommended. While we have described many steps in the process of designing scenarios, in our experience, it is important to stay focused and tend to simplicity rather than complexity. Avoid too many learning objectives and keep revisiting them throughout the design process. Scenarios evolve so be open to feedback from all those working with them.

We have oriented readers to key concepts in scenario design. We have introduced foundational concepts, navigated simulation language, and offered considerations in broad educational design in scenario-based learning. We recommended resources for further developing your practice. While wide knowledge user consultation and codesign add complexity, it can also lead to more authentic scenarios and is an exciting process. We hope that the NHET-Sim phases have illustrated a systematic approach to scenario design referring to Smith et al. pre-, during, and postsimulation to provide meaningful experiences for learners and the older adults who contribute to our field [6].

Resources

Overall Simulation Design

- INACSL Standards Committee (2016). INACSL Standards of Best Practice: Simulation Design. *Clinical Simulation in Nursing* 12: S5–S12. https://doi.org/10.1016/j.ecns.2016.09.005.
- Smith, C. M., Sokoloff, L. G., & Alsaba, N. (2020). Collaborative framework for working with older simulated participants (SP). *BMJ simulation & technology enhanced learning*, *7*(2), 112–115. https://doi.org/10.1136/bmjstel-2020-000613.
- Nestel, D., & Gough, S. (2018). Designing healthcare simulation learning experiences. In D. Nestel, M. Kelly, B. Jolly, & M. Watson (Eds.), *Healthcare simulation: Theory, Evidence & Practice* (pp. 135–142): John Wiley & Sons.

Writing Learning Objectives

- Chatterjee D, Corral J. How to Write Well-Defined Learning Objectives. J Educ Perioper Med. 2017 Oct 1;19(4):E610. PMID: 29766034; PMCID: PMC5944406. https://www.ncbi.nlm.nih.gov/pmc/articles/PMC5944406/
- INACSL Standards Committee. (2016). INACSL Standards of Best Practice: SimulationSM: Outcomes and Objectives. *Clinical Simulation in Nursing, 12*, S13–S15. https://www.nursingsimulation.org/article/S1876-1399%2816%2930127-X/fulltext

Debriefing and/or Feedback

- INACSL Standards Committee (2016, December). INACSL standards of best practice: SimulationSM Debriefing. *Clinical Simulation in Nursing*, 12(S), S21–S25. https://doi.org/10.1016/j.ecns.2016.09.008.
- Bajaj, K., Meguerdichian, M., Thoma, B., Huang, S., Eppich, W., & Cheng, A. (2018). The PEARLS Healthcare Debriefing Tool. *Acad Med, 93*(2), 336. https://doi.org/10.1097/ACM.0000000000002035.
- Jaye, P., Thomas, L., & Reedy, G. (2015). 'The Diamond': a structure for simulation debrief. *Clin Teach, 12*(3), 171–175. https://doi.org/10.1111/tct.12300Pendleton.

Reflecting

- Reflection Toolkit—https://www.ed.ac.uk/reflection [Accessed April 2022].

Acknowledgement Eileen Webb (EW) worked as a simulated patient with DN over several years. She passed away aged 91 during the production phase of this book. She has shared some of her experiences highlighted in this chapter.

References

1. The NHET-Sim Monash Team. The National Health Education and Training—Simulation (NHET-Sim) program. 2012. http://www.nhet-sim.edu.au.
2. World Health Organization. Ageing [Internet]. Geneva: World Health Organization; 2023. https://www.who.int/health-topics/ageing#tab=tab_1.
3. Lewis KL, Bohnert CA, Gammon WL, Hölzer H, Lyman L, Smith C, Thompson TM, Wallace A, Gliva-McConvey G. The association of standardized patient educators (ASPE) standards of best practice (SOBP). Adv Simul. 2017;2(1):1–8. https://doi.org/10.1186/s41077-017-0043-4.
4. INACSL Standards Committee. INACSL standards of best practice: simulation SM simulation design. Clin Simul Nurs. 2016;12(S):S5–S12. https://doi.org/10.1016/j.ecns.2016.09.005.
5. Purva M, Nicklin J. ASPiH standards for simulation-based education: process of consultation, design and implementation. BMJ Simul Technol Enhanc Learn. 2018;4(3):117–25. https://doi.org/10.1136/bmjstel-2017-000232.
6. Smith CM, Sokoloff LG, Alsaba N. Collaborative framework for working with older simulated participants (SP). BMJ Simul Technol Enhanc Learn. 2020;7(2):112–5. https://doi.org/10.1136/bmjstel-2020-000613.
7. Davies EL, Pelentsov LJ, Montagu A, Gordon AL, Hooper KJ, Esterman AJ. "Who Am I and Why Am I Here?" A scoping review exploring the templates and protocols that direct actors in their roles as simulated (standardized) patients. Simul Healthc. 2021;16(3):190–8. https://doi.org/10.1097/SIH.0000000000000470.
8. Kim S, Phillips WR, Pinsky L, Brock D, Phillips K, Keary JA. Conceptual framework for developing teaching cases: a review and synthesis of the literature across disciplines. Med Educ. 2006;40:867–76. https://doi.org/10.1111/j.1365-2929.2006.02544.x.
9. Reedy GB. Using cognitive load theory to inform simulation design and practice. Clin Simul Nurs. 2018;11(8):355–60. https://doi.org/10.1016/j.ecns.2015.05.004.
10. Davitadze M, Ooi E, Ng CY, Zhou D, Thomas L, Hanania T, Blaggan P, Evans N, Chen W, Melson E, Arlt W, Kempegowda P. SIMBA: using Kolb's learning theory in simulation-based learning to improve participants' confidence. BMC Med Educ. 2022;22(116):1–11. https://doi.org/10.1186/s12909-022-03176-2.
11. O'Brien BC, Battista A. Situated learning theory in health professions education research: a scoping review. Adv Health Sci Educ Theory Pract. 2020;25(2):483–509. https://doi.org/10.1007/s10459-019-09900-w.
12. Husebø SE, O'Regan S, Nestel D. Reflective practice and its role in simulation. Clin Simul Nurs. 2015;11(8):368–75. https://doi.org/10.1016/j.ecns.2015.04.005.
13. Ní Chianáin L, Fallis R, Johnston J, McNaughton N, Gormley G. Nothing about me without me: a scoping review of how illness experiences inform simulated participants' encounters in health profession education. BMJ STEL. 2021;7(6):611–6. https://doi.org/10.1136/bmjstel-2021-000886.
14. O'Regan S, Molloy E, Watterson L, Nestel D. Observer roles that optimise learning in healthcare simulation education: a systematic review. Adv Simul. 2016;1(4):1–10. https://doi.org/10.1186/s41077-015-0004-8.
15. Ker JS, Dowie A, Dowell J, Dewar G, Dent JA, Ramsay J, Benvie S, Bracher L, Jackson C. Twelve tips for developing and maintaining a simulated patient bank. Med Teach. 2005;27(1):4–9. https://doi.org/10.1080/01421590400004882.
16. Busselle K. De-roling and debriefing: essential aftercare for educational theatre. Theatre Topics. 2021;31(2):129–35.
17. Cowperthwait A. NLN/Jeffries simulation framework for simulated participant methodology. Clin Simul Nurs. 2020;42(C):12–21. https://doi.org/10.1016/j.ecns.2019.12.009.
18. Nestel D, Gough S. Educating for professional practice through simulation. In: Delany C, Molloy E, editors. Learning and teaching in clinical contexts: a practical guide. Chatswood: Elsevier; 2018. p. 175–92.
19. Gough S, Yohannes A M. And Murray J. Using video-reflexive ethnography and simulation-based education to explore patient management and error recognition by pre-registration physiotherapists. Adv Simul 1, 9 (2016). doi:https://doi.org/10.1186/s41077-016-0010-5.
20. Nestel D, Bearman M, Fleischman C. Simulated patients as teachers: the role of feedback. In: Nestel D, Bearman M, editors. Simulated patient methodology: theory, evidence, and practice. London: Wiley; 2015.
21. Gibbs G. Learning by doing: a guide to a teaching and learning methods. Oxford: Oxford Polytechnic; 1988.

4 Training Older Adult Simulated Participants for Role Portrayal

Leanne Picketts, Anne Woll, and Claudia Schlegel

Key Messages

1. Older adult SPs are valuable team members in simulation, and Universal Design provides an inclusive strength-based approach to training to optimize SPs' engagement, performance, and retention.
2. Consider factors that might affect training and role portrayal with older adult SPs: physical, sensory, and cognitive changes, changes in health history, and life transitions.
3. When preparing to train older adult SPs, consider how the written text is formatted and how the training will be scheduled, accessed, and delivered.
4. Throughout the simulation, provide in-person support and frequent breaks to accommodate changing stamina levels and to prevent fatigue and cognitive overload.
5. Create a relationship with each SP that promotes their well-being from recruitment and training through role-play and debriefing, and utilize multiple strategies to solicit their feedback to improve their experience as an SP.

Box 4.1 Vignette

Your role: You are part of an educational team who has been tasked with creating an interprofessional simulation focused on the care of older adults.

The simulation scenario: The team decides to focus the scenario on elder abuse; the patient is a 76-year-old person experiencing psychological, physical, and financial abuse by their caregiver, who is the patient's adult son. The scenario the team has written is lengthy and complex, containing an extensive health history. The patient is taking many medications, each with different dosing information.

The simulation schedule: The event will require seven hours of active simulation with multiple interprofessional team encounters, including an hour break for lunch. Due to the complexity of scheduling an interprofessional simulation, you cannot change the schedule.

SP recruitment: You need to recruit SPs for this role who can believably portray a 76-year-old patient.

SP training: You often train SP scenarios in one three-hour session but you can adjust the training duration. You train either onsite in your simulation center or virtually using an online platform.

Your objectives: In addition to meeting the learning objectives of the scenario and working within the policies of your institution, your objective is to recruit and prepare SPs for safe, effective, and authentic role portrayal.

Introduction

There has been a significant focus on SP training practices [1–4] which have guided SP educators toward safe, effective, and authentic role portrayal during simulation. While these guidelines have established clear and practical training frameworks, working with older adult SPs highlights considerations for accessibility and inclusion that SP educators must take into account—specifically, physical, sensory, and cognitive changes in older adult SPs that might affect their partici-

L. Picketts (✉)
Centre for Collaborative Clinical Learning & Research, Dalhousie University, Halifax, NS, Canada
e-mail: Leanne.Picketts@dal.ca

A. Woll
M Simulation, University of Minnesota, Minneapolis, MN, USA
e-mail: wollx003@umn.edu

C. Schlegel
Berner Bildungszentrum Pflege, Bern, Switzerland
e-mail: Claudia.schlegel@bzpflege.ch

C. M. Smith et al. (eds.), *Comprehensive Healthcare Simulation: Geriatric Simulation*, Comprehensive Healthcare Simulation,
https://doi.org/10.1007/978-3-031-65742-9_4

pation [5]. Changes associated with an individual's health history and life transitions (e.g., retirement, care or death of loved ones) may also impact older adult SPs' comfort with specific scenarios, and their ability to participate may change [6]. Understanding these changes may come from an SP's self-disclosure or through observation by an SP educator during training and role-play. It is important to acknowledge the continuous changes that occur in SPs over time and to foster a safe, compassionate, respectful, and confidential environment for disclosure and discussion while finding ways to enable SPs' continuous and successful participation.

SP educators have an obligation to maintain safe, effective, and authentic role-play and work under guiding ethical principles and values of physical and psychological safety, respect, and trust [1, 7]. This includes avoiding generalizations about any community; when working with older adult SPs, it is important to acknowledge potential discrimination and stigmatization from ageism and ableism. Older adult SPs offer valuable contributions to simulation-based education, and SP educators must honor the value and vulnerability of SPs [7, 8]. Adopting an inclusive strength-based approach in place of a deficit discourse benefits both SPs and simulation. This includes acknowledging and supporting the changing physical, sensory, and cognitive function of older adult SPs (within aging as part of the continuum of human development), while simultaneously empowering older adult SPs to succeed and find value in their contributions to simulation-based education.

Older adult SPs are valuable to health professions education; their participation benefits our learners as community representation is required in simulation to effectively train healthcare learners to provide care for diverse patients. They have a breadth of life experience and embodied knowledge, including personal experience as patients within our healthcare systems, which is an important contribution to their collaboration with simulation-based education. Older adult SPs are motivated to participate in simulation-based education and have cited many benefits to participating beyond financial gain, including having a sense of purpose, meaningful involvement and contribution, social interaction, altruism, and feeling appreciated [6, 9]. Although the motivation of SPs may shift depending on country, institution, culture, and individuality, the mutual value simulation and older adult SPs share can be fostered and enhanced through training practices that acknowledge and support their unique needs.

Other chapters within this text specifically discuss considerations that should be given to simulation scenario development (see Chap. 3) and recruitment of older adult SPs (see Chap. 9); this chapter focuses on inclusive practices when training older adult SPs for role portrayal—how SP educators might prepare for training with older adult SPs, important considerations for the training session itself, ways to minimize psychological and physical harm during role-play while maintaining effective and authentic simulation, and finally the debrief and evaluation postsimulation. Although the focus of this chapter is on working with older adult SPs, the inclusive training practices we suggest should not be limited to older adult SPs; inclusive training practices have relevance to all SPs.

Preparation for the Training Process

SP role training is well described in the literature, reflecting a variety of training methods [1–4]. Importantly, the *Association of SP Educators Standards of Best Practice* [1] outline principles for training preparation, including consideration of the training plan and schedule, preparatory materials, and the physical environment. However, SPs are diverse, and SP educators must consider which method is most appropriate for the individual and the specific learning context. Creating a training process that is inclusive and effective requires preparation and the acknowledgment that individual learners have unique learning needs. *Universal Design for Learning* [10] provides guidance to support the diversity of learning preferences by considering multiple ways to deliver the same information. While the physical and cognitive changes of aging can create specific training needs for older adult SPs, differing training needs are not exclusive to any one demographic.

Recruiting older adult SPs to a specific role requires screening for physical, sensory, and cognitive ability (e.g., mobility, hearing, vision, memory, stamina) and psychological safety (e.g., lived experience and comfort with role) [6]. SPs should be screened for any emotional challenges of the role, ensuring they are comfortable with the content and whether they have personal experience that might affect them in role. Once SPs understand the psychological risks and other demands of the role, they can provide informed consent for their participation which supports their safety and encourages autonomy and empowerment.

SP educators need to consider how the training schedule and plan will support the needs of the participating SPs. Often, the temptation is to accomplish as much as possible in training in a limited amount of time. When considering cognitive and physical overload for SPs, the training may be best accomplished with more time, with breaks, or across more sessions to maintain focus and engagement. Advance communication about the time, duration, and expectations of the training may help older adult SPs anticipate any modifications they might need and to arrive prepared and ready to collaboratively engage in the training activities. Sending scenario materials in advance and scheduling the training session close to the event day can also enhance memory retrieval [5].

Layout and presentation of training materials can support memory retention and retrieval, notably by using larger font, keywords, chunking information, and developing references to highlight specific content, like a medication list [5, 11].

Older adult SPs may have changing physical abilities that may impact their access to physical space. Create a barrier-free environment that allows individuals of all abilities to access the space; consider the accessibility from different entrances and the challenges of navigating distances, complex facility layouts, and heavy or self-closing doors. Proactively provide maps and anticipate staffing needs to escort individuals, hold doors, and move chairs. Within the training space, identify any acoustic challenges such as ambient noise, echoing, and distance from the audio source, and identify mitigation strategies. Ensure the physical setup is appropriate and has good lighting. Provide stable, comfortable seating options suitable for the duration of training.

The training plan and schedule should allow ample time for practice and feedback to calibrate role portrayal and to allow for questions. Training should allow for any physicality in the portrayal to be practiced, to ensure any movement required is physically safe for each SP. This includes specific movements in the scenario (e.g., a patient transfer from hospital bed to chair) as well as restricted movements (e.g., lying motionless on a highly sensitive bed alarm).

If the training takes place online, ensure that SPs have training to the platform being used and, prior to training, have adequate familiarity with the relevant technology. Consider how to make any or all portions of the training reviewable by the SP by recording the session, providing narrated presentations, or sharing additional training notes.

Knowing the learner is a fundamental tenet in education, and the approach to SP training preparation must balance thinking broadly about best practices with all SPs and anticipating needs specific to the individuals being trained. Consider the range of ages, abilities, and anticipated learning needs of the SPs. Are there individuals in the training that can benefit from specific approaches? How can the SP trainer help the SPs accept and be supportive of another SP's unique needs in the training? Approaching training with adequate levels of preparation, support, and flexibility may require more resources—time, human, and technical—but this commitment is essential to achieving the inclusivity in human simulation programming that healthcare education requires.

Box 4.2 Preparation for the Training Process

SP Scenario Considerations

During your scenario review, you recognize that there is a lot of detail for SPs to remember.

- You remove redundant information and limit paragraph size.
- You chunk the content into relevant sections, using headings, bullets, and short lists [11].
- You decide to provide SPs with a medication list (which they can hand to the learners) to eliminate some memorization.
- You ensure the font is at minimum 12-point [11].
- You share the updated scenario document and your rationale with your co-authors, recognizing that they also can benefit from understanding how to better collaborate with the SPs on this project.

Simulation Schedule Considerations

During review of the simulation day schedule, you realize that a 7-h simulation day, with an emotionally demanding role, may be tiring for SPs.

- You decide to put the SPs on a rotation, giving them every second hour off to rest and recharge. This means you need to recruit double the number of SPs, which has budget implications. To create a sustainable work environment and for the SPs, this budget increase is approved.

Training Schedule Considerations

You are concerned that there is too much content for one training session. However, you also want to minimize possible transportation issues, as you know some SPs may need to schedule specialized transportation services to come to your center.

- You schedule two 90-min training sessions: the first will be virtual, and the focus will be to situate the SPs into the educational context within which they will be working and to review the scenario together. The second will be in-person, at the event day location, to familiarize SPs with the site, the equipment, and props (e.g., wheelchair and medication list), and to provide time to role-play.
- The two training sessions both take place within ten days of the simulation day.
- You decide that for this scenario, it is important that all SPs be present for each training, so that they can learn from observing one another in role.

SP Recruitment Considerations

Elder abuse may be a triggering topic, and you are concerned about SPs' comfort and psychological safety. You need to consider whether SPs may have personal experiences that might affect their psychological safety in role. You also know some SPs have mobility challenges.

- In addition to the project details you typically share when recruiting SPs for a role (e.g., details about logistics, dates, times, SP responsibilities, and payment), you also explain that there will be two separate trainings–one virtual and one in-person. You explain what technical requirements they would need for the virtual training.

- You decide you should screen the SPs for their comfort with the topic of elder abuse and for any mobility challenges they might have that would make it difficult for them to get in and out of a wheelchair. You do this by telling them, during the initial recruitment, the general content of the role (elder abuse) and by explaining that they will need to move in and out of a wheelchair during the simulation. You explain that some SPs may be uncomfortable with the content or the physicality of the role and normalize being able to decline work on this basis. You offer to send them the scenario to consider the role further and offer to follow up with a telephone call.
- You explain the duration of the day, and that they will be on a rotation. You also offer them the opportunity to work only half the day.
- You send the scenario to the SPs one week prior to training, letting them know they should review it fully prior to training and to prepare any questions they might have. You tell them you will pay them for 30-min for this home review.
- You include instructions on how to access the virtual training and offer two virtual "drop-in" sessions where they can test their connection to the training platform.
- You also include directions and a map so they know where the in-person training is taking place. These directions include details about accessibility, like whether there are stairs or elevators that need to be accessed.

Training Delivery Considerations

You are concerned about cognitive overload and the emotional challenges of the scenario. You also know that some SPs have mobility challenges and portraying the role from a wheelchair (as per the scenario) may be difficult due to the physical movement of getting in and out of the chair throughout the day.

- You identify training strategies to prevent cognitive overload and enhance memory retention: you simplify the number of scripted lines the SPs need to memorize and plan to incorporate role-play and round robin exercises into training. You plan to suggest to SPs that after training, they could frequently review the material and recite sections of the role throughout regular daily activities (e.g., bathing, meal preparation, commuting).
- You arrange to have a wheelchair available during the second training to practice getting in and out of the wheelchair and to ensure SPs know how to use and lock the wheels.
- You secure two training spaces: a large room where there is ample space to practice physical movements with the wheelchair, and the smaller space where the simulation will take place on event day.

Training for Role Portrayal

The training session provides the opportunity to cocreate the role portrayal with the SPs, and SP educators can create a space that allows SPs to contribute by fostering training as collaborative practice. Each SP brings their own personal experience and embodied knowledge to training, and for some, sharing their experience—whether similar to or different from the specific scenario details—may help the entire group understand the role better. In addition to what the SP trainer has anticipated and prepared, embracing a stance of curiosity and a willingness to codiscover new approaches during training is beneficial to all.

SP educators should give thoughtful attention to the beginning of the SP training session with all SPs to establish an environment that supports psychological safety, like the prebrief that occurs at the beginning of a simulation [12]. Introductions help build relationships and provide a sense of belonging. The introduction also provides an opportunity to establish expectations for SPs and to highlight the support that the trainer and SP program will provide. SP educators should deliberately provide mechanisms through which any SP can reveal any concerns, both in the moment and privately. The goal is to normalize challenges and create a shame-free, respectful environment. The introduction should also review the process the training session will follow, and the context within which the simulation event takes place (e.g., level of learner, type of assessment, review of notification/timing signals, duration of each encounter, etc.).

Many of the same communication skills that learners develop in simulation are also important for SP educators to increase engagement and participation with SPs: enunciating clearly, avoiding speaking too fast, projecting volume appropriately, pausing for questions, summarizing, and checking for understanding. These skills are especially important with older adult SPs who may require more time to process information or rely on lip reading to supplement hearing loss.

Measured verbal delivery paired with the effective design of training materials is essential for increased understanding of training content.

During the training session, SP educators must carefully observe SPs' verbal and physical cues that suggest challenges or successes and actively engage with SPs, using multiple strategies, to assess understanding, comfort, and safety. This ensures appropriate SP preparation as a measure of quality assurance and collaboration with each SP to assess their own capacity to fulfill the assignment. By the end of the training session, some SPs may benefit from additional, customized training, and some SPs may be feeling increasingly concerned about participation. Assuring open communication during and after the training helps navigate these needs.

Box 4.3 Training for Role Portrayal

In addition to implementing your training plan, you decide to do the following:

- During the virtual training, ask SPs if you can record the session so they can review it afterward if they choose. Disclose who else will have access to the video recordings.
- Start with a pre-brief of the session:
  - Begin with introductions to create a sense of belonging.
  - Review what will happen in the 90-min virtual training: "First we will review the context of the simulation, then we will talk about the scenario, and finally we will do one or two role-plays."
  - Discuss the simulation objectives and logistics.
- Encourage SPs to ask questions during the training sessions and create space for questions.
- Review the role.
- Do a round robin exercise and one or two role-plays, where the SPs can have the role in-hand.
- To conclude the first training:
  - Review your expectations for the upcoming in-person 90-min training: review the location and ask SPs to come prepared to role-play without their role in hand.
  - Encourage SPs to reach out to you between the first and second training session (and after!) if they have any questions or concerns about the role.
- During the second [in-person] training:
  - Role-play with each SP, using the full encounter time, while everyone else observes.
  - Because this is an interprofessional simulation, ask a simulationist colleague to join so that the SPs can navigate answering questions from different people during the role-play.
  - Calibrate the role portrayal to the required level of accuracy, ensuring the role is consistent and the affect is similar across SPs. This shared understanding can be achieved by having each SP role-play while all others observe, followed by targeted feedback and the opportunity to practice again. This leads to a collective understanding of the role and ensures each SP is role-ready.

Simulation

During the simulation event, it is important for SP educators to be present during the simulation to observe and support SPs. SPs should be free to opt out at any time for their own psychological and physical safety. Frequent breaks and rotations may help support stamina levels and prevent fatigue and cognitive overload [5, 6].

Once the simulation has ended, SP educators have an immediate responsibility to acknowledge the emotional impact on SPs and any unintended consequences of the simulation [7]. This can be achieved through debriefing—allowing participants to reflect on their actions, impact, and feelings of the simulation. Debriefing is an important and effective component of simulation [13], and different debriefing methods are well documented in the literature [14, 15]. Debriefing helps SPs derole and reflect on the simulation activity.

Using the vignette from the beginning of this chapter as an example, an SP may feel emotionally drained after portraying a victim of psychological, physical, and financial abuse by their caregiver. They may want to talk about how they feel with the content of the scenario and how they felt during role-play. They may have some uncertainty about their role portrayal and whether it was accurate and authentic. They may have some discomfort from sitting in a wheelchair throughout the day and may want to have an opportunity to be led through some stretches. A debrief can allow SPs to step out of the role, examine the emotional impact of the role portrayal, and receive ongoing constructive feedback from their SP educators.

Finally, it is important to evaluate SPs' experience with the simulation to find ways the scenario, training, and role portrayal may be improved. This could be part of the debrief or done separately. SP educators themselves should also reflect on the training and role portrayal and how the simulation event unfolded. When thinking specifically about engaging and supporting older adult SPs, they should consider how the training session challenged assumptions or expectations. What does the SP educator understand better about how specific SPs in their program learn, and how can they adapt the training process to better support anticipated and unanticipated needs to create a more effective and inclusive training experience? Evaluation and reflection on the success and limitations of the simulation can benefit and improve future simulation.

Box 4.4 Simulation

You remind yourself that you have an important role in supporting the SPs in-person during the simulation:

- Remind SPs how they can speak to you throughout the day if they have any concerns. Continue to establish safety by letting them know you will also be available to them during their off-rotation.
- Observe SPs in role, if possible (e.g., using cameras in the room, one-way windows, etc.). If you notice changes in affect, proactively check in with the SP.
- During each "shift change" (each hour when SPs rotate out of role), check in with the SPs, and give them the opportunity to debrief—to discuss their portrayal or how the encounters made them feel. Provide opportunities for them to stretch and hydrate.
- After the simulation, facilitate a full group debrief. Evaluate their experience with the role. Did they feel the role was too emotionally challenging? Too complex? How did the rotation schedule work for them?

Closing

As SPs progress through the aging process, it is important to collaboratively find strategies to support their ongoing simulation work. Older adult SPs bring tremendous skill to simulation, and their involvement in education benefits learners and patients. At the same time, participating in simulation-based education provides personal value to older adult SPs, and it is imperative to acknowledge the importance of older adult SPs maintaining an ongoing connection to SP work. Simulation-based education that collaborates with SPs places the patient and community at the center of healthcare education. The mutual benefit of this work is our commitment as SP educators.

While the focus of this chapter is on creating an inclusive approach to training that recognizes and responds to human changes during aging, these practices should be applied to all SPs to ensure we are supporting SPs in alignment with recognized practices for diversity, inclusion, equity, and accessibility. Any training for SP role portrayal should acknowledge that all SPs have unique preferences and styles of learning. This acknowledgment will make training more accessible and valuable for all SPs and will normalize human differences.

References

1. Lewis KL, Bohnert CA, Gammon WL, Hölzer H, Lyman L, Smith C, Thompson TM, Wallace A, Gliva-McConvey G. The association of standardized patient educators (ASPE) standards of best practice (SOBP). Adv Simul. 2017;2(1):1–8.
2. Nestel D, Bearman M. Introduction to simulated patient methodology. In: Nestel D, Bearman M, editors. Simulated patient methodology: theory, evidence and practice. Chichester: Wiley Blackwell; 2015. p. 1–4.
3. Nestel D, Fleishman C, Bearman M. Preparation: developing scenarios and training for role portrayal. In: Nestel D, Bearman M, editors. Simulated patient methodology: theory, evidence and practice. Chichester: Wiley Blackwell; 2015. p. 63–70.
4. Smith C, Gliva-McConvey G, Chapin A. Training SPs for authentic role portrayal. In: Gliva-McConvey G, Nicholas C, Clark L, editors. Comprehensive healthcare simulation: implementing best practices in standardized patient methodology. Cham: Springer Nature; 2020. p. 73–104.
5. Smith CM, Sokoloff LG, Alsaba N. Collaborative framework for working with older simulated participants (SP). BMJ Simul Technol Enhanc Learn. 2021;7(2):112.
6. Schlegel C, Smith CM. "Please let me know when I do not realize it myself": a qualitative analysis of senior simulated patients' experiences. Adv Simul. 2019;4(1):1–1.
7. Park CS, Murphy TF, Code of Ethics Working Group; Society for Simulation in Healthcare. Healthcare Simulationist Code of Ethics; 2018. http://www.ssih.org/Code-of-Ethics.
8. Nestel D, McNaughton N, Smith C, Schlegel C, Tierney T. Values and value in simulated participant methodology: a global perspective on contemporary practices. Med Teach. 2018;40(7):697–702.
9. Thompson J, Tiplady S, Hutchinson A, Cook G, Harrington B. Older people's views and experiences of engagement in standardised patient simulation. BMJ Simul Technol Enhanc Learn. 2017;3(4):154.
10. CAST [Internet]. Universal design for learning guidelines, version 2.2; 2018. http://udlguidelines.cast.org.
11. Office of Disease Prevention and Health Promotion, U.S. Department of Health and Human Services [Internet]. Health Literacy Online; 2016. https://health.gov/healthliteracyonline/display/.
12. Rudolph JW, Raemer DB, Simon R. Establishing a safe container for learning in simulation: the role of the presimulation briefing. Simul Healthc. 2014;9(6):339–49.
13. Levett-Jones T, Lapkin S. A systematic review of the effectiveness of simulation debriefing in health professional education. Nurse Educ Today. 2014;34(6):e58–63.
14. Kolbe M, Eppich W, Rudolph J, Meguerdichian M, Catena H, Cripps A, Grant V, Cheng A. Managing psychological safety in debriefings: a dynamic balancing act. BMJ Simul Technol Enhanc Learn. 2020;6(3):164.
15. Sawyer T, Eppich W, Brett-Fleegler M, Grant V, Cheng A. More than one way to debrief: a critical review of healthcare simulation debriefing methods. Simul Healthc. 2016;11(3):209–17.

Fostering Psychological Safety in Learning Conversations

5

Nemat Alsaba, Lisa Guttman Sokoloff, Cathy M. Smith, and Debra Nestel

Key Messages

1. Learning conversations are often complex, cultural, and relational.
2. Learning conversations are informed by theories from education.
3. Psychological safety is an important goal for faculty to foster in everyone involved in learning conversations—for learners, simulated participants (SPs), and faculty.
4. Learning conversations involve conversations before, during, and after simulation activities.

Introduction

While this book is framed as one that promotes learning through working with older adults as simulated participants (SPs), learning opportunities arise in conversations before, during, and after the simulation that include all those involved in SP-based work. In this chapter, we start by outlining three theories that inform learning conversations—experiential learning, reflective practice, and cognitive load. We then shift focus to exploring psychological safety for all those involved as key to creating a productive learning culture. We refer to "faculty" as the teacher, educator, briefer, debriefer, and/or facilitator. While we view SPs as coteachers, in this chapter, our focus is on faculty who facilitate SP-based work. We refer to *briefing* as information shared before the simulation. While the term *feedback* is commonly used to describe the sharing of information on performance gaps, it also has different meanings in different contexts [1] and, in some disciplines, is used interchangeably with *debriefing*. We use the umbrella term of *debriefing* as the facilitated conversations that occur between participants after a simulation and conversations that explore what happened in the simulation, why things happened and goals to improve future performance. To support this, the chapter focuses on supporting faculty to facilitate learning conversations in simulation-based education (SBE).

Theories Informing Learning Conversations

While many theories inform SBE, we have chosen to outline three commonly referenced theories. While the theories all inform simulation design, our illustrations relate to their relevance to learning conversations, especially in briefing and debriefing.

Experiential Learning Theory

Kolb's [2, 3] experiential learning cycle describes a four-stage process, and as the name suggests, it is cyclical with no specific start or end point, as learning is continuous and can happen across anywhere in the cycle (Fig. 5.1). The theory describes how we acquire, develop, and use knowledge,

N. Alsaba (✉)
Faculty of Health Sciences and Medicine, Bond University, Gold Coast, QLD, Australia
e-mail: nalsaba@bond.edu.au

L. G. Sokoloff
Faculty of Applied Health and Community Studies, Sheridan College, Brampton, ON, Canada

Department of Speech Pathology, Temerty Faculty of Medicine, University of Toronto, Toronto, ON, Canada
e-mail: lisa.sokoloff@sheridancollege.ca

C. M. Smith
Baycrest Academy for Research and Education, Baycrest Centre for Geriatric Care, Toronto, ON, Canada
e-mail: CSmith4@baycrest.org

D. Nestel
School of Clinical Sciences, Faculty of Medicine, Nursing & Health Sciences, Monash University, Clayton, VIC, Australia

Department of Surgery (Austin Precinct), University of Melbourne, Parkville, VIC, Australia
e-mail: debra.nestel@monash.edu

C. M. Smith et al. (eds.), *Comprehensive Healthcare Simulation: Geriatric Simulation*, Comprehensive Healthcare Simulation,
https://doi.org/10.1007/978-3-031-65742-9_5

Fig. 5.1 Kolb's experiential learning cycle and learning conversations

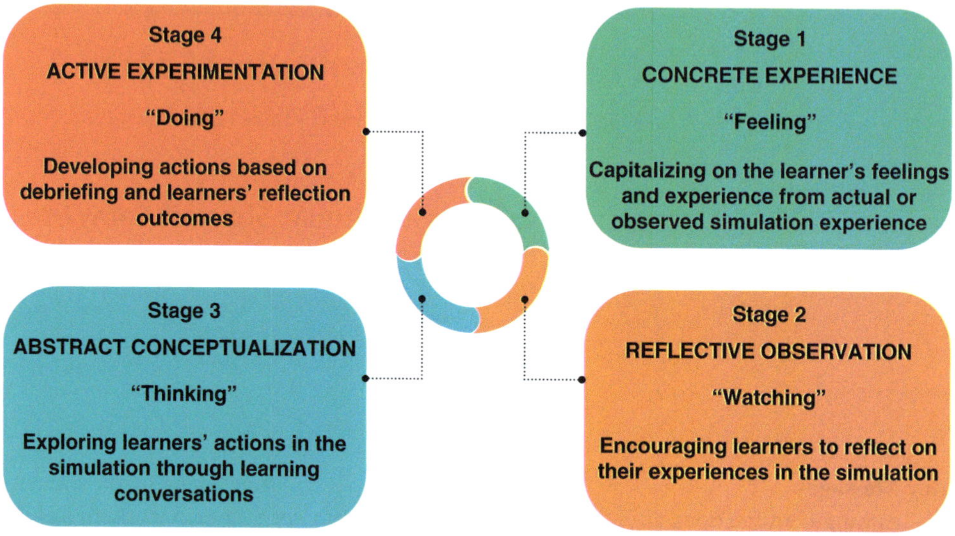

especially as it relates to *experience*. The stages are the following:

1. **Concrete experience** (feeling): This may be illustrated with learners taking part in a simulation or the experience of observers in a simulation. Participating in a simulation or observing a simulation may evoke emotions. Both are examples of concrete experience that represent some form of embodiment for the learner.
2. **Reflective observation** (watching): This can be illustrated by a facilitator encouraging learners and observers to reflect on their thoughts and feelings during the concrete experience. A facilitator may ask directly about how learners felt during the simulation. Observation is a key clinical skill that takes on an especially important role in SBE. Further, the opportunity for learners to observe their own performance through video can be a powerful additional prompt for reflection as learners can see how they appeared to others.
3. **Abstract conceptualisation** (thinking): In SBE, this can be illustrated by a facilitator encouraging learners to explore their actions, to self-assess against a given standard of performance, to recognise strengths and gaps, and to connect their performance with underlying concepts or principles. In SBE, stages 2 and 3 together usually form the basis of the debriefing.
4. **Active experimentation** (doing): This can take different forms in SBE and usually occurs in the debriefing, for example, by giving learners another opportunity to go through the simulation to apply the newly learned actions from stages 1, 2, and 3 or by supporting or encouraging learning in developing action plans for future improvement. However, it may also relate to the briefing of a new SBE activity where prior learning and experiences are surfaced and then applied in a simulation designed to respond to the recent learning. This brings the facilitator and learners back to stage 1.

Reflective Practice Theories

While several scholars have proposed theories of reflective practice, Bolton [4] describes the process of reflection as "… an in-depth consideration of events or situations outside of oneself: solitary, or with critical support. The reflector attempts to work out what happened, what they thought or felt about it, why, who was involved and when, and what these others might have experienced and thought and felt about it. It is looking at whole scenarios from as many angles as possible: people, relationships, situation, place, timing, chronology, causality, connection, and so on, to make situations and people more comprehensible. This involves reviewing or reliving the experience to bring it into focus" [4]. This description positions reflective practice as an individual act. Without structure and guidance for learners, this process of reflection may be descriptive and superficial. In debriefing following SP-based scenarios, the role of the facilitator is to offer structure and guidance to foster reflective practice. Schön [5, 6] has written extensively about reflective practice and proposes that it is a defining characteristic of professional practice. Schön introduced the term "reflection-on-action" to refer to the process of individuals later making sense of what happened during an "action" (usually a critical event), how the actions led to the outcomes, and alternative actions and outcomes. Implicit in the process is the desire for continuous learning. Gibbs [7] proposed a six-step cycle of reflection that has been widely adopted in health professions' education, especially in nursing programmes. The steps include (1) description, (2) feelings, (3) evaluation, (4) analysis, (5) conclusion, and (6) action plan. Later in this chapter, we refer to debriefing frameworks, each of which mirrors these steps. Husebo et al. [8] offer a detailed description of Gibbs' reflective cycle for debriefing frameworks.

Cognitive Load Theory

Cognitive load theory was first described in the context of problem-solving [9], and in health professions, education has been further developed and applied by Van Merrienboer and Sweller [10]. Based on earlier research on information processing and the limitations of working memory, the theory considers the importance of encoding and storing information to enable retrieval as required. When information is relevant, meaningful, and presented at an appropriate level, it will be retained more easily. There are three types of cognitive load:

1. **Intrinsic load** refers to the level of complexity or difficulty of a task.
2. **Extraneous load** refers to how information is presented and how difficult or easy it is for individuals to process it.
3. **Germane load** refers to how information is processed, moved into long-term memory, and mapped with information already in long-term memory.

Cognitive overload can occur if a task is too difficult, has too much information, or is provided in an unstructured or meaningless way. While Reedy [11] shares considerations of cognitive load theory for designing SBE, in this chapter, our attention is focused on cognitive load theory and key features of learning conversations. Using the briefing to explore learners' prior experiences relevant to the planned simulation, what they have found easy or hard and why, and then adjusting the scenario to an appropriate level of complexity can ensure learners are well prepared for the simulation. Orienting learners to the learning environment, including the simulators and their tasks, can assist in balancing intrinsic and extraneous loads. It is during the debriefing that the germane load is largely addressed. A facilitator who explores learners' explanations for their actions during a simulation can highlight what information the learner has drawn on and how the expected standard of performance resonates with what they already know relative to the simulation focus. The conversation during debriefing is intended to raise learners' awareness of their *cognitive schema* or *mental frames* and seeks to align any discord to achieve the expected standard of performance.

Psychological Safety

Psychological safety has surfaced as a key feature for promoting learning in organisations. Edmondson [12] describes psychological safety as "a shared belief held by members of a team that the team is safe for interpersonal risk taking". While the concept comes from management literature, Edmondson has popularised it in healthcare. The phrase has become a God term in health professions' education and specifically in simulation. This is likely to relate to the pressure that some SBE places on learners requiring them to perform in the moment as they would be expected to in real clinical settings. Bearman et al. [13] explored educators' own experiences of simulation. While mainly overwhelmingly positive learning experiences were reported, it was not uncommon for educators to recall deeply negative and unhelpful emotions that had endured for decades. That simulation can have profoundly positive and negative impacts and can influence how learners see their identity highlights the importance of considering the psychological safety of everyone involved. In related literature, Kahn [14] referred to psychological conditions for personal engagement and disengagement at work as "the sense of being able to show and employ one's self without fear of negative consequences to self-image, status or career". This is a critical consideration in SBE where learners may choose to engage or disengage in the activity depending on how psychologically safe they feel. Inevitably, learning involves exploring ideas, expressing uncertainty, and making mistakes. A feature of SBE is the opportunity to create these conditions for learning, for making mistakes without consequences for actual patients. Learners new to SBE may be more familiar with organisational cultures that do not genuinely foster curiosity, questioning, and uncertainty. Facilitators in SBE need to consider these experiences of different working and learning cultures. Conversations with all those involved in SBE as part of the learning process are critical to fostering psychological safety. It is also important to remember that each learner determines whether they feel psychologically safe and that this feeling is dynamic.

Strategies to Foster Psychological Safety

A skilled facilitator will seek to foster the psychological safety of all participants throughout the simulation activity. Somerville et al. [15] describe strategies to foster psychological safety for learners before the simulation. These include ensuring that the design of the simulation activity is appropriate for the learners (e.g. relevance, level of challenge, etc.), that the learning objectives are addressed in the scenario, and that learners are oriented to the simulation activity (e.g. the space, the task, the expectations of performance, the process for observation and feedback, etc.). These strategies are intended to create a culture where learners will feel "safe" to explore ideas, ask questions, express concerns, and make mistakes. When learners feel psychologically safe, they can participate in frank and open discussions of their performance. It is important to remember that feeling psychologically safe may still evoke feelings of discomfort, frustration, stress, and anxiety in learners.

Learners may approach simulation activities with some level of discomfort that is not witnessed with other educational activities. As a facilitator, exploring learners' feelings (e.g. How are you feeling about today's session? etc.) and experiences of simulation (e.g. Have you worked with SPs before?, How did it go?, etc.) can be a helpful way to connect with learners as they arrive. These rapport-building conversations can help foster psychological safety for learners. These strategies can also be applied to the simulation faculty, and older adult SPs in the briefing phase, to foster psychological safety through exploring their attitudes and experiences about the simulation activity and the scenario, knowing who the learners they will be engaging with and what learning objectives they will be working around and connecting with the faculty and their cofacilitators.

Somerville et al. [15] refer to *The Basic Assumption* developed at the Center for Medical Simulation, Boston, MA, which is commonly adopted in SBE. The statement "We believe that everyone participating in activities at (Insert Organization Name) is intelligent, capable, cares about doing their best, and wants to improve" can be displayed as a poster to remind learners and faculty that they are in an environment that is intended to promote learning [16].

Kolbe et al. [17] summarise strategies for fostering psychological safety across a simulation event. They emphasise the dynamic nature of psychological safety and the challenges it poses for faculty before, during, and after a simulation. They outline implicit and explicit strategies, some of which are outlined above. They also emphasise two concepts. First, the importance of holding others in "positive regard" and second "behavioural integrity" which refers to the consistency of faculty in doing what they say they will do. Table 5.1 outlines strategies adapted from Kolbe et al. [17] to foster psychological safety of older adult SPs in simulation activities.

Preparing faculty and learners for a productive debriefing starts before or during the briefing. The briefing sets the stage for learners and faculty on how to reach the goal of the simulation while fostering psychological safety.

In 2021, the International Association for Clinical Simulation and Learning (INACSL) created standards for *preparation* and *briefing* [18]. Many of the actions described for faculty are designed to foster psychological safety. The standards also consider specific actions when the simulation activity is a high-stakes assessment.

Table 5.1 Strategies for faculty to foster psychological safety of older adult SPs in simulation activities

Before the simulation	During the simulation	After the simulation
Before the day	• Where possible, ensure the older adult SP knows that they can stop/pause a scenario and how they can do so.	***During the debriefing***
• Match the older adult SP skills with the requirements of the scenario (e.g. less experienced SPs with less complex scenarios).	• Where possible, observe the older adult SP for any signs that they may need assistance.	• Invite the older adult SP to come out of role and welcome them by name to the debriefing.
• Ask the older adult SP if they feel comfortable portraying specific scenarios (e.g. end-of-life discussions, elder abuse, etc.) or with specific task trainers (e.g. urinary catheterization, etc.).	• Try to ensure that the logistics plan is followed (e.g. observers, video capture, timing, etc.)	• Seat the older adult SP at the debriefing circle in the learning space to optimize their contribution; ensure they can see and hear group members.
• Provide training for role portrayal for the older adult SP.		• Check how they are feeling before proceeding.
• Provide training in feedback and debriefing for the older adult SP.		• Give the older adult SP some time to gather their thoughts after the simulation.
• Send a group email to all faculty including the older adult SP with the simulation activity information and logistics (e.g. date, time, breaks, scenario, clear learning objectives, targeted learners, etc.).		• Invite the older adult SP to share their thoughts openly (e.g. "I am interested in your thoughts.") and to use open-ended questions.
On the day including briefing		• Pause after a question to give time for the older adult SP to process and respond.
• Arrive early to ensure starting on time.		• Listen attentively to their reflections and feedback.
• Welcome the older adult SP.		• Apply positive affect through body language (e.g. leaning forward, open posture, head nodding, and culturally appropriate eye contact
• Include the older adult SP in the faculty briefing.		• Use paraphrasing and active listening in response to older adult SP contributions (e.g. "I hear you.")
• Ask the older adult SP to introduce themselves with a focus on their SP practice during the faculty briefing.		• Include the older adult SP in the take-home messages at the end of the debriefing.
• Discuss with the older adult SP their ideas about being present during the learner briefing; Some SPs prefer not to meet the learners until the scenario.		• Express appreciation of the contribution and participation of the older adult SPs. (e.g. *"Thank you for sharing your thoughts during the debriefing."*)
• Clarify expectations of feedback and debriefing for learners with the older adult SP.		• Convey positive regard through a calm voice tone and kind, empathic facial expressions.
• Use inclusive and respectful language.		• Honor any older adult SP specific requests raised before the simulation to give feedback on their portrayal or participation in the learning conversation.
• Set expectations of feedback to older adult SPs on their contribution (e.g. role portrayal, feedback technique).		• Finish on time.
• Model behaviours that convey gratitude to the older adult SPs.		***After the debriefing***
		• Invite feedback from the older adult SPs (written or verbal) on their experience of the simulation with a view to improving the simulation activity (and follow up on suggestions).
		• Offer support and make yourself available.

Adapted from Kolbe et al. [17]

Debriefing and Feedback

Debriefing has been identified as a crucial feature of SBE. Debriefing and feedback are related concepts and in some professional disciplines may even mean the same thing. Commonly, in SBE, debriefing and feedback are seen as processes intended to improve learner's knowledge and performance. Van der Ridder et al. [19] describe feedback as information shared on the gap between an observed and expected performance. More recent descriptions of feedback acknowledge the importance of exchanging information between those involved, which aligns with the notion of a learning conversation. Cheng et al. [20] define debriefing as a "discussion between two or more individuals in which aspects of a performance are explored and analyzed with the aim of gaining insights that impact the quality of future clinical practice". Debriefing and feedback are also described as "experience-informed dialogues upon which experiential models of learning often depend" [21]. This resonates with the idea of learning conversations. They all share similar objectives and draw on similar educational theories, but each has distinct theoretical roots leading to variations in the literature [21]. This explains why the terms—feedback, learning conversations and debriefing—have been used interchangeably, although the boundaries can sometimes be blurred [22].

Debriefing Frameworks

There are several frameworks to guide debriefing following simulations [23]. Two common approaches are PEARLS (Promoting Excellence and Reflective Learning in Simulation) [24] and the Diamond Debrief [25]. However, there are many others, including the Calgary-Cambridge Observation Guide (CCOG) [26, 27], GAS (Gather-Analyze-Summarize) [28], the 3D Model (Defusing, Discovering, Deepening) [29], TALK (Target, Analysis, Learning point, Key actions) [30], and Plus-Delta [31]. Common to many of the frameworks is an opportunity for learners to "vent", draw explicit attention to the learning goals, and include some recall of what happened in the simulation, enabling faculty, SPs, and learners to share judgements of performance (what worked well and why and what can be improved and how) and identify some future focus of key learning points. Even though the approaches focus on the conversation that happens after the simulation, some of the frameworks also acknowledge the importance of establishing rapport during briefings and of setting expectations for who will be involved in the debriefing and the way in which the debriefing will be conducted. Although the literature outlines many frameworks, little evidence supports one method over another [32]. What is apparent are the factors that assist in choosing a specific framework—what is taught, the level of the learner's previous experiences, the facilitator skills, and the learning space. These factors can sometimes create a "blended debriefing" approach from the published frameworks [32], resulting in a dynamic and creative approach regarded as much an art as a technical process. Links to additional resources are provided at the end of the chapter.

PEARLS Approach

The approach known as PEARLS offers a structure for postsimulation discussions between faculty and learners. Eppich and Cheng [24] provide detailed guidance on using the approach, including scripted examples for faculty at each stage of the debriefing. Features of the approach include an invitation to learners to make judgements about their performance (self-assessment), strategies for faculty to facilitate exploration of the learners' performance, and techniques for directive feedback, especially as it relates to the learning objectives. The approach is flexible, acknowledging time constraints, and it has relevance to all domains of practice, including "clinical decision-making, improving technical skills, teamwork training, and interprofessional collaboration".

Diamond Approach

This approach, named for its diamond "shape", was developed by Jaye et al. [25] and has three phases—description, analysis, and application. Between each phase, there are transition tasks that assist faculty and learners in progressing the discussion. The debriefing commences with a factual recollection of what happened in the simulation instead of starting with learners sharing their emotions, which differs from most other approaches. Learning goals are revisited, and then the performance is analysed using examples of scripted prompts. The authors include techniques such as advocacy-inquiry, which is outlined later in the chapter.

The Calgary-Cambridge Observation Guide

We also draw attention to the Calgary-Cambridge Observation Guide (CCOG) [26, 27] that was developed for application in patient-centred consultations, especially for general practice/family medicine. Given that many scenarios in which older adult SPs will participate are likely to include patient-centred consultations, it is a valuable reference point. Unlike PEARLS and Diamond, the CCOG is more focused on content of a consultation rather than the process of debriefing.

Assessing Debriefer Performance

While there are instruments available to assess debriefing skills, these are mainly used formatively to support debriefers developing their practice. For example, the Objective

Structured Assessment of Debriefing (OSAD) [33] was developed based on literature synthesis and expert opinion and has relevance in clinical and simulation settings. The instrument covers eight core elements each with behavioural markers on a five-point scale. The elements include the debriefer's approach to the learners, including establishing a psychologically safe environment, clarity about the purpose of the debriefing and setting expectations, encouragement of learner participation through the use of open-ended questions, inviting their reactions, etc. Another example is the Debriefing Assessment for Simulation in Healthcare (DASH) [34], developed in the specific context of healthcare simulation that has both learner and instructor versions. The instrument was developed based on theory and multiple expert observations. Using a seven-point scale of behavioural markers, six elements are included. Examples include establishing and maintaining an engaging learning environment, structuring the debriefing, etc. Both the OSAD and DASH instruments have documents that describe their development and application and are valuable tools for healthcare simulation.

Receiving and Providing Feedback During Learning Conversations

Feedback is essentially information that is shared with the intent of improving future performance [35]. We share some tips that learners and educators can use to improve learning cultures. These tips are adapted from Ramani et al. [36]:

Receiving Feedback

Most of the feedback literature is focused on how to train faculty to give meaningful and impactful feedback, with less emphasis on how to train and upskill learners to receive, accept, and value feedback.

The following tips on how to foster a learner-initiated feedback culture align with the notion of feedback literacy [37], "a psychological construct residing within individuals".

(a) **Fostering a Learner Growth Mindset**

A growth mindset allows learners to seek feedback and be more receptive to feedback while ensuring they incorporate ideas into everyday performance. This could be achieved by embedding feedback in all interactions and encounters and making it the norm rather than the exception while ensuring feedback culture becomes embedded in learners' curricula and part of their professional development.

(b) **Encouraging Active Feedback-Seeking Behaviour**

Learners can self-assess their performance by identifying their strengths and gaps. Learners who focus on learning goal orientation instead of performance goal orientation are more likely to solicit and accept feedback that impacts their growth. This could be achieved by encouraging and training learners to identify their learning goals and seek specific goal-directed feedback accordingly.

(c) **Supporting Learner-Initiated Feedback Action Plans**

Feedback should include an achievable and practical performance improvement plan, at minimum codeveloped with the learner. This can foster a change in the learner's feedback behaviour as they self-assess their learning needs and performance gaps, decide on actions to achieve them, and bridge the performance gaps.

Providing Feedback

The following are educator-initiated tips to promote a safe, impactful feedback culture that fosters psychological safety in learning conversations.

(a) **Establishing a Positive Learning Environment**

This could be achieved by setting expectations for the learning activity and meeting the learners' needs while establishing a respectful learning conversation. Further, educators can be role models, providing and receiving respectful learning conversations and making that ingrained in daily interactions and every learning encounter.

(b) **Ensuring Credibility of the Feedback**

This could be supported by establishing a respectful relationship in the learning environment, utilising observational skills to provide feedback on specific performances, and providing feedback aligned with the learner's self-assessment.

(c) **Applying the Johari Window Framework to Enhance Self-Awareness and Reflection**

Learner's self-reflection and self-assessment are starting points to support feedback and learning conversation. The Johari Window [38] consists of four quadrants: (1) Open, what is known to self and others; (2) Blind, unknown to self but known to others; (3) Hidden, known to self and unknown to others; and (4) Unknown, unknown to self and others. Figure 5.2 highlights the Johari window's four quadrants and how to use them in feedback to promote learner self-awareness and self-assessment.

Faculty should employ this framework with caution to expand the "open" window while addressing the "blind" window while ensuring the application of some of the psychological safety strategies mentioned in this chapter. This will ultimately narrow the "hidden" and the "unknown" window, leading to boosting the learner's self-awareness and reflection.

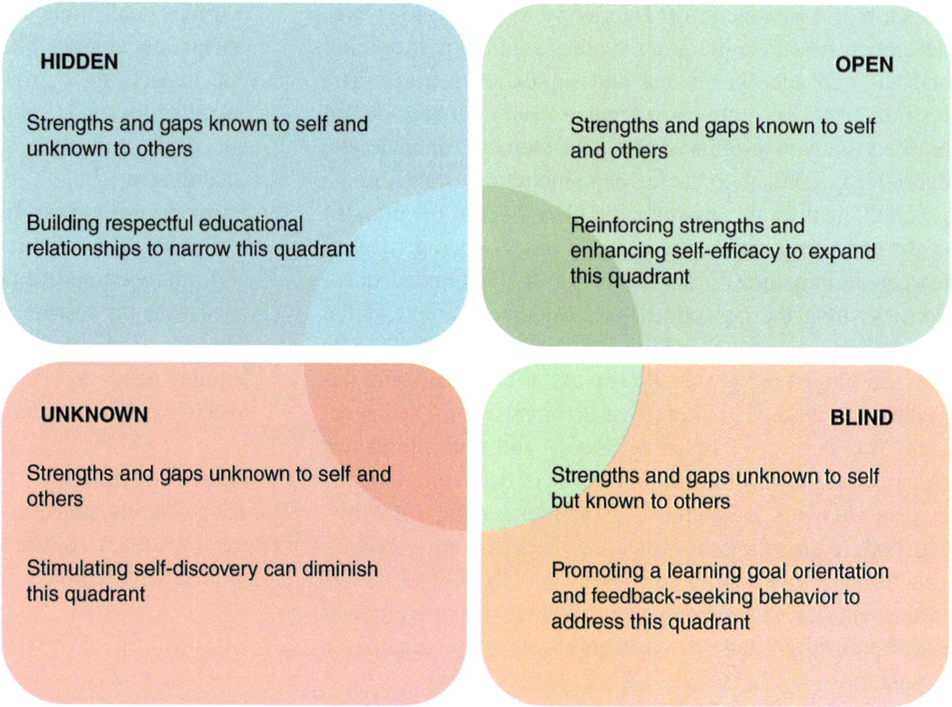

Fig. 5.2 Using the Johari window framework in improving feedback literacy

Key Skills for Debriefing and Learning Conversations

When reflecting on what makes a learning conversation effective, it is not about recounting or sharing facts but rather helping to create a deeper understanding of thoughts, actions, and attitudes that have surfaced in the learning conversation [39]. This could be achieved by carefully crafting curious questions, creating an intimate learning space, attentively listening to verbal language, and observing body language and facial expressions. In this section, we share key skills to create effective learning conversations while highlighting the principles of these techniques and how we can apply them to provide debriefing and feedback more widely. We share a summary of these skills in (Table 5.2).

Observational and Listening Skills

Active, intentional, and attentive listening, combined with observing and detecting subtle body language, is a crucial skill for learning conversations. In learning conversations, one listens to understand instead of listening to respond, therefore building trust and respectful relationships. Being aware of gestural/nonverbal communication (e.g. body language paralinguistic cues such as tone of voice, rate of speech, volume, etc.) can help the debriefer gain valuable information and understanding of learners' actions and behaviours, ultimately establishing a psychologically safe learning conversation. It has been noted that gestural/nonverbal communication comprises 60% of what has been conveyed and absorbed by the receiver in any conversation [40, 41]. As a facilitator, being aware of your own verbal and gestural/nonverbal communication is important to foster respectful engagement. This can include using strategies such as nodding, scanning gaze to all participants, maintaining culturally appropriate eye-to-eye contact, and open posture.

The Art of Crafting Questions

The artistry of crafting questions can be challenging and intriguing to simulation educators. There are well-known and established conversational techniques and strategies in SBE to support the acquisition and maintenance of this skill. The Plus/Delta technique uses simple and linear questions [42]. The Plus/Delta is best framed in the improvement language (e.g. what would you do differently or how you could improve next time) [36].

While the "advocacy and inquiry" strategy helps the debriefer to position a curious question with "good judgement" [43, 44], it also allows the debriefer to gain insight into the learner's thoughts or mental frames by advocating or stating their observation of the learner's action and then inquiring about the learner's underlying frame of mind that led to their action [45].

Example of advocacy and inquiry question is given as follows:

Table 5.2 An overview of core skills useful in learning conversations

Core skill	What is it?	Why do it?	How?
Observing and listening	The ability to actively listen, observe, and detect subtle gestural/nonverbal communications, such as facial expressions, body positioning, and paralinguistic cues, such as tone of voice, volume, rate of speech, etc.	It fosters remembering and reinforces essential details and ideas to build trust and respectful relationships. It also supports gaining valuable information and understanding about learners' behaviours and actions and helps identify engagement or interaction issues to support a psychologically safe learning conversation.	By being present and attentive during the entire learning conversation.
Crafting questions	There are different styles of questions.	Questions explore individuals' reasons, explanations, justifications, and rationales.	Choosing and blending conversation techniques and different styles of questions to suit learners and the focus/goal of the learning conversation.
	• *The Plus/Delta* Simple linear question	• *The Plus/Delta* To explore learners' actions.	• *The Plus/Delta* What would you change next time?
	• *Advocacy and Inquiry* Positioning a curious question in the learning conversation with "good" judgment	• *Advocacy and Inquiry* To allow the debriefer to gain insight into the learners' mental frames.	• *Advocacy and Inquiry* *"**I heard** you raise your voice during your interaction with the older adult SP; **I am concerned** that you may be stereotyping all older people to have hearing difficulties without establishing if this information is correct. This might risk the relationship with your patient. **I am interested** to hear your thoughts on this".*
	• *Circular questions* A questioning technique that helps the learners to explore others' thoughts and feelings to understand their actions	• *Circular questions* To explore the dynamic relationship in the learning conversation and to bring clarity while offering a valuable shift in learner perspective	• *Circular questions* *"What do you think the team leader experiences when they get into a situation like this?"*
Paraphrasing	The ability to repeat learners' comments in a different style while using your own words, sometimes to provide more clarity, without implying agreement or disagreement.	Reinforces the statement shared by the learner while often providing clarity to encourage ongoing learning conversations.	*"What I am hearing is that the transference of bias in looking after this patient started from the triage phase and has affected the treating team's clinical judgment. Does that sound about right?"*
Establishing a shared mental model	A shared belief and mutual understanding of the why, what, and how of the simulation activity with learners and faculty.	Reduces ambiguity and stress of the unknown; it brings everyone involved back to the learning conversation to meet the activity goals/objectives and learners' expectations.	Explicitly share with learners and faculty in the briefing why we are doing the simulation and what the logistics of the simulation activity are.
Normalizing	The ability to relate learners' behaviour and feelings to a social norm without implying approval or rejection of the behaviour. It also includes sharing personal experiences when relevant and appropriate.	It builds trust and dissipates fear, frustration, and embarrassment while fostering psychological safety.	*"This is a complex scenario. It is really tough to navigate the complexity and the atypical presentation of an older person presenting to ED, which makes it easy to miss a diagnosis; I had this problem happen to me last week as well."*

(continued)

Table 5.2 (continued)

Core skill	What is it?	Why do it?	How?
Validating	The ability to recognize and accept learners' thoughts and feelings without implying approval.	It makes the learner feel seen and heard and it builds a supporting, respectful and safe learning conversation.	*"I hear you! It is not easy to tackle difficult conversations with the family."*
Adapting	Allowing flexibility in changing the debriefing framework and structure in an evolving and dynamic learning conversation.	This helps provide learner-centered learning conversations and promotes learner engagement.	Blend multiple debriefing frameworks and improvise the learning objectives and discussion points based on the learners' actions in the simulation.
Pausing	Deliberately utilizing and embedding intentional pausing and silence in the learning conversation.	Pausing *after* a question gives the learner time to reflect, gather their thoughts, and analyze the information.	Example, pausing at the end of the learning conversation and asking the learners to share their "take-home messages."
		Pausing *before* asking a question or moving to a new topic attracts the learner's attention to what is coming.	
Signposting/previewing	Explicitly stating that a phase or statement is about to occur	It helps bring everyone back into the learning conversation and cultivate their attention and engagement.	*"I would like to move on and focus our discussion on teamwork in the simulation."*
Understanding learning spaces and debriefing choreography	Recognizing and understanding the impact of learning spaces seating arrangements, distractions, and noise levels on the learning conversations.	Provides comfort and confidentiality while fostering psychological safety.	Hanging a sign on the door indicating "Simulation debriefing in progress" prevents interruption.
		Allows better observation of body language.	Arranging the seating in a circular fashion allows conversations to happen at the same eye level.

- **Advocacy** *"I saw/noticed*—state what you observed objectively. *"I think/I am concerned*—your perspective and the impact of the observed behaviour or action.
- **Inquiry** *"I wonder/I am interested*—ask the learner their frame of mind at the time of the action.

Circular questions have been introduced in debriefing but are harder to master. Initially developed in systemic family therapy, they can be used in simulation debriefing, especially with teams, to explore a relationship/interaction between two people as a third person sees it by inviting the third person to describe the relationship/interaction [46]. Circular questions should not be the sole strategy used in debriefing but rather an adjunct and extension to other conversational techniques. The aim is to master exploring the dynamic relationship in the learning conversation, to generate information, and to put actions into a relational context [46] by bringing clarity and offering a valuable shift in our perspective. Circular questions simply help the learners to be in the shoes of other learners/members of the team by exploring what they think and feel, thus allowing them to understand their behaviour or actions. Unlike *linear questions*, which are ideal for obtaining definitive facts and content and determining information about the situation (e.g. How long does it take to get the required analgesia?), *circular questioning* promotes reflection to explore how the issue relates to others within the learning conversation (e.g. What do you imagine the team leader experiences when they get into a situation like this?)

Certain factors and considerations support the successful application of circular questions in debriefing. These factors include ensuring a psychologically safe and respectful learning environment, holding the learners in high regard, previewing and signposting to the learner that circular questions will be used [46].

Paraphrasing

Paraphrasing is the art of saying the same thing but in a different way. For example, the debriefer repeats the learner's comment but instead uses their own words and phrases to interpret them [40]. Paraphrasing does not imply agreement or disagreement but rather reinforces the statement by choosing words and phrases that highlight the learner's comments and reflections to encourage ongoing learning conversation while providing clarity and supporting psychological safety [47].

Shared Mental Model

A shared mental model is an important element of thriving learning conversations [45]. Shared mental models establish a joint understanding and cultivate shared awareness of the simulation activity—"why?, what?, how?, and who?" It is a road map for all involved, signalling where they are currently and how to reach their destination goal. A shared mental model helps the faculty and learners share a mutual understanding of the simulation activity objectives and goals. This reduces ambiguity and stress of the "unknown" and helps bring everyone on the same page, all of which foster psychological safety in any learning conversation.

Normalisation

Normalisation in debriefing is when facilitators relate the learners' "behaviours, feelings, or attitudes to a societal norm" and genuinely share their personal experience that aligns with the current situation [40, 48]. It does not denote approval of the behaviour or attitude but rather shows an understanding of the situation while communicating that such feeling or attitude is common or considered normal [40]. Normalisation also builds trust and dissipates fear and other unwanted emotional situations, such as being upset, frustrated, or embarrassed, which ultimately fosters psychological safety in the simulation activity.

Validation

Validation is acknowledging and accepting that learners' thoughts and feelings are real and understandable [40] while supporting and building respectful and effective learning conversations. Validation occurs when learners feel they have been seen and heard, their feelings understood and accepted, and their perspectives valued. Similar to normalisation, it does not denote approval of the behaviour or feeling but rather acknowledges learners' emotional responses while giving them a safe space to process their feelings and attitude. An emotionally validated learner is more likely to have a solid sense of identity and self-worth while being able to regulate their emotions effectively [40, 49]. This is integral to fostering psychological safety in any learning conversation.

The Art of Flexibility

Although multiple debriefing frameworks exist, they should not take away the debriefer's discretion to change and alter the framework to suit an evolving and dynamic learning conversation [32]. The art of flexibility helps debriefers meet learner's needs and match their interactions and reactions [32], which ultimately fosters psychological safety and learner engagement. Debriefing frameworks are mind maps to show the debriefer the way, but they do not dictate the pace and flow of how they navigate this path nor when to pause or take a shortcut. This is an advanced skill that Krogh et al. [32] describe as the art of "thinking on your feet".

The Power of Pause

The art of deliberately using pausing and silence in learning conversations is a powerful tool [45]. A pause allows those involved in the learning conversation to hear, understand, and process what is being said. It is important to know when to pause and for how long to make pausing an attention-grabbing act. Pausing for too long can make learners uncomfortable, while too short a pause might not achieve its intended aim of giving the learners time to reflect, gather their thoughts, and analyse the information. A pause can be used before asking a question to gather your thoughts and consider the emphasis you want to share with learners; it can also be used after asking a question to allow learners enough time to reflect on their experience and actions in the simulation, formulate their thoughts, and critically analyse their mental frames. An example of a deliberate pause and silence is the conclusion or "take-home" pause at the end of a debriefing.

Signposting

Known also as previewing, signposting is a technique to indicate explicitly that a phase or statement is about to occur [40]. It helps create order and structure and can bring everyone back into the learning conversation, gaining their attention and engagement.

Learning Spaces and Debriefing Choreography

Learning spaces or environments that provide comfort and confidentiality for all involved in the simulation activity are preferred [40]. Seating arrangements can impact learners. Circular seatings enable optimal "choreography". They reflect an inviting and intimate learning space that allows conversations to happen at the same eye level while mitigating power differences. It also allows for better observation of body language compared to debriefing while standing. Signage can be used outside the space to ensure the debriefing process is not disrupted by outside noises or distractions (e.g. simulation debriefing in progress).

Closing

Learning conversations are complex. Understanding the significance of fostering psychological safety in learning conversations is crucial. We have shared theories, approaches, and several strategies to inform decisions you might make to support faculty and learners in undertaking their roles in debriefing and learning conversation safely and effectively.

Resources

Many resources support learning conversations. The following resources include podcasts, educational videos, blogs, and websites:

- **Academic Life in the Emergency Department (ALiEM)** is a website that serves as a digital connection for medical educators and academics to provide free open access medical education (FOAMed) and education beyond classroom walls. **SimLIFE-EM** is a subsection of ALiEM and has created simulation videos that educators can use to view, practise, and reflect on debriefing skills. https://www.aliem.com/2014/simlife-em-challenge/
- **Injectable Orange** is a website created and run by Jess Spurr, an enthusiastic nurse educator. The website is home to multiple posts and discussions around simulation and debriefing. http://injectableorange.com/2013/07/debriefing-careful-you-dont-just-give-carrot-a-little-stick-is-sometimes-needed/
- **St. Emlyn's** is one of the early FOAMed digital platforms led by a team of emergency medical and critical care specialists to improve medical education and the care and outcomes of patients. The website has a rich repertoire of simulation-based education and its tools. http://stemlynsblog.org/good-to-talk-debrief-in-the-emergency-department/
- **The Intensive Care Network (ICN)** is a digital network developed to educate and connect healthcare professionals delivering critical and acute care; however, some of their resources, especially those based on medical education and simulation principles, are transferable to all other professions. http://intensivecarenetwork.com/radford-vandyke-simulation/
- **EM Sim Cases** is a fantastic simulation website filled with resources, shares peer-reviewed simulation cases and templates, and tackles some simulation topics. https://emsimcases.com/2015/06/30/debriefing-techniques-the-art-of-guided-reflection/
- **The Debriefing Academy**—https://thedebriefingacademy.com/—is the home of the **PEARLS** approach to debriefing. While the website promotes its courses, it shares great tips and strategies for debriefers and simulation educators.
- **Simulcast podcast**—http://simulationpodcast.com/Jesse Spurr, Vic Brazil, and Ben Symons work their magic in getting interesting materials into podcasts while covering the fundamentals of SBE. They have a monthly journal club. Listen to them all—they are mainly excellent and engaging.
- **The Objective Structured Assessment of Debriefing (OSAD)** Arora S, Ahmed M, Paige J, Nestel D, Runnacles J, Hull L, Darzi A, Sevdalis N. Objective structured assessment of debriefing: bringing science to the art of debriefing in surgery. Annals of surgery. 2012 Dec 1;256(6):982–8.
- **The Debriefing Assessment for Simulation in Healthcare (DASH)** Brett-Fleegler M, Rudolph J, Eppich W, Monuteaux M, Fleegler E, Cheng A, Simon R. Debriefing assessment for simulation in healthcare: development and psychometric properties. Simulation in Healthcare. 2012 Oct 1;7(5):288–94.
- **TALK Foundation** is an organisation that supports debriefing after clinical or educational events. It also promotes team reflexivity, aligning with patient safety principles. The TALK website shares tools and a framework named (TALK) including videos. https://www.talkdebrief.org/talkframeworkbackground

References

1. Bearman M, Eppich W, Nestel D. How debriefing can inform feedback: practices that make a difference. In: The impact of feedback in higher education: improving assessment outcomes for learners. Cham: Springer International Publishing; 2019. p. 165–88.
2. Kolb DA. Experiential learning: Experience as the source of learning and development. Englewood Cliffs: Prentice Hall; 1984.
3. Kolb AY, Kolb DA, Passarelli A, Sharma G. On becoming an experiential educator: the educator role profile. Simul Gaming. 2014;45(2):204–34.
4. Bolton G. Reflective practice: writing and professional development. Sage; 2010.
5. Schön DA. The reflective practitioner: how professionals think in action. Avebury [Ashgate]; 1991.
6. Schön DA. Educating the reflective practitioner. Jossey-Bass; 1987.
7. Gibbs G. Learning by doing: a guide to teaching and learning methods. Further Education Unit; 1988.
8. Husebø SE, O'Regan S, Nestel D. Reflective practice and its role in simulation. Clin Simul Nurs. 2015;11(8):368–75.
9. Sweller J. Cognitive load during problem solving: effects on learning. Cogn Sci. 1988;12(2):257–85.
10. van Merriënboer JJG, Sweller J. Cognitive load theory in health professional education: design principles and strategies. Med Educ. 2010;44(1):85. https://doi.org/10.1111/j.1365-2923.2009.03498.x.
11. Reedy GB. Using cognitive load theory to inform simulation design and practice. Clin Simul Nurs. 2015;11(8):355–60. https://doi.org/10.1016/j.ecns.2015.05.004.
12. Edmondson A. Psychological safety and learning behavior in work teams. Adm Sci Q. 1999;44(2):350–83.

13. Bearman M, Greenhill J, Nestel D. The power of simulation: a large-scale narrative analysis of learners' experiences. Med Educ. 2019;53(4):369–79. https://doi.org/10.1111/medu.13747.
14. Kahn WA. Psychological conditions of personal engagement and disengagement at work. Acad Manag J. 1990;33(4):692–724.
15. Somerville SG, Harrison NM, Lewis SA. Twelve tips for the prebrief to promote psychological safety in simulation-based education. Med Teach. 2023;18:1–8.
16. Center for Medical Simulation. 2023. http://www.harvardmedsim.org/. [Internet. Cited 2023 Dec 26].
17. Kolbe M, Eppich W, Rudolph J, Meguerdichian M, Catena H, Cripps A, Grant V, Cheng A. Managing psychological safety in debriefings: a dynamic balancing act. BMJ Simul Technol Enhanc Learn. 2020;6(3):164.
18. McDermott DS, Ludlow J, Horsley E, Meakim C. Healthcare simulation standards of best practice™ prebriefing: preparation and briefing. Clin Simul Nurs. 2021;58:9–13.
19. Van De Ridder JM, Stokking KM, McGaghie WC, Ten Cate OT. What is feedback in clinical education? Med Educ. 2008;42(2):189–97.
20. Cheng A, Eppich W, Grant V, Sherbino J, Zendejas B, Cook DA. Debriefing for technology-enhanced simulation: a systematic review and meta-analysis. Med Educ. 2014;48(7):657–66.
21. Tavares W, Eppich W, Cheng A, Miller S, Teunissen PW, Watling CJ, Sargeant J. Learning conversations: an analysis of the theoretical roots and their manifestations of feedback and debriefing in medical education. Acad Med. 2020;95(7):1020–5.
22. Voyer S, Hatala R. Debriefing and feedback: two sides of the same coin? Simul Healthc. 2015;10(2):67–8.
23. Decker S, Alinier G, Crawford SB, Gordon RM, Jenkins D, Wilson C. Healthcare simulation standards of best practice™ The debriefing process. Clin Simul Nurs. 2021;58:27–32.
24. Eppich W, Cheng A. Promoting Excellence and Reflective Learning in Simulation (PEARLS): development and rationale for a blended approach to health care simulation debriefing. Simul Healthc. 2015;10(2):106–15.
25. Jaye P, Thomas L, Reedy G. 'The diamond': a structure for simulation debrief. Clin Teach. 2015;12(3):171–5.
26. Kurtz SM, Silverman J, Draper J, Silverman J. Teaching and learning communication skills in medicine. Radcliffe Medical Press; 1998.
27. Silverman J, Kurtz S, Draper J. Skills for communicating with patients. Radcliffe Medical Press; 1999.
28. Phrampus PE, O'Donnell JM. Debriefing using a structured and supported approach. In: The comprehensive textbook of healthcare simulation. New York: Springer; 2013. p. 73–84.
29. Zigmont JJ, Kappus LJ, Sudikoff SN. The 3D model of debriefing: defusing, discovering, and deepening. Semin Perinatol. 2011;35(2):52–8.
30. Diaz-Navarro C, Leon-Castelao E, Hadfield A, Pierce S, Szyld D. Clinical debriefing: TALK© to learn and improve together in healthcare environments. Trends Anaesth Crit Care. 2021;40:4–8.
31. Fanning RM, Gaba DM. The role of debriefing in simulation-based learning. Simul Healthc. 2007;2(2):115–25.
32. Krogh K, Bearman M, Nestel D. "Thinking on your feet"—a qualitative study of debriefing practice. Adv Simul. 2016;1:1–1.
33. Arora S, Ahmed M, Paige J, Nestel D, Runnacles J, Hull L, Darzi A, Sevdalis N. Objective structured assessment of debriefing: bringing science to the art of debriefing in surgery. Ann Surg. 2012;256(6):982–8.
34. Brett-Fleegler M, Rudolph J, Eppich W, Monuteaux M, Fleegler E, Cheng A, Simon R. Debriefing assessment for simulation in healthcare: development and psychometric properties. Simul Healthc. 2012;7(5):288–94.
35. Boud D, Molloy E. What is the problem with feedback? In: Feedback in higher and professional education. Routledge; 2012. p. 1–10.
36. Ramani S, Könings KD, Ginsburg S, van der Vleuten CP. Twelve tips to promote a feedback culture with a growth mind-set: swinging the feedback pendulum from recipes to relationships. Med Teach. 2019;41(6):625–31.
37. Nieminen JH, Carless D. Feedback literacy: a critical review of an emerging concept. Higher Educ. 2023;85(6):1381–400. https://doi.org/10.1007/s10734-022-00895-9.
38. Luft J. Of human interaction. National Press Books; 1969.
39. Launer J. Narrative-based practice in health and social care: conversations inviting change. Routledge; 2018.
40. Grant VJ, Robinson T, Catena H, Eppich W, Cheng A. Difficult debriefing situations: a toolbox for simulation educators. Med Teach. 2018;40(7):703–12.
41. Macdonald E, editor. Difficult conversations in medicine. Oxford University Press; 2004.
42. Cheng A, Eppich W, Epps C, Kolbe M, Meguerdichian M, Grant V. Embracing informed learner self-assessment during debriefing: the art of plus-delta. Adv Simul. 2021;6(1):1–9.
43. Rudolph JW, Simon R, Dufresne RL, Raemer DB. There's no such thing as "nonjudgmental" debriefing: a theory and method for debriefing with good judgment. Simul Healthc. 2006;1(1):49–55.
44. Rudolph JW, Simon R, Rivard P, Dufresne RL, Raemer DB. Debriefing with good judgment: combining rigorous feedback with genuine inquiry. Anesthesiol Clin. 2007;25(2):361–76.
45. Sawyer T, Eppich W, Brett-Fleegler M, Grant V, Cheng A. More than one way to debrief: a critical review of healthcare simulation debriefing methods. Simul Healthc. 2016;11(3):209–17.
46. Kolbe M, Marty A, Seelandt J, Grande B. How to debrief teamwork interactions: using circular questions to explore and change team interaction patterns. Adv Simul. 2016;1:1–8.
47. Patterson KD, Grenny J, Mcmillan R, Switzler A. Crucial conversations: tools for talking when stakes are high. 2nd ed. McGraw-Hill; 2012.
48. Gallagher RS. How to tell anyone anything: breakthrough techniques for handling difficult conversations at work. 1st ed. American Management Association; 2009.
49. Hall KD, Cook MH. The power of validation: arming your child against bullying, peer pressure, addiction, self-harm & out-of-control emotions. 1st ed. New Harbinger Publications; 2012.

Supporting Older Adult Simulated Participants to Provide Feedback to Learners

6

Cathy M. Smith, Nemat Alsaba, Debra Nestel, and Lisa Guttman Sokoloff

Key Messages

1. Feedback as part of a dynamic exchange between older adult SPs and learners can make a valuable contribution to developing person-centred care.
2. There are benefits and challenges for older adult SPs in providing feedback to learners.
3. Providing feedback is a complex task that can increase cognitive load for older adult SPs.
4. The Association of SP Educators (ASPE) Standards of Best Practice provides guidelines for training SPs to provide feedback.
5. A collaborative framework for supporting older adult SPs considers possible age-related cognitive, physical, and sensory changes that may need to be considered when applying the ASPE SOBP.
6. It is important for SP educators and facilitators to consider the psychological safety of older adult SPs when they provide feedback.

C. M. Smith (✉)
Baycrest Academy for Research and Education, Baycrest Centre for Geriatric Care, Toronto, ON, Canada
e-mail: CSmith4@baycrest.org

N. Alsaba
Faculty of Health Sciences and Medicine, Bond University, Gold Coast, QLD, Australia
e-mail: nalsaba@bond.edu.au

D. Nestel
School of Clinical Sciences, Faculty of Medicine, Nursing & Health Sciences, Monash University, Clayton, VIC, Australia

Department of Surgery (Austin Precinct), University of Melbourne, Parkville, VIC, Australia
e-mail: debra.nestel@monash.edu

L. G. Sokoloff
Faculty of Applied Health and Community Studies, Sheridan College, Brampton, ON, Canada

Department of Speech Pathology, Temerty Faculty of Medicine, University of Toronto, Toronto, ON, Canada
e-mail: lisa.sokoloff@sheridancollege.ca

Introduction

What is the most challenging part of my work? Giving feedback. (Leonie Tuite)

Simulated participant (SP) feedback is a nuanced, complex, and multilayered task. Traditionally, feedback in health professional education was thought of as a one-way process focused on providing "… specific information about the comparison between a trainee's observed performance and a standard, given with the intent to improve the trainee's performance" [1, p. 27]. Accordingly, in this approach, the SP's feedback would be structured so the SP might provide two or three points to learners about what worked well and what could be changed from their perspective, and the encounter between the learner and SP would end. Increasingly, feedback is seen as part of a dynamic process within a debriefing, "… the conversation about the simulation experience that traditionally occurs post event (i.e. after the simulation ends)" [2, p. 158]. In this context, SPs are part of a rich learning conversation [3] in which they are often guided by a faculty facilitator to provide feedback and engage meaningfully with learners [4, 5]. Facilitators are responsible for fostering an atmosphere of psychological safety, that is, "… the belief that speaking up with ideas, questions, concerns, or mistakes is expected and feasible, and is best summarised as a sense of permission for candour " [6, p. 271] for SPs as well as learners during this process (see Chap. 5).

The feedback an SP offers is usually connected to the role they have just portrayed. While the chapter mainly positions the SP in clinician-patient interactions, we recognise that SPs may play other roles. SP feedback requires the same careful training as role portrayal [4, 7]. It can be considered an advanced skill because it increases the cognitive load of

C. M. Smith et al. (eds.), *Comprehensive Healthcare Simulation: Geriatric Simulation*, Comprehensive Healthcare Simulation,
https://doi.org/10.1007/978-3-031-65742-9_6

an SP by requiring them to simultaneously be in role, as the person they are portraying, and out of role as they make judgements about their experience. Further, the SP will then share these judgements with the learner. SPs can provide verbal or written feedback, in activities designed to support learning (formative) or assess learning (summative). SPs are commonly involved in scenarios with a focus on communication competencies and person-centred care [4, 7–10].

Benefits of SP Feedback to Learners and for SPs

In work with undergraduate learners, Berenson (2012) notes that SP feedback "fills a critical educational role in the interpersonal and affective domains" [11, p. e27]. It offers learners invaluable perspectives from SPs, as proxies for the people they represent, that they might not have when working with real patients. This feedback can allow learners the opportunity to reflect and apply lessons learned in future interactions [8, 12]. In a systematic review of feedback by SPs in undergraduate medical education, Bokken et al. (2009) note that medical students value SP feedback "equally or more positively" than feedback provided by tutors [8, p. 203]. The authors report one study in which medical students who received SP feedback were able to perform skills better at 6 months than those that did not and suggested that feedback received by SPs may have contributed to this outcome.

Research also indicates that SPs value supporting learners through feedback [13, 14]. Older adult SPs also report that they can derive great satisfaction from sharing their life experiences with learners in the hope that this will improve future healthcare for older adults [15, 16].

Challenges SPs Identify Related to Providing Feedback

SPs have reported that they find various aspects of feedback challenging and stressful [4, 5, 7, 8, 12, 17], including the following:

- Feeling pressure to provide feedback that is specific, authentic, and meaningful to a learner
- Feeling unsafe to articulate their experience
- Feeling uncertain about how to balance communicating what worked well for them versus what did not work well
- Being unsure about how to provide honest feedback to a learner who is struggling
- Feeling unsupported by others in the room, such as a faculty member

In addition, older adult SPs report concerns related to possible changes in their cognitive, physical, and sensory abilities [15, 16, 18, 19], including the following:

- Anxiety about being able to remember what feedback to give
- Feeling overly fatigued from portraying a role and then participating in a feedback session
- Not being able to clearly hear the learner during the interaction

> Giving feedback to doctors and nurses brings the stress of giving feedback to another level. They may have saved your life (in a scenario), and been rough or abrupt in doing so, but how do you balance that feedback when at the end of the day they kept me alive? (Robyn Vinodolac)

Ways in Which SPs Provide Feedback

There are considerable variations in the ways that SPs, including older adult SPs, can provide feedback. SP feedback can be verbal or written (e.g. free text, rating scale, structured checklist) and provided in person, via audio or visual recording or electronically. Written feedback can take more time for an SP to formulate and provide than oral feedback [20].

Additionally, the feedback can be formative, which is intended to support learning, or summative, which is part of an assessment that measures learning. SPs may also function as assessors in high-stakes summative exams where decisions are made related to licensure or certification [21].

The focus of feedback can relate to the impact an encounter had on the SP or to a learner's clinical or communication skills [5, 8, 13]. The SP may be asked to link their feedback to tools such as the Calgary-Cambridge Observation Guide, developed for application in patient-centred consultations [22, 23], rating scales [10], or checklists specifically linked to a scenario [24]. SPs who are assessing learners in a high-stakes assessment with checklists usually require targeted and longer training times, to ensure that they are using the tool as intended [25–27].

There are wide variations reported in how SP feedback is integrated into teaching sessions [4, 12, 17]. It usually occurs in the debriefing phase of a simulation and is often led by faculty [5]. There is incomplete documentation of the ways in which SPs, including older adult SPs, are supported in providing feedback to learners and there is little research to indicate that one way is better than another [5, 12, 17, 28]. There is evidence-informed guidance to support SPs to provide feedback, such as the Association of SP Educators (ASPE) Standards of Best Practice (SOBP) [27]. In a scoping review on training SPs for role portrayal and feedback, Doyle et al.

(2023) ask "… if SPs engage in suboptimal feedback practices, does this deny learners valuable learning?" [17, p. 2] For example, asking older adult SPs to provide feedback that might include details from their own lives as a way to promote authenticity [28] may have nothing to do with the learning objectives and therefore prove to be a distraction.

A Strategic Approach to Supporting Older Adult SPs in Providing Feedback

As we have established, the content and process of SP feedback varies widely. To illustrate a systematic way of supporting older adult SPs to provide verbal feedback to learners in an education session, we use three reference points. First, the NHET-Sim phases, developed for a national training programme in Australia [29], provide a structure for this approach. These phases include preparing, briefing, simulating, de-roling, feedback/debriefing of learners, reflecting, and evaluating (see Chap. 3). Second, we apply the ASPE SOBP [27] within these phases with particular focus on Domain 1, Safe Work Environment; Domain 3, Training SPs; and Domain 4, Program Management. Third, through a vignette, we embed a collaborative framework for supporting older adults [18]. This Framework considers possible age-related cognitive, physical, and sensory changes that may need to be considered when applying the ASPE SOBP.

Considerations when working with older adult SPs: Vignette (Part 1)

Imagine that you are an SP educator. You have been asked to work with colleagues to implement a scenario for senior undergraduate healthcare learners (e.g. from medicine, nursing, physiotherapy, occupational therapy, social work). The scenario focuses on an interaction between the healthcare learner and an 82-year-old person who has been diagnosed with dementia. Learning objectives include the demonstration of person-centred care and communication competencies such as empathy.

This session is designed to support learning and takes place over a day. SPs will be required to portray this person and provide feedback to learners up to ten times and within small groups. One learner will interview the SP about their history and the other learners will observe the interaction. A facilitator will guide the process. Each interaction with a learner will take 15 minutes, and then there will be 15 minutes for a debrief in the format of a learning conversation that includes SP feedback. You will be required to recruit several SPs who will portray this person simultaneously in different rooms.

You discuss with your colleagues the importance of recruiting SPs who appear close to the age of this person (rather than a much younger person) to promote authentic and respectful interactions with learners. There are older adult SPs in your programme who would be ideal for this activity. They have all had previous training and experience providing feedback to learners. In preparing to support them, and as you review the scenario, you consider relevant sections of the ASPE SOBP. You also consider factors related to "knowing" the SPs, drawn from a framework for supporting older adult SPs. You recognise that some of the SPs may need additional support related to age-related changes.

NHET-Sim Phase: Preparing

This preparing stage often takes the most time. It is worth the investment and includes steps related to preparing for and then leading the SP training. Note that all of these steps are done in addition to training SPs for role portrayal (see Chap. 4).

Preparation for Training (ASPE SOBP 1.1, 3.1, 4.2 and 4.5)

Reviewing the Scenario (ASPE SOBP 1.1.1, 3.1.1, and 4.2.4)

The scenario is the blueprint that guides SPs to provide feedback, so it is essential that the SP educator reviews it thoroughly to understand the educational details such as who the learners are, what the objectives are, and how they relate to the feedback from SPs, the type of SP feedback, and how it is being incorporated into a session (e.g. unidirectional, part of a learning conversation). Logistical details can include understanding how many times the SP is required to provide feedback and the length of the feedback session. Box 6.1 lists questions that an SP educator can consider when reviewing a scenario to determine the involvement of SPs in providing verbal feedback.

Box 6.1 Questions an SP Educator May Consider When Planning for SPs to Provide Verbal Feedback

Education questions

- Who are the learners?
- Are the learning objectives clearly articulated?
- What is the complexity of the role that the SP is required to portray prior to providing feedback?
- What kind of feedback is the SP required to provide? (e.g. based on their experience, linked to a guide or ratings form?)
- Does the feedback the SP is asked to provide align with the learning objectives?
- What is the feedback/debriefing approach? (e.g. unidirectional, multi directional)
- What is the feedback/debriefing framework? (e.g. PEARLS, GAS)
- Is there a facilitator guiding the feedback/debriefing?
- How are learners and facilitators briefed about the nature of the SP feedback?

Logistic questions

- How long is the entire session?

- How many times will the SP have to portray the role and provide feedback?
- Will the SP be working with one learner or with a group of learners?
- How much time does the SP have to provide feedback?
- How much feedback is required from the SP?
- When will the SP feedback be provided in the session? (e.g. after each learner, once)
- Does the budget include time to train SPs to provide feedback and to debrief them about this process?

This type of review can be an exciting, productive, and creative opportunity to clarify understanding and expectations, optimise SP involvement, and consider psychological safety for all.

Addressing Any Knowledge Gaps (ASPE SOBP 3.1.2)

The SP educator must address any lack of knowledge related to the feedback/debriefing model or communication tool within which the SPs will provide feedback.

Creating a Training Plan (ASPE SOBP 1.1.3, 1.1.4, 3.1.3, and 4.5.2)

Creating a training plan allows you to set goals for the training, prioritise key points, and manage your time efficiently. At the same time, this plan needs to have some flexibility built in to respond to the needs and questions of the SPs being trained. Ideally, this training takes place in conjunction with training for role portrayal as the two tasks are intertwined. It is helpful to train SPs portraying the same role in a group, so they can learn from and with each other and calibrate their collective understanding of what is required.

Creating a Schedule

The number of trainings is dependent on a number of factors, including whether the session is for educational or assessment purposes, the complexity and length of the simulation scenario, the number of times the SP has to portray the role, the level of learners, the skill of the facilitator, the type of feedback required and how it is going to be integrated into the educational session, the experience and skill level of the SPs in providing the required feedback, and the amount allocated in the training budget. If an SP is expected to fill in an assessment form or to participate within a format that is new to them, further training time may be required.

Recruiting SPs

Recruiting SPs to provide feedback for a specific session necessitates that the SP educators have familiarity with their knowledge, skills, and attitudes. A group of SPs can have many different understandings because they often come from different backgrounds [12]. Orientation to feedback workshops can provide SP educators with insight to the suitability of SPs for providing feedback, including their ability to actively listen, to move in and out of role as required, to report on their experience in the role, and to demonstrate openness to receiving feedback themselves and flexibility in adapting to different feedback approaches (see Chap. 9 for additional guidance related to recruiting older adult SPs).

Gathering and Organising Resources Needed for Training (ASPE SOBP 3.1.4)

Resources can include scenario-specific materials such as rating forms the SPs might use to guide their verbal or written feedback, as well as practical details such as securing training rooms. Other training aids such as videos of learner performances can be used to illustrate different learner approaches that SPs might encounter and provide opportunities for them to practise providing feedback.

Considerations when working with older adult SPs: Vignette (Part 2)

During the review, you anticipate that some older adult SPs will be fatigued by participating in a full day session. You propose and receive budget approval to hire two groups of older adult SPs who will each come for a half day, to recruit an additional alternate SP for each group who can relieve anyone who gets fatigued, and to include additional training time if SPs require it. You suggest a health break for everyone after three interactions with learners with light refreshments, which is built into the schedule. You also arrange for the SPs to have a private room with comfortable seating where they can gather before and after the simulation activity and during the break.

You consider the psychological safety of the SPs. When you recruit them, you explain the role they will be required to portray and confirm that they are comfortable portraying someone in the early stages of dementia. You also make it clear that if, at any point after they have agreed to participate, for whatever reason, they do not feel they are able to continue, they can withdraw from the activity.

Since some of the SPs are less experienced providing feedback, you decide to have two trainings to offer the opportunity for further practice and reinforcement. The trainings will be a maximum of two hours as you notice that some SPs get fatigued if the trainings go longer.

You also recognise that some of the SPs may have challenges with memory retention, so you schedule the first training online about ten days ahead of the simulation activity (to review the role, feedback model, and logistics involved on the day) and an in-person dry run three days ahead of the session. The SPs are comfortable with technology and using an online platform to train.

The next step in your preparation is leading the actual training.

Leading the Training (ASPE SOBP 3.2, 3.3 and 4.2.5)

Reviewing with SPs the Fundamental Principles of Feedback Related to the Planned Activity (ASPE SOBP 3.3.1 and 3.3.4)

At the heart of what an SP does when providing feedback is to voice their perspective to a learner about the impact of this learner's behaviour on them while in the role of the person they have just portrayed. They are the only one in the room with this perspective.

Effective SP feedback addresses the learning objectives of a scenario as well as being meaningful to learners and promoting their growth; effective feedback also means that the feedback is provided in a manner consistent with how the SP has been trained. We present some fundamental principles of effective SP feedback adapted from those identified by Bokken et al. [8] and for feedback related more broadly to health professions education [30–32].

1. *Specific*
   SP feedback is based on what the SP perceives they heard a learner say or saw a learner do.
2. *Related to the impact on the* SP
   SP feedback is related to the impact on them of what the learner said or did rather than on clinical content (unless SPs are specifically trained to give feedback in this area).
3. *Balanced*
   SP feedback is balanced. The SP provides information about what worked well for them and what did not work.
4. *Measured*
   The amount of information the SP is required to provide varies depending on the learning activity. Too much feedback can overwhelm both a learner and the SP.
5. *Addresses something that can be changed*
   SP feedback addresses behaviour that can be changed, should the learner decide to do so.
6. *Respects each learner as an individual*
   SP feedback is respectful in that it considers each learner as an individual, rather than comparing one learner to another.

Here is an example of feedback that demonstrates these principles:

> At the beginning of the interview, I really appreciated how you maintained eye contact with me. When we started, you asked me how I was and left silence for me to answer. It was hard for me to tell you why I had come in and you left the space to let me talk in my own time and I felt so encouraged to go on. And hopeful that I could get help for this issue. Later in the interview, I noticed that you started to ask me questions where I could only answer yes or no, and I started to feel frustrated and a bit worried. There was so much I wanted to tell you that I thought would be important for you to know in order to help me.

Structuring Feedback: Completing the Sentence

It can be helpful for SPs to practise feedback using a simple structure such as this exercise called "Completing the Sentence" that reinforces the principles of SP feedback described above.

In this structure, the SP starts by identifying something that they heard or saw the learner do during the simulation activity:

When you said ______________.
or
When you did _________________________.

Then the SP links this information to the impact it had on them:

I felt ____________________.
I was ____________________.
*I experienced*____________________.
I noticed I _________________________.

For example:

> When you said, "Do I want sleeping pills?", I was confused because I did not think we had really explored why I've been sleeping poorly.

Words Matter

Even though this approach may seem very straightforward and simple, it can be trickier than it looks. Sometimes SPs have identified that part of the stress they feel providing feedback is in finding the right words [4, 13, 17]. Some trainers supply SPs with a list of "feeling" words [33]. Regular ongoing practice supports SPs in developing this skill. A series of prompting questions can be helpful for SPs to consider in thinking about how they have been affected by an interaction with a learner [5] (see Box 6.2).

Box 6.2 Questions an Older Adult SP May Consider in Preparation for Feedback to Learners

- How did I feel throughout the encounter?
- What did the learner do or say that led to my satisfaction?
- What did the learner do or say that led to my dissatisfaction?
- Did I feel able to tell my "story"?
- Did I get a chance to share my ideas?
- Was I able to share my concerns?
- Was I given a chance to ask questions?
- Did I feel comfortable enough to ask questions?
- Was I given the opportunity to make specific requests?
- Were my feelings acknowledged?
- Did I have a clear idea of the next steps?

Adapted from Nestel et al. [5]

> It's sometimes difficult to find the correct words to describe the impact of a scenario and this is something I strive to find every time. However, when I feel I get it right, the satisfaction makes my heart sing. (Karenne Marr)

Behaviour Matters

As well as being aware of the words they use, SPs must also be conscious of their behaviour when giving feedback including their posture, gestures, facial expressions, and paralinguistic elements such as their tone of voice, rate of speech, and volume. Berenson (2012) points out that learners are taught the importance of behaviour in building rapport with and promoting a sense of psychological safety for patients. In turn, when SPs provide feedback to learners, this dynamic is flipped, and the SP's behaviour can help to build rapport and promote psychological safety for learners through not just what they say but how they say it [11]. Berenson further notes that there needs to be a congruence between the SP's words and actions.

Troubleshooting (ASPE SOBP 3.2.3)

Discussing potential challenges involved in providing feedback can be helpful in making SPs feel more comfortable. Proactively equipping SPs with troubleshooting strategies for these "what-if" situations and practising them during training can be empowering (see Table 6.1).

Ensuring SP Readiness (ASPE SOBP 3.3.5)

A SP feedback-readiness criteria form provides an SP educator and SPs with guidelines to assess SP readiness for the task. Sharing the form with SPs promotes psychological safety with them, by making expectations explicit and transparent. It also takes an SP educator out of the position of making subjective decisions about whether or not an SP is ready to provide feedback. In addition, if an SP is not meeting the criteria, the SP educator has a tool that they can use to work with the SP to hopefully close the gap. SPs who are observing can also benchmark their understanding by referring to the form when watching other SPs provide feedback. See Table 6.2 for a simple feedback-readiness form that can be adapted to specific contexts and feedback criteria.

Keep in mind that no matter how much training some SPs have, they may still report feeling challenged by certain aspects of the task and a lack of feedback readiness because there are so many unknowns and pressures involved with the task [4, 7, 8, 12, 13].

Considerations when working with older adult SPs: Vignette (Part 3)

During the training, some SPs express a concern that they will not be able to remember what to say in the feedback. They identify that some of their anxiety would be alleviated if they could jot down feedback points. Together, you incorporate this modification into the training.

You model how the facilitator will interact with them and provide them with a number of expected learner approaches in the simulation, so they are prepared for these variations. You draw on the experiences of some of the more experienced SPs to suggest possible learner behaviours in this interaction, based on their past involvement.

You point out to the SPs that if they are not fully ready to provide feedback after the second training; you still have the option of meeting with them again. You normalise for them that additional practice is an opportunity for them to fully integrate all the steps involved in giving feedback and you are there to support them in that process.

Using a Feedback Readiness Form (see Table 6.2), you sign off the SPs as being ready to provide feedback.

Table 6.1 Troubleshooting related to SP feedback

Issue	Solution(s)
• SP cannot think of anything to provide feedback about.	• SP can ask the learner or facilitator if there is a specific part of the session that they could provide feedback about: *"Is there a particular point in the scenario that you think would be helpful for me to comment on?"*
	• SP can ask facilitator for a bit more time to formulate feedback: *"I just need a few more minutes to formulate my feedback."*
	• SP educator can provide SPs with paper or a template that they can use to jot down notes as a memory aid
• Learner or facilitator challenges or disagrees with the SP's feedback.	• SP educator can provide SPs with a strategy to move away from the impulse to argue or defend. *"It is interesting there are different views. I wanted to share my experience of what happened."*
• SP provides feedback that is focused on something other than their experience (e.g. tells the learner what clinical content they should have covered).	• If the SP recognizes that they have done this, they can step back and reformulate their feedback. *"I'd like to reframe my feedback by giving you information about my experience."*
	• The facilitator can redirect the SP by asking them to reframe their feedback. "*Thanks and can you focus on the impact on you of the moment in the simulation that you are describing?"*
• Learner asks SP the "right" way to do something.	• The SP educator can provide the SPs with a response they might use: *"There is no single right way to do this. I wonder if we can discuss strategies together and how they might have played out in the scenario."*
• The SP is not able to release a high emotional affect (e.g. frustration, grief, despair) before giving feedback.	• SP can leave the room if they are so upset that they might not provide feedback in a way that is safe for a learner to hear.
	• Facilitator can call a time out if they sense that the SP is not able to de-role.
	• SP educator can provide the SP with strategies such as asking for more time to de-role before providing feedback. *"I just need a few more minutes to formulate my feedback."*

Table 6.2 Example of a simple SP feedback-readiness form based on principles of feedback related to the simulation activity

SP feedback readiness form				
SP Name:				
SP Educator:				
Date:				
Project:				
SP Role:				
	Principles	*Not done*	*Partially Done*	*Done correctly*
1	Specific			
2	Related to the impact on the SP			
3	Balanced			
4	Measured			
6	Addresses behaviour that can be changed			
7	Respects each learner as an individual			
8	De-roles before providing feedback			
9	Other:			
Notes:				

NHET-Sim Phase: Briefing (ASPE SOBP 1.1.5, 1.1.6, 1.1.7, 3.3.2, and 3.3.3)

Immediately prior to the simulation activity, SPs should be briefed related to the logistics (e.g. number of learners they will see, break times, format of feedback) and offered the opportunity to ask any further questions. Similarly, learners and faculty should be briefed about the nature of SP involvement related to feedback on the day. Strategies such as creating a one-page guide for faculty that they can refer to during the feedback, especially if they are not used to working with SPs, are helpful. SPs have noted that having a supportive working relationship with faculty during the simulation and feedback/debrief session is imperative [17]. The briefing phase helps to create this supportive environment.

Considerations when working with older adult SPs: Vignette (Part 4)

You schedule a short briefing with SPs before the sessions. You review the educational aspects such as who the learners are, the purpose of their feedback, and logistics and orient SPs to their rooms and the washrooms. You remind them that if they become tired, they can request that an alternate SP take their place. You also note that you will be observing and available for any support or questions.

You also create a briefing guide for facilitators to remind them about how they might have to adapt when working with older adult SPs. For example, if an SP has hearing loss, you could offer some suggestions for room setup (e.g. facilitators placing themselves in the room in such a way that the SP can clearly hear them; light levels in the room allow the SP to refer to their notes).

NHET-Sim Phase: Simulation Activity (ASPE SOBP 1.1.9 and 3.5.1)

Although this phase does not involve SP feedback, it is helpful to observe how SPs are portraying the role (e.g. behind a two-way mirror, viewing a video feed, within the room) to get a sense of how this interaction relates to their feedback after the simulation is over.

NHET-Sim Phase: De-roling (ASPE SOBP 1.1.8)

Once the simulation ends and prior to giving feedback, it is essential for an SP to de-role or separate from the role that they have just portrayed [34]. This step happens each time the SP moves into providing feedback to a learner. De-roling frames that the simulation activity is over and promotes psychological safety for learners, SPs and the facilitator by signalling that the SP is now out of role. If the SP has had a strong emotional affect, de-roling allows them to release the emotion, so they can engage in feedback with the learner in a more grounded and thoughtful manner. If the SP has portrayed someone who is really angry or challenging, for example, and they fail to de-role, providing feedback in this heightened emotional state can be confusing and upsetting for a learner. In addition, if an SP has to portray their role and then provide feedback a number of times with a number of different learners, there is a risk that, if they do not de-role, their affect can start to heighten and become distorted from the original intention of the role.

There are SP de-roling techniques discussed in this book (see Chap. 14). The facilitator can support this process once the simulation activity has been completed by introducing the SP to the learners out of role, thanking them for playing the SP role and asking them how they are feeling now (see Chap. 3).

NHET-Sim Phase: Feedback/Debriefing (ASPE SOBP 3.3.1 and 3.3.4)

Here are two examples of how SP feedback might unfold in the feedback/debriefing phase in a small group setting with a facilitator, a learner who has interacted with an SP and 3–4 learner observers.

Example 1
If there is only a short amount of time for SPs to provide feedback (e.g. 5 min), then a unidirectional structure might be used:

1. The facilitator signals the simulation is over and the SP de-roles.
2. The SP and learners move into the debriefing space.
3. The facilitator checks that the SP is okay and introduces the SP to the learners, reinforcing the act of de-roling.
4. The facilitator gives the SP some time to formulate feedback for the learner who just interacted with them.
5. The facilitator checks in with the learner that they are okay and to get an initial sense of their reactions to the encounter. As the SP listens to the learner's response, they may think about adjusting their feedback to meet the learner's needs.

The facilitator invites the SP to provide feedback to the learner. This is usually in the form of general and then specific questions that relate to the learning objectives and the SP's experience of the learner (e.g. what worked well for them and what needs development).

Example 2
When SP feedback is framed as part of a longer debriefing or learning conversation, it can be part of a process that provides opportunities for more in-depth exploration and processing by the learner (see Chap. 5). Here is an example of how SP feedback might unfold in a small group setting with 15 min for feedback, once steps 1–5 (above) have been completed.

6. Once the SP has provided some initial feedback, the facilitator checks in with the learner to ask them for their response to or reflection on the SP's comments.
7. From here, the facilitators might encourage conversation between the learner and the SP to establish further understanding and/or ask observers to comment.
8. The facilitator might ask the learner if they wish to try part of the simulation over again.
9. The facilitator ends the session by asking the SP if they have any final observations.
10. The facilitator asks the learner and observers for their take home points.

You will notice that in example 2, the learner is being asked to reflect, analyse, and make sense for themselves rather than to be offered immediate solutions by either the facilitator, the SP, or other learners who are observing. Here is one SP's perspective on participating in this kind of session.

> I think the thing that is helpful is having a great facilitator who creates a space where the learner has time to reflect on my feedback and make sense of it. It becomes a conversation between the learner and me then. (Susan Greenfield)

In certain situations, though, feedback (from the SP, observers, and facilitator) may become more directive (e.g. next time you may want to try doing things this way). Often this kind of SP feedback is related to a communication tool (e.g. the Calgary Cambridge Guide) to which they are linking their feedback (see Chap. 5). It is essential that those who prepare SPs understand and communicate the scope of feedback SPs are being asked to provide [4, 12, 17].

Considerations when working with older adult SPs: Vignette (Part 5)
Drawing further from the Framework, you offer your full support to the older adult SPs by observing the feedback they offer (e.g. behind a two-way mirror). You make sure that everyone involved in the simulation knows that you are observing in this way and that your purpose is to support the SPs. You check in with them periodically to see how they are doing, offer feedback, and/or address any questions or concerns. You also make notes about what they are doing well and where there might be areas for improvement.

NHET-Sim Phase: Reflection (ASPE SOBP 3.5.1)

As noted in Chap. 3, in this phase, the focus is on reflection, and it offers the opportunity to support SPs to maintain and further develop their feedback skills. SPs indicate they greatly value the opportunity to reflect [12]. It can be helpful to provide SPs with questions as follows: How was that experience of feedback for you?; What do you think you did well?; Where were you challenged?; What did you do to overcome the challenge?; Is there anything you need to have clarified?; and What can you take forward or improve upon next time? In addition, an SP educator can reflect on their own strengths and areas for growth in supporting SPs to provide feedback.

Debriefing SPs (ASPE 1.1.8 and 3.5.1)
Just as with learners, debriefing allows SPs to process, make sense of, and learn from their experiences providing feedback [35].

NHET-Sim Phase: Evaluation (ASPE SOBP 3.5.1, 4.6.2, 4.6.3, 4.6.4, and 4.6.5)

SPs can offer valuable judgements about how well feedback training supported their ability to provide feedback and if there are things that would be helpful to include in future trainings.

Ongoing Quality Management
The ASPE SOBP notes that ongoing quality management is important for all aspects of an SP programme including SP

feedback practices [27]. Several instruments have been developed to assess verbal SP feedback in educational sessions [36–39]. Doyle et al. (2023) remind us that it is imperative that SP educators provide ongoing feedback to SPs to promote their growth [17]. In turn, SPs have indicated that they also desire this kind of feedback [12, 16, 20]. In addition, encouraging SP self-assessment and peer assessment can be a powerful way for SPs to develop their feedback capabilities and support one another [40]. Further strategies an SP educator might use to promote quality feedback practices involve scheduling ongoing SP feedback trainings [4, 17].

Considerations when working with older adult SPs: Vignette (Part 6)

Through the reflection and evaluation phase, you draw on the Framework to "invest and integrate," supporting the older adult SPs to maintain and develop their feedback skills. You ask them to reflect on and make sense of their experiences providing feedback to learners. You ask them to evaluate the session in terms of how they felt supported and if there were any cognitive, sensory, or physical challenges they might have experienced. You reflect on how you might apply their feedback to your future work with them.

Moving forward, you highlight how their feedback specifically contributes to the development of the scenario and refinements in your training approach. You also share other relevant feedback from the learner and faculty evaluations about their participation.

Several SPs note that they would appreciate a refresher training on the general principles of verbal feedback in an education context, so you plan a general training session. You ask each SP to provide you with one goal they would like to achieve in this training.

> I think the biggest thing for me is practice, practice, practice. It's got to be part of the training process. … That's the only way we really get better at providing feedback. (Susan Greenfield)

Closing

Older adult SPs can provide great value to learners through the authenticity of the feedback they offer by virtue of their lived experience coupled with careful training. This chapter provided an overview of SP feedback, both in general and related to older adult SPs, including benefits and challenges as well as the ways in which SPs provide feedback. We then presented a foundational, evidence-informed way to support older adult SPs in providing feedback to learners in educational contexts. While the practices reflect those of the wider SP population, consideration was also given to adaptations drawn from a Framework for working with older adult SPs related to potential age-related cognitive, sensory, and physical changes as well as to fostering their psychological safety.

> Being an SP has given me a broader understanding and keen interest in the importance and value of succinct, kind and honest communication in the health domain. I've learned to really listen and be aware of the vulnerability of my fellow human beings. (Kareene Marr)

Acknowledgements Susan Greenfield, Karenne Marr, Leonie Tuite, and Robyn Vinodolac share their perspectives as older adult SPs through this chapter.

References

1. Van de Ridder J, Stokking KM, McGaghie WC, Ten Cate OTJ. What is feedback in clinical education? Med Educ. 2008;42(2):189–97.
2. Cheng A, Eppich W, Sawyer T, Grant V. Debriefing: the state of the art and science in healthcare simulation. In: Nestel D, Michelle K, Jolly B, Watson M, editors. Healthcare simulation education: evidence, theory and practice. Hoboken: Wiley Blackwell; 2017. p. 158–64.
3. Tavares W, Eppich W, Cheng A, Miller S, Teunissen PW, Watling CJ, et al. Learning conversations: an analysis of the theoretical roots and their manifestations of feedback and debriefing in medical education. Acad Med. 2020;95(7):1020–5.
4. George RE, Wells H, Cushing A. Experiences of simulated patients in providing feedback in communication skills teaching for undergraduate medical students. BMC Med Educ. 2022;22(1):1–11.
5. Nestel D, Bearman M, Fleishman C. Simulated patients as teachers: the role of feedback. In: Simulated patient methodology: theory, evidence and practice. Oxford: Wiley; 2015. p. 71–8.
6. Edmondson AC, Besieux T. Reflections: voice and silence in workplace conversations. J Change Manage. 2021;21(3):269–86.
7. Lovink A, Groenier M, van der Niet A, Miedema H, Rethans J-J. The contribution of simulated patients to meaningful student learning. Perspect Med Educ. 2021;10:341–6.
8. Bokken L, Linssen T, Scherpbier A, Van Der Vleuten C, Rethans JJ. Feedback by simulated patients in undergraduate medical education: a systematic review of the literature. Med Educ. 2009;43(3):202–10.
9. Dugmore H, Carr S, Saunders R. Interpreting the value of feedback: older adult voices in nursing education. Nurse Educ Pract. 2020;48:102868.
10. Clark L, Gliva-McConvey G, Richards A. Cultivating compassionate communication with clinical competence: utilizing human simulation to provide constructive feeedback to learners. In: Gliva-McConvey G, Nicholas C, Clark L, editors. Comprehensive healthcare simulation: implementing best practices in standardized patient methodology. Cham: Springer; 2020. p. 117–68.
11. Berenson LD, Goodill SW, Wenger S. Standardized patient feedback: making it work across disciplines. J Allied Health. 2012;41(1):27E–31E.
12. Sullivan C, Doyle AJ, O'Toole M, Mulhall C, McNaughton N, Eppich W. 'How can we help the students learn?' A grounded theory study of simulated participants as educators. Med Teach. 2023;45:1047–53.
13. Nestel D, Clark S, Tabak D, Ashwell V, Muir E, Paraskevas P, et al. Defining responsibilities of simulated patients in medical education. Simul Healthc. 2010;5(3):161–8.
14. Sullivan C, Condron CM, O'Connor L, Pawlikowska T, Murray JM. Their OSCE, not your Oscar: simulated patients' perspectives. Clin Teach. 2021;18(6):596–601.
15. Schelgel C, Smith CM. "Please let me know when I do not realize it myself": a qualitative analysis of senior simulated patients' experiences. Adv Simul. 2019;4(1):18.
16. Thompson J, Tiplady S, Hutchinson A, Cook G, Harrington B. Older people's views and experiences of engagement in stan-

dardised patient simulation. BMJ Simul Technol Enhanc Learn. 2017;3(4):154–8.
17. Doyle AJ, Sullivan C, O'Toole M, Tjin A, Simiceva A, Collins N, et al. Training simulated participants for role portrayal and feedback practices in communication skills training: a BEME scoping review: BEME Guide No. 86. Med Teach. 2024;46:162–78.
18. Smith CM, Sokoloff LG, Alsaba N. Collaborative framework for working with older simulated participants (SP). BMJ Simul Technol Enhanc Learn. 2021;7(2):112.
19. Shawler C. Palliative and end-of-life care: using a standardized patient family for gerontological nurse practitioner students. Nurs Educ Perspect. 2011;32(3):168–72.
20. Nelson G, Swenson J, Kozmenko V, Thompson P. Training standardized patients to provide effective feedback: development, implementation, and its effect on the efficacy of medical students' education. Aesculapius J. 2022;3(1):1.
21. Smith C, O'Byrne C, Nestel D. Simulated patient methodology and assessment. In: Nestel D, Bearman M, editors. Simulated patient methodology: theory, evidence and practice. Chichester: Wiley-Blackwell; 2015. p. 85–92.
22. Silverman J, Kurtz S, Draper J. Skills for communicating with patients. Boca Raton: CRC Press; 2016.
23. Kurtz SM, Silverman JD. The calgary—Cambridge referenced observation guides: an aid to defining the curriculum and organizing the teaching in communication training programmes. Med Educ. 1996;30(2):83–9.
24. Sarzynski E, Foley K, Riekse R, Laird-Fick H, Keilman L, Barnikow T, et al. An OSCE to assess trainee management of complex older adults and to teach documentation, coding, and billing. MedEdPORTAL. 2014;10:9903.
25. Wallace P. Coaching standardized patients: for use in the assessment of clinical competence. New York: Springer; 2007.
26. May W. Training standardized patients for a high-stakes clinical performance examination in the California consortium for the assessment of clinical competence. Kaohsiung J Med Sci. 2008;24(12):640–5.
27. Lewis KL, Bohnert CA, Gammon WL, Hölzer H, Lyman L, Smith C, et al. The association of standardized patient educators (ASPE) standards of best practice (SOBP). Adv Simul. 2017;2(1):10.
28. Smith CM, Alsaba N, Nestel D, Sokoloff L. Older adults as simulated participants: a scoping review. Int J Healthc Simul. 2023; https://doi.org/10.54531/bocf7225.
29. The NHET-Sim Monash Team. The National Health Education and Training—Simulation (NHET-Sim) Program. 2012. http://www.nhet-sim.edu.au.
30. Ende J. Feedback in clnical medical education. JAMA. 1983;250(6):777–81.
31. Lehner GF. Aids for giving and receiving feedback. Los Angeles: University of California; 1987.
32. Ramani S, Könings KD, Ginsburg S, van der Vleuten CP. Twelve tips to promote a feedback culture with a growth mind-set: swinging the feedback pendulum from recipes to relationships. Med Teach. 2019;41(6):625–31.
33. Rosenberg M. Center for non violent communciation—how expansive is your emotional vocabulary? [Internet]. Encinitas: PuddleDancer Press; 2023. https://www.nonviolentcommunication.com/learn-nonviolent-communication/feelings/
34. Busselle K, Fazio H. Windows into Revolutionary Recovery: Check-Ins, De-Roling, and Debriefing Practices for Rehearsal and Performance. Theatre/Practice. 2023;12:1–20.
35. Clark L, Woll A, Owens TL, Shropshire D, Kiser B, Gephardt G, et al. SP safety, autonomy and healthcare simulation practice in the COVID-19 era. BMJ Simul Technol Enhanc Learn. 2021;7(5):450.
36. Wind LA, Van Dalen J, Muijtjens AM, Rethans JJ. Assessing simulated patients in an educational setting: the MaSP (Maastricht Assessment of Simulated Patients). Med Educ. 2004;38(1):39–44.
37. Schlegel C, Woermann U, Rethans J-J, van der Vleuten C. Validity evidence and reliability of a simulated patient feedback instrument. BMC Med Educ. 2012;12(1):6.
38. May W, Fisher D, Souder D. Development of an instrument to measure the quality of standardized/simulated patient verbal feedback. Med Educ Dev. 2012;2(1):e3.
39. Bouter S, van Weel-Baumgarten E, Bolhuis S. Construction and validation of the Nijmegen Evaluation of the Simulated Patient (NESP): assessing simulated patients' ability to role-play and provide feedback to students. Acad Med. 2013;88(2):253–9.
40. Perera J, Perera J, Abdullah J, Lee N. Training simulated patients: evaluation of a training approach using self-assessment and peer/tutor feedback to improve performance. BMC Med Educ. 2009;9(1):37.

7 Programme Evaluation and Quality Improvement Approaches in Older Adult Simulated Participant Methodology

Alexis Battista and Debra Nestel

Key Messages

1. Programme evaluation (PE) enables judgements about a programme's quality, value, or need, whether it has met its intended purpose or if there are any unintended consequences. It is also commonly used for quality improvement of programmes.
2. Conducting evaluations is a systematic and methodical approach like conducting research.
3. Articulating the purpose of the PE is vital to determining the relevant parties or knowledge users for the evaluation, the type of data to be collected, when and how, the approach to the data analysis, and the reporting of findings, recommendations, and dissemination.
4. An evaluation may occur at the programme level or focus on programme elements (e.g. the quality, value, or need of a scenario). Evaluating more minor aspects of a programme (e.g. a scenario) may inform a larger-scale evaluation (e.g. a whole SP programme).
5. Few published programme evaluations report the inclusion of SPs during the evaluation process; however, they should be considered important contributors to the PE of an SP programme, depending on the purpose of the evaluation.

A. Battista
The Henry M Jackson Foundation for the Advancement of Military Medicine, Center for Health Professions Education, F. Edward Hébert School of Medicine, "America's Medical School", Uniformed Services University of the Health Sciences, Bethesda, MD, USA
e-mail: alexis.battista.ctr@usuhs.edu

D. Nestel (✉)
School of Clinical Sciences, Faculty of Medicine, Nursing & Health Sciences, Monash University, Clayton, VIC, Australia

Department of Surgery (Austin Precinct), University of Melbourne, Parkville, VIC, Australia
e-mail: dnestel@unimelb.edu.au; debra.nestel@monash.edu

Introduction

Programme evaluation (PE) of simulated participant (SP) programmes is crucial given the field's rapid growth and the evolving understanding of how to employ simulations best. Evidence of effective practices is developing at pace, including developing guidelines for working with SPs of different ages [1, 2]. PE is a crucial component of professional simulation practice regardless of whether a simulation programme is under development or well established, as it measures the need for, value, or impact of a programme. PE can focus on programme outcomes, the need for a programme, or the structure and processes of a programme. Some examples include the following:

- Conducting a needs assessment to determine if a new simulation programme is needed and what its focus should be.
- Evaluating participants' learning experiences in an established SP programme to determine if the programme is working as intended and to identify unanticipated ill effects and/or benefits.
- Evaluating how adding a new simulation programme impacts faculty and student workload, learning, and well-being [3].
- Evaluating an established SP programme impacted by organisational changes (e.g. funding, staffing) to determine whether the programme's scope needs modification.

This chapter outlines what PE is, who does it, and how, using SP programmes as our context. Within the scope of an introductory chapter like this, we can only cover foundational concepts. At the end of the chapter, we share examples of hypothetical and published PEs and offer resources for developing PE skills.

C. M. Smith et al. (eds.), *Comprehensive Healthcare Simulation: Geriatric Simulation*, Comprehensive Healthcare Simulation,
https://doi.org/10.1007/978-3-031-65742-9_7

What Is Programme Evaluation (PE)?

Simulation knowledge users (e.g. simulationists, programme directors, and programme administrators) may be asked to decide whether an SP programme is needed, whether it is effective, or how it might be improved or modified. The practice of PE is the process that underlies these efforts. PE involves the systematic use of social research methods to investigate the effects of a programme to provide evidence that can inform future decision-making about the programme [4].

Whether the evaluation is smaller in scale (e.g. a formative simulation-based curriculum, an Objective Simulated Clinical Exam (OSCE), an SP training programme), or a larger scale (e.g. a graduate nursing education programme, a medical specialty training programme), the efforts of evaluation are similar. Each involves articulating the purpose of the evaluation, planning for, designing the evaluation, collecting and analysing data, and reporting findings and recommendations and dissemination. Programme directors or those able to effect change should consider actions/decisions based on the recommendations in the evaluation report. Evaluators rely on diverse methods, including qualitative, quantitative, or mixed-method approaches, and therefore also use a range of analytic techniques to collate and interpret data.

Although PE relies on the same systematic approaches as research, some key differences exist. For example, a feature of PE is that it leads to recommendations for improvement in response to the purpose of the evaluation [4]. Additionally, PE may not require human research ethics/institutional review board approval because the results are used locally for quality improvement. However, sometimes PE has a research angle and/or the findings are disseminated beyond the institution; therefore, human research ethics/institutional review board approval is needed. Professional programme evaluators also work to professional standards (see resources), like those expected of researchers.

Why Conduct PE?

PE can provide valuable feedback about a programme and its operations that help relevant parties make informed decisions about its future while promoting institutional value. For example, aggregating learner outcomes, such as licensure pass rates, provides insight into broader programme outcomes [5]. Additionally, PE findings can inform curricular revisions and improvements as part of a designing, implementing, evaluating, and revising cycle to ensure continuous improvement of a programme [4, 5]. Results from a PE may also provide information to administrators, support staff, and others responsible for maintaining a programme's structure and logistic operations (e.g. library, technology, assessment).

Further, programme evaluation can play a role in accreditation and reaccreditation efforts because accrediting bodies often require a demonstration of continued programme improvement [6]. Accreditation of healthcare simulation programmes and other awards clearly state PE requirements (see resources).

Moreover, although many programmes are designed for reasons that appear compelling, they may not consistently achieve their intended outcomes. For example, programme designers may find that the original circumstances have changed due to new technology, new demands previously unaccounted for, or changes in practice guidelines. Factors undermining a programme's success include faculty or programme support limitations, budgetary constraints, unanticipated outside forces (e.g. pandemic [7]), and organisational changes [4, 5, 8]. PE can help identify gaps in these situations so those invested in the programme can revise the programme. Consider the case study in Box 7.1.

Box 7.1 A Hypothetical Case Study

A government agency has funded a new older-adult SP programme that will support the development of communication skills of the care workforce in residential aged care facilities in your community. The skills will focus on interpersonal communication between the healthcare workforce and older adult residents.

1. **What is the goal of PE?**

   To evaluate the impact of a new older adult SP programme designed to support development of communication skills of the care workforce in residential aged care facilities.
2. **Who are the knowledge users and/or relevant parties?**
   - The care workforce in the aged care facilities
   - Residents in the aged care facilities
   - A government agency funding the programme
   - The community served by the aged care facility (e.g. families, support agencies or organizations)
   - The residential aged care facilities, including management
3. **What data might you collect? When and how?**

   (a) Performance data on observed communication skills of the care workforce in simulated encounters

   SP and observer judgments on care workforce communication skills in simulated encounters before and after the programme (digital forms)

(b) Performance data on observed communication skills of the care workforce in real encounters
 Aged care resident judgments on care workforce communication skills in real encounters before and after the programme (digital forms, satisfaction surveys)
(c) Care workforce experiences of participating in the programme (digital forms)
(d) Written complaints and expressions of gratitude relevant to the communication skills of the care workforce from users of the aged care facilities (collection of artifacts with permission)
(e) Faculty and older adult SP experience of the programme, including views on maintenance of participants' communication skills

4. **How will you analyse the data?**
   - Data analysis for a) and b) will compute scores before and after and apply statistical approaches to reveal broad patterns in the care workforce performance
   - Data analysis for c) may include content analysis of participants' written comments
   - Data analysis for d) and e) will include content analysis
5. **What will you do with the findings?**
   - Share findings with funders (e.g. a government agency), including considerations for programme maintenance
   - Share a summarised version of the findings with faculty, including SPs (if they request access)
   - Share a summarised version of the findings with participants (if they request access)

Additional information to consider before designing the PE

- What access will the care workforce have to the programme?
- Will this be a one-off programme, or will maintenance programmes be offered?
- Who will pay for the programme beyond the initial funding?

Who Is Involved in PE, and What Are Their Contributions?

A PE involves numerous participants, including individuals, departments, and organisations, with a vested interest in the programme and who may be impacted by the evaluation findings and recommendations. These individuals and entities can be referred to as relevant parties or knowledge users. This includes persons who are responsible for making decisions about the direction of the programme (e.g. starting, continuing, or discontinuing), programme sponsors who provide funding for the programme, participants such as SPs or learners, programme managers, and programme staff and even evaluation and research communities [4].

Common considerations include those who have authority over the programme (e.g. clerkship director, simulation lab director), who are responsible for the delivery of the programme (e.g. faculty, simulationists, SPs), who are the intended beneficiaries of the programme (e.g. learners, patients, community members), and funders [4]. However, it is also important to consider seeking out those who may be silent, marginalised, or overlooked (e.g. simulated participants, adjunct faculty) [9], taking the time to develop a good relationship with the programme and pursuing an understanding of the context in which the programme functions can help evaluators identify relevant parties [9].

Knowledge users play a vital role in determining the focus and direction of an evaluation [4, 10]. For example, knowledge users or beneficiaries are likely to know about the underlying mechanisms and processes that moderate programme outcomes and what outcomes might be beneficial to examine [11]. They can also provide critical insight into what evaluation questions might be the most useful and what resources might be available to help conduct the evaluation. Engaging knowledge users in this process can also help ensure the evaluation results are understood and the findings are employed more effectively [4, 10].

PEs may also involve research or evaluation professionals to help guide or lead the evaluation, collect data, and provide methodological and analytic expertise. Medical librarians can play a crucial role in evaluations by supporting and guiding the conduct of a literature review. For those charged with conducting an evaluation, it is essential to consider the existing capabilities and expertise of the evaluation team and identify additional support if significant gaps are identified.

Designing and Conducting PE

When embarking on a PE, it is essential to take the time to determine the purposes of the evaluation before advancing to other stages of the evaluation design. Choosing the purposes will, in turn, shape the evaluation questions, methodological approaches, data collection strategies, and analytic choices. Some of the earliest efforts of an evaluation include developing a programme description, which involves an in-depth understanding of the programme and its context [4]. This step involves reviewing programme documentation, interviewing key informants, and examining external sources, such as conducting a literature review and examining guidelines from governing or accreditation bodies (see resources).

One way to approach and frame a programme description involves creating a logic model. Logic models highlight the importance of a systematic approach to PE and flag considerations of the 'inputs, activities, outputs and outcomes in any programme'. For example, Kaba et al. (2023) describe using a logic model to frame their approach to PE in their healthcare simulation programme [12]. By using a model, PE can be focused and scalable. The authors argue that this approach 'can contribute to both *demonstrating value* and *impact* to healthcare teams, in addition to establishing a growing culture of evaluation at any health system level' [11, p. 1].

Once the evaluator has a better understanding of the programme, they can work with relevant parties to determine the overarching purpose of the evaluation. For example, many PEs are conducted to improve a programme's impact. Another common goal of evaluation is to examine a programme's processes and design. Evaluations can also focus on accountability, determining the need for a programme or taking a continuous quality improvement approach [4] (Table 7.1).

The language of PE is often complex, and some professional groups have adopted their ways of describing PE

Table 7.1 Types of evaluations, operational definitions, when to use, guiding questions, and why useful

Type of evaluation	Operational definitions, when to use, guiding questions, and why they are helpful/useful.
Needs assessment	Needs assessments include systematic approaches to identifying a community's nature, magnitude, and distribution to identify current conditions and desired services or outcomes for a programme [4]. Needs assessments are usually conducted during the development of a programme or when an existing programme needs modification.
	Guiding questions may include:
	• What are the needs of the population? What caused or created the need?
	• What kinds of assistance or support might address the identified needs?
	• What are the characteristics of the population in need?
	Needs assessments are helpful because they help identify what the gaps are between what is, what is desired, and what solutions may help close the gap. Conducting a careful needs assessment helps increase the likelihood that the programme will succeed.
Assessment of programme theory and design	Assessment of programme theory and design is an approach used to examine whether the underlying assumptions of the programme are valid and feasible and support the program's efforts to achieve its intended outcomes [4]. Programme theory assessment may occur as a first step to any other evaluation approaches (e.g. programme process, cost) when a programme has never been formally evaluated or persisted for years without evaluation or if a programme has experienced significant changes.
	Guiding questions may include:
	• What outcomes did the programme set out to affect? Do the outcomes relate to the problem or situation the programme is expected to change? If so, how?
	• Does the programme focus on the appropriate population, given the needs and goals the programme is intended to address? How does the programme reach the people it is intended to support?
	• How is the programme organized, resourced, and staffed, and is it adequate given its goals?
	Assessing programme theory can help identify how realistic, reasonable, and feasible the programme is.
Assessment of program process	Assessing programme processes includes evaluating the quality of the programme's implementation fidelity [4]. Evaluations of programme processes are ideally conducted as soon as the programme begins and as an ongoing practice to monitor existing programmes.
	Guiding questions may consist of the following:
	• Is the programme being delivered to the intended population?
	• Are the recipients of the programme satisfied with the services they are receiving?
	• Is the programme well managed (e.g. administrative functions, organizational functions)?
	Assessing a programme's processes can serve as an early warning for future problems. They also allow the programme to monitor how well it is doing.
Impact evaluation	Impact assessments examine whether the programme is achieving its ultimate goals [4]. Impact evaluations are ideally conducted when programmes have matured and are stable or at the end of a programme [4]. They are also typically performed at appropriately designated intervals.
	Guiding questions may include:
	• Are the goals and objectives being met?
	• Are the trends in the outcomes trending in the desired direction?
	• Are there any adverse effects on participants? What are they? What is causing them?
	• Are some participants affected for better or worse? Who are they? Why?
	Impact assessments provide evidence that can be used to inform others about the programme's value and for policy and funding decisions.

(continued)

Table 7.1 (continued)

Type of evaluation	Operational definitions, when to use, guiding questions, and why they are helpful/useful.
Efficiency assessment/cost analysis/cost-effectiveness evaluation	Efficiency and cost analysis provide information about the specific costs incurred by a programme, including what resources are being used and their costs compared to outcomes [4]. These evaluations may be conducted when designing the programme or in ongoing intervals once the programme has started. Guiding questions may include: • What are the total costs of operating the programme? • Is the programme using the resources efficiently without excessive waste?

approaches. For example, clinicians are likely familiar with the Plan-Do-Study-Act quality improvement approach, sometimes applied in health professions' education evaluations [13]. Other common languages used in health professions education include decision-oriented, outcomes-oriented, or expertise-oriented and evaluation frameworks (e.g. Kirkpatrick model) [14, 15]. While evaluators and researchers in health professions' education have relied heavily on the Kirkpatrick model, challenges to its status as the *gold standard* are increasing [16, 17]. We strongly recommend that readers review the work of professional programme evaluators (Table 7.1, Resources).

Developing Evaluation Questions

Like identifying the purpose of an evaluation, developing evaluation questions should also be done with care. Additionally, this stage needs time for programme evaluators and key knowledge users to negotiate and refine the evaluation questions. For example, even if evaluators are familiar with the programme and context, they can only be expected to partially understand the experiences of all key knowledge users [8, 18]. Similarly, key knowledge users may need to be made aware of common evaluation strategies or approaches [8]. Collaboratively developing evaluation questions can help increase the chances that evaluation findings will be understood and appreciated and increases the chances of the findings and recommendations being used to improve the programmee [8, 10].

Evaluation questions should be tailored to the purpose of the evaluation. For example, for needs assessments, questions should focus on understanding why a programme is needed or what problem a programme is intended to solve (e.g. What are the needs of the population? What are the characteristics of the people the programme will serve? What are the gaps in knowledge/skill that the programme is intended to fill?) [4, 8]. Alternatively, if the goal of the evaluation relates to programme operations or delivery, questions might include: Are the intended services reaching the target population? Are there needful but underserved persons that the programme is not reaching? [4, 8]

Evaluation questions should also specify the group or population under evaluation rather than being overly generalised [8]. Identify specific measures and cut-off values where needed and consider how feasible it will be to gather and analyse the required data [8]. Evaluation questions may also be shaped by drawing from best practice guidelines (e.g. ASPE Best Practice Standards, the Joint Committee on Standards for Educational Evaluation or the Higher Learning Commission's Culture Matrix) [6, 19–22] (Box 7.2).

Box 7.2 Example Evaluation Questions Informed by Practice Guidelines from the ASPE Standards of Best Practice

Is the programme well designed?

Question: How do SP educators engage SPs when preparing them to portray their roles for the interprofessional geriatric simulation programme?

ASPE Standard: 3.2.2 Engage SPs in discussing and practicing role portrayal features (e.g. affect, signs and symptoms, behaviors).

Question: What strategies are SPs taught to help them manage unanticipated learner questions and behaviors for the interprofessional geriatric simulation programme?

ASPE Standard: 3.2.3 Provide SPs with strategies for unanticipated learner questions and behaviors.

Is the programme implemented effectively?

Question: Do most simulated participants supporting the geriatric simulation course feel satisfied with the ratio of rotations to breaks when portraying a role?

ASPE Standard: 1.1.1 Ensure safe working conditions in the design of the activity (e.g. number of rotations, number of breaks, physical, cognitive, and psychological challenges in the role portrayal).

Question: Do simulated participants report experiencing potential occupational hazards, such as exposure to allergic or infectious substances, sharps, or air quality hazards?

ASPE Standard: 1.1.2 Anticipate and recognize potential occupational hazards, including threats to SP safety in the environment (e.g. allergenic substances, exposure to sharps, air quality, and live defibrillators).

Selecting Evaluation Methods, Data Collection Strategies, and Analysis

Credible evaluation requires evaluators to identify measures and data collection approaches and then collect them in a way that is consistent with the chosen approaches and measures [4, 8]. Choosing evaluation methods involves considering methodological approaches and how, when, and where data will be collected and how and who will analyse it [8]. Selecting evaluation methods should also consider the purpose and goals of the evaluation, the evaluation context, and the resources available to conduct the evaluation.

For example, if the goal and purpose of the evaluation are to examine programme outcomes (e.g. OSCE performance), then quantitative approaches may be ideal. Quantitative approaches often rely on numeric data forms. They are analysed using descriptive or inferential statistics to predict or confirm how regular or widespread a phenomenon is (e.g. examination of performance scores and survey results). Typical data collection tools include the use of assessments or scales and surveys.

Conversely, qualitative approaches should be considered if the goals of the PE focus on understanding learners' or instructors' experiences, determining whether the programme is causing harm, or understanding the causal process that led to learner or programme outcomes. Qualitative approaches are ideal when describing evaluation contexts, understanding people's perspectives and experiences, and identifying the underlying causal processes that lead to specific outcomes. Common data collection methods when using qualitative approaches include interviews, focus groups, observations, and analysis of relevant artifacts, such as instructional design documents or documentation about how the programme or curriculum has changed over time.

Sometimes, evaluators rely on both qualitative and quantitative approaches, called mixed- or multiple methods. Mixed methods involve integrating the qualitative and quantitative approaches to generate a more informative meta-inference than single-method approaches [23]. Integration can occur during study implementation, such as using one approach to inform sampling decisions about the other approach or at the analysis stage [23]. There are also instances when evaluators may want to use qualitative and quantitative approaches without taking the additional integration step, an approach referred to as multiple methods [24]. For more detail regarding mixed- and multiple-methods, see Teddlie and Tashakori (2009), and Fetters (2020) [23, 25].

The evaluation context, which includes the broader environment of the evaluation and the immediate circumstances in which the evaluation is to be conducted, also influences methodological, data collection, and analytic choices [4, 8, 18]. For example, some programmes may routinely collect and aggregate information or data about their programme, and thus, relevant parties and evaluators may choose to start the evaluation process using existing data [4]. Another consideration involves considering the accessibility of participants—it may be relatively easy to schedule interviews with key programme relevant parties (e.g. programme director, SP educators) while scheduling interviews or focus groups with faculty or SPs, who often have diverse schedules or work in different locations, might be more challenging. Here, evaluators might consider employing a survey to ensure their perspectives are included. Evaluation expertise is another consideration. If this is the first time a team is conducting an evaluation, or if there are gaps in the team's expertise (e.g. methodological, analytic approaches), it may be best to table some components of the evaluation until another team member with that expertise can join the project [18].

Disseminating Findings

Dissemination involves making the information learned during a PE available and usable to various audiences, including knowledge users, the broader organisation where the evaluation was conducted, and external entities (e.g. professional organisations and funding agencies). Depending on the purpose of the PE, interim reporting of findings to selected knowledge users may also be considered. Our focus here is on the end of PE dissemination. Dissemination is a way to communicate the findings, make recommendations to practise policy, clarify what the programme does and the issues or problems it addresses, clarify the resources needed, and ultimately help promote change in programmes, policies, and practices [26].

Dissemination can take many formats (e.g. verbal, written, visual), such as formal reports, memos, executive summaries, brochures, newsletters, and websites [26, 27]. Channels or mediums in which information is sent to its intended audience may include local meetings and conferences, professional conferences, and professional and peer-reviewed literature [26, 27].

When considering a dissemination strategy, appraise *who the audience is and what information they might need or desire* [27]. For example, professional simulation staff who work for the evaluated programme may want a detailed report of the evaluation findings and recommendations because it directly impacts their roles in the organisation. Staff meetings, workshops, or retreats may be ideal for professional SP employees to ask questions, consider what recommendations to start with, and reflect on the impact changes may have when being implemented. It is also important to think through interpersonal and other challenges if PE reveals underperformance of individuals or at the programme level.

Conversely, senior leadership may prefer an executive summary outlining key findings and recommendations or a brief oral presentation. If presenting the evaluation at a professional conference, attendees may be interested in the evaluation *methods, findings, and any lessons learned* or *what kinds of challenges or tensions were encountered* so that they might consider them when pursuing an evaluation in their organisation. Ideally, much of this information is identified during the planning process of the evaluation; however, it is still a good idea to double-check with relevant parties to determine if there are changes.

Examples of PE in Older Adult SP Programmes

In this section, we share published examples of PE in SP methodology (Table 7.2); however, it is notable that there are very few published examples of older adult SP programmes. This may be because PE is not conducted as research, making it harder to publish in conventional sources. They may also not have human research ethics approval to publish beyond the reading of relevant parties. On looking at broader SP programme evaluations, SPs were rarely reported as having a role in the evaluation. Depending on the purpose of the evaluation, it is hard to understand why SPs would be excluded.

One exception is by Smith et al. (2021), who report on older adult SPs' experiences of a change to their SP programme implemented during COVID-19 [28]. While the article is presented as research, it is an evaluation of an innovation in their older adult SP programme. The authors used focus groups to gather data in their exploratory change investigation. They used thematic analysis to analyse and report their findings. The article content would inform a larger-scale evaluation of their SP programme.

In another example, Fisher and Walker (2013) see a commonly used approach to evaluation [29]. The authors sought to evaluate the effect of a newly designed simulation-based intervention on the participants' knowledge and their attitudes towards geriatric medicine [29]. The authors also sought feedback on the learners' experiences of the simulation-based intervention. The PE included three testing points, pre-, immediately post-, and again 1 month later. The authors then compared the test scores with a group of learners who received 'usual' teaching in geriatric medicine. While the authors do not explicitly express a specific evaluation purpose, Fisher and Walker (2014) include goals and foci that are consistent with impact evaluations (Table 7.1) because they examine whether the desired outcomes for the programme were affected (e.g. participant knowledge) [29].

Braude et al. (2015) evaluated a short multimodality two-site simulation-based programme designed for medical and nursing staff working in elderly care [30]. The paper's framing suggests that the evaluation examined simulation as an acceptable method for learners to address deficits in specific aspects of elderly care and that the programme was effective. Data were only collected from learners and included pre- and postprogramme 'validated semistructured questionnaires' that requested self-report of confidence in managing a diverse range of clinical scenarios involving older adults and participants' experiences of the simulation-based programme. The questionnaires were not included in the reporting, so only an interpretation of the format can be inferred. It is unclear in what context the 'validation' occurred. Statistical tests were used to determine the change in confidence, and thematic analysis was used for the free text comments. Few recommendations were made concerning improving the programme. While the authors acknowledge some limitations in the design of their evaluation, they somewhat boldly recommend national adoption of such programmes.

Moving away from older adult SP programmes, the fourth example is from Yilmaz et al. (2022) [31]. The authors used data that had already been collected on the 'quality of SPs', their role portrayal, and the scenario. This is data that had been collected systematically over many years. The forms were used regularly to provide development opportunities for SPs. Cumulatively, this data is a valuable indicator of local practices, at least as perceived by instructors and SP trainers. Again, the study did not include SPs' perspectives, but the findings may be used to create standardised forms for data collection for future evaluations. The authors positioned their work in a broader framework using a logic model for PE to develop a quality management culture in SP programmes. The logic model was not embedded in the main focus of their reported data, but it demonstrates how their focused evaluation informs a more extensive PE of their programme.

The final example is also of an SP programme, not specifically for older adults. Vordenberg et al. (2018) used an approach familiar to many clinicians involved in clinical quality improvement activities (Plan-Do-Study-Act) [32]. The authors offered several examples of implementing the PDSA cycle. The authors report multiple data sources that were collected over time. SPs were included from the outset, which appeared to be a feature of the approach. Like Yilmaz et al. [31], the authors wanted to promote a quality improvement culture for their SP programme.

These examples demonstrate diverse ways these programmes tailored their evaluations by including specific knowledge users and using different PE purposes, methods, and data sources, which helped them determine the value of their SP programmes.

Table 7.2 Examples of PE in SP methodology

	Author/s	Evaluation goal/s	Description of approach
1.	Smith et al. (2021) [28]	To evaluate SPs' perspectives on the effectiveness of weekly virtual 1-h meetings during COVID-19 and the impact of the shift from in-person to virtual meetings on their well-being and SP skill development.	SPs were invited to participate in a focus group (~45–60 min). Focus group questions and probes 1. Do you feel that social distancing during COVID-19 has affected you? (a) In what way(s)? (b) Please share some examples. 2. Concerning social distancing, how do you feel about our weekly SAGE ZOOM get-togethers? (a) Do they add value? (b) Do they have an effect on your mental health/well-being/social connectedness? 3. How do you feel about the following components of the weekly sessions? (a) Mindfulness activities? (b) Weekly assignments? (c) Social conversation? 4. Have you taken anything from this that you can use as an SP? 5. Is there anything else you would like to share?
2.	Fisher and Walker (2013) [29]	To evaluate the effect of a newly designed simulation-based intervention on students' knowledge and their attitudes toward geriatric medicine.	Three points of testing, pre-, immediately post-, and again 1 month later.
		To obtain feedback on students' experiences of the simulation-based intervention.	The knowledge test comprised free text comments on falls, delirium, and elder abuse. Each question/prompt was closely aligned with the simulation activities: 1. You are the F1 (Year 1 doctor) on call. You have been called to the ward to see an elderly gentleman who has fallen over. Please list as many things as possible that you would do, look for, consider, and document in the medical notes as part of your assessment of this patient. 2. You are the F1 on call. You are bleeped to the ward at 2 am to review an elderly lady who is distressed, agitated, and hallucinating. You review her notes. She has been diagnosed with delirium. She has a proven UTI and is on appropriate antibiotics. What steps might you take to manage this patient? 3. Please list five different forms of elder abuse. Describe what steps you would take, or consider taking, if you were clerking in an elderly patient who you suspected was being abused. Students were asked to rate their level of agreement (Strongly Agree, Agree, Neither Agree nor Disagree, Disagree, Strongly Disagree) with 11 statements. 1. The teaching today was of a high standard. 2. The day was well organised. 3. The acting by the role-players was of a high standard. 4. Simulation activities provided valuable learning opportunities. 5. The cases were realistic. 6. The day was enjoyable. 7. The day has had a positive impact on how I think about geriatric medicine. 8. After the session, I feel better equipped to deal with a delirious patient. 9. After the session, I feel better equipped to deal with a patient who has fallen. 10. After the session, I feel better equipped to deal with a patient who I suspect may be subject to abuse. 11. After the session, I feel better equipped to deal with breaking bad news to a patient

	Author/s	Evaluation goal/s	Description of approach
3.	Braude et al. (2015) [30]	To evaluate a multi-modality simulation-based course for "medical and nursing staff working in elderly care."	Participants were asked to complete a semi-structured questionnaire about their learning and experience of specific skills (not supplied).
		The aims of the course were "to facilitate experiential learning of both technical and non-technical abilities with a focus on human factor skills, interprofessional geriatric medicine and challenging aspects of geriatric care such as elder abuse, continence, and end-of-life care."	Participants also completed pre- and post-course questionnaires to rate their confidence (on a scale from 0% to 100%) in managing geriatric clinical scenarios (e.g. entering new clinical situations, leadership, emergency management, continence management, multi-disciplinary meetings, communication, managing agitated patients, end-of-life decisions, end-of-life communication, deploying 'non-technical' skills.
4	Yılmaz et al. (2022) [31]	To determine programmatic and systematic issues in the scope of quality assurance and improvement through trainer and instructor feedback on SP performance.	Analysis of instructors' and SP trainers' ratings of the *quality of the SP* [Feedback given by SP; Professionalism (e.g. preparedness and punctuality)], *SP portrayal* [Knowledge of case information, appropriate responses, affect (e.g. experience and consistency)] and *quality of scenario* [Adequacy of case details; suitability and use of equipment). Retrospectively collected data (over 6 years) was included. The numerical data were summarised descriptively, and content analysis was conducted on free text.
5	Vordenberg et al. (2018) [32]	To describe the use of a continuous quality improvement process for strengthening the SP program and the initial steps that have been implemented.	Example 1:
			Plan: Informally identified opportunities for improvement in the SP programme.
			Do: Organized SP faculty workgroup—collaboration of five faculty with experience working with SPs.
			Study: Faculty successfully identified opportunities for improvement, tested and refined ideas
			Act: Continue to have faculty workgroup but the composition of members will change based on teaching responsibilities; composed manuscript about the process.
			Example 2:
			Plan: New or established faculty with a new teaching assignment must prepare to work with SPs.
			Do: Developed faculty and graduate student instructor handbook—created checklist of crucial steps, including requesting SPs, logistics, the content of cases, and debriefing with students and SPs.
			Study: Handbook developed and need identified for easily accessible and living document.
			Act: Exploring page on the internal College of Pharmacy website to house information, continuing to develop plans for maintaining content.

Considerations When Collaborating with Older SPs

We have already shared that SPs have had minimal involvement in published evaluations of SP programmes. While the purpose of PE will always be the decisive influence, we propose that SPs should be included in PE until there is a reason to exclude them. There may be good reasons to exclude older adult SPs, but our default position is that they be included.

The following considerations may have relevance for older adult SPs but should be considered for any SP. Sociocultural and economic factors may influence the power distance (real or perceived) between SPs, other relevant parties, and the evaluator(s). It is important to emphasise to older SPs the value of their input to evaluation by verbally stating so and creating time within a session (or at some other designated time) to participate in evaluation activities. Older SPs may fear that criticism of the programme could result in less or no work for them or cause trouble for programme staff. Privacy, anonymity, and confidentiality may all be important in gaining genuine feedback from SPs.

Making varied formats available for older adult SPs to participate in evaluation—paper and pencil forms, digital forms, individual interviews, group interviews, and focus groups—may all increase participation. Informal data collection can also occur during individual or group discussions after sessions. Considerations such as larger font size, providing written questions in advance of interviews and focus groups, physical positioning of chairs to facilitate communication, and minimising background noise may also assist older adult participation. It is essential to collect and feed this data into the evaluation cycle systematically.

Closing

Throughout this chapter, we have addressed what a PE is and who does it and introduced essential concepts, such as how to approach an evaluation's design, implementation, reporting, and dissemination. We have also reported how PE in health professions' education has sometimes evolved without reference to the professional work of programme evaluators. It is important to remember that PE is ideally viewed as an area of specialised practice and ideally warrants a methodical approach and the willingness to develop or recruit individuals with the experience and expertise to do evaluation well. We have shared examples of published PEs related to simulation programmes and noted the exclusion of SPs from PE. We strongly encourage exploring and utilising the resources below for developing PE skills.

Disclaimer The views expressed in this chapter do not necessarily reflect the official policy or position of the Uniformed Services University of the Health Sciences, the Department of Defense, the Henry M. Jackson Foundation, or the US Government.

Resources

There are many excellent resources on PE linked with public health. Explore this site from the Center for Disease Control and Prevention for guidance. https://www.cdc.gov/evaluation/index.htm [Accessed July 30, 2023]

Competencies for evaluators. https://www.eval.org/About/Competencies-Standards/AEA-Evaluator-Competencies [Accessed July 30, 2023]

The many different types of evaluation. https://www.eval.org/Policy-Advocacy/Evaluation-Policy-Initiative/Practices-and-Methodology [Accessed July 30, 2023]

Ethical practices for educational programs. https://education.nsw.gov.au/teaching-and-learning/professional-learning/pl-resources/evaluation-resource-hub/evaluation-design-and-planning/ethical-conduct-in-evaluation [Accessed July 30, 2023]

Association of Standardized Patient Educators (ASPE) Standards of Best Practice (SOBP). https://advancesinsimulation.biomedcentral.com/articles/10.1186/s41077-017-0043-4 [Accessed July 30, 2023]

Healthcare Simulation Standards of Best Practice. https://www.nursingsimulation.org/article/S1876-1399(21)00093-1/fulltext [Accessed July 30, 2023]

Accreditation requirements for simulation programs. https://www.ssih.org/Credentialing/Accreditation [Accessed July 30, 2023]

https://www.sesam-web.org/accreditation/ [Accessed July 30, 2023]

https://www.facs.org/for-medical-professionals/education/programs/accredited-education-institutes/accreditation-standards-and-criteria/ [Accessed July 30, 2023]

Association for Medical Education in Europe (AMEE) ASPIRE Award for Simulation. https://www.amee.org/news/aspire-to-excellence-award#Simulation [Accessed July 30, 2023]

Additionally, you may find valuable resources from the websites of professional organizations that provide access to guidelines, standards, a code of ethics, and other helpful materials for conducting PE.

American Evaluation Association (AEA) https://www.eval.org/, [Accessed July 30, 2023]

European Evaluation Society (EES) https://europeanevaluation.org/ [Accessed July 30, 2023]

Australasian Evaluation Society (AES) https://www.aes.asn.au/ [Accessed July 30, 2023]

References

1. Smith CM, Sokoloff LG, Alsaba N. Collaborative framework for working with older simulated participants (SP). BMJ Simul Technol Enhanc Learn. 2021;7(2):112.

2. Gamble A, Nestel D, Bearman M. Children and young people as simulated patients: recommendations for safe engagement. Int J Healthc Simul. 2022; https://doi.org/10.54531/erqf8206.
3. Richardson H, Goldsamt LA, Simmons J, Gilmartin M, Jeffries PR. Increasing faculty capacity: findings from an evaluation of simulation clinical teaching. Nurs Educ Perspect. 2014;35(5):308–14.
4. Rossi PH, Lipsey MW, Henry GT. Evaluation: a systematic approach. 8th ed. Thousand Oaks: Sage; 2019.
5. Lovato C, Wall D. Programme evaluation: improving practice, influencing policy and decision-making. In: Swanwick T, editor. Understanding medical education: theory and practice. 2nd ed. Hoboken: Wiley; 2014.
6. Ingersoll GL, Sauter M. Integrating accreditation criteria into educational program evaluation. Nurs Health Care Perspect. 1998;19(5):224–30.
7. Clark L, Woll A, Owens TL, Shropshire D, Kiser B, Gephardt G, Park CS. SP safety, autonomy and healthcare simulation practice in the COVID-19 era. BMJ Simul Technol Enhanc Learn. 2021;7(5):450–1.
8. Newcomer KE, Hatry HP, Wholey JS, editors. Handbook of practical program evaluation. 4th ed. San Francisco: Jossey-Bass & Pfeiffer Imprints, Wiley; 2015.
9. Ryan K, Greene J, Lincoln Y, Mathison S, Mertens DM, Ryan K. Advantages and challenges of using inclusive evaluation approaches in evaluation practice. Am J Eval. 1998;19(1):101–22.
10. Onyura B. Useful to whom? Evaluation utilisation theory and boundaries for programme evaluation scope. Med Educ. 2020;54(12):1100–8.
11. Griffiths S, Weston L, Morgan-Trimmer S, Wheat H, Gude A, Manger L, Oh TM, Clarkson P, Quinn C, Sheaff R, Clark M. Engaging stakeholders in realist programme theory building: insights from the prospective phase of a primary care dementia support study. Int J Qual Methods. 2022;21:16094069221077521.
12. Kaba A, Cronin T, Tavares W, Horsley T, Dube M, Grant VJ. Improving team effectiveness using a program evaluation logic model: case study of the largest provincial simulation program in Canada. Int J Healthc Simul. 2022; https://doi.org/10.54531/fqzq4032.
13. Cleghorn CD, Headrick LA. The PDSA cycle at the core of learning in health professions education. Jt Comm J Qual Improv. 1996;22(3):206–12.
14. Blanchard RD, Torbeck L, Blondeau W. AM last page: a snapshot of three common program evaluation approaches for medical education. Acad Med. 2013;88(1):146.
15. Kirkpatrick JD, Kirkpatrick WK. Kirkpatrick's four levels of training evaluation. Alexandria: ATD Press; 2016.
16. Yardley S, Dornan T. Kirkpatrick's levels and education 'evidence'. Med Educ. 2012;46(1):97–106.
17. Allen LM, Hay M, Palermo C. Evaluation in health professions education—is measuring outcomes enough? Med Educ. 2022;56(1):127–36.
18. Robson C. Small-scale evaluation. Thousand Oaks: Sage; 2017.
19. Lewis KL, Bohnert CA, Gammon WL, Hölzer H, Lyman L, Smith C, Thompson TM, Wallace A, Gliva-McConvey G. The association of standardized patient educators (ASPE) standards of best practice (SOBP). Adv Simul. 2017;2(1):1–8.
20. Yarbrough DB, Shulha LM, Hopson RK, Caruthers FA. The program evaluation standards: a guide for evaluators and evaluation users. Thousand Oaks: Sage; 2010.
21. Genereaux M, Nguyen M, Bostwick JR, Vordenberg SE. Using the higher learning commission's assessment culture matrix to support continuous quality improvement of a simulated patient program. Innov Pharm. 2021;12(2) https://doi.org/10.24926/iip.v12i2.3684.
22. Balmer DF, Riddle JM, Simpson D. Program evaluation: getting started and standards. J Grad Med Educ. 2020;12(3):345–6.
23. Teddlie C, Tashakkori A. Foundations of mixed methods research: integrating quantitative and qualitative approaches in the social and behavioral sciences. Thousand Oaks: Sage; 2009.
24. Anguera MT, Blanco-Villaseñor A, Losada JL, Sánchez-Algarra P, Onwuegbuzie AJ. Revisiting the difference between mixed methods and multimethods: is it all in the name? Qual Quant. 2018;52:2757–70.
25. Fetters MD. The mixed methods research workbook: activities for designing, implementing, and publishing projects. Thousand Oaks: Sage; 2019.
26. Mueller NB, Burke RC, Luke DA, Harris JK. Getting the word out: multiple methods for disseminating evaluation findings. J Public Health Manag Pract. 2008;14(2):170–6.
27. Centers for Disease Control and Prevention. Disseminating program achievements and evaluation findings to garner support. Evaluation Briefs. 2009;9.
28. Smith CM, Sokoloff LG, Gallucci CE. 'It's like a shot in the arm': evaluating the experiences of older simulated participants in structured virtual meetings during COVID-19. Int J Healthc Simul. 2021;1(1):33–40.
29. Fisher JM, Walker RW. A new age approach to an age old problem: using simulation to teach geriatric medicine to medical students. Age Ageing. 2014;43(3):424–8.
30. Braude P, Reedy G, Dasgupta D, Dimmock V, Jaye P, Birns J. Evaluation of a simulation training program for geriatric medicine. Age Ageing. 2015;44(4):677–82.
31. Yılmaz DU, Last N, Harvey J, Norman L, Monteiro S, Sibbald M. Quality in standardized patient training and delivery: retrospective documentary analysis of trainer and instructor feedback. Cureus. 2022;14(1):e21022.
32. Vordenberg SE, Smith MA, Diez HL, Remington TL, Bostwick JR. Using the plan-do-study-act (PDSA) model for continuous quality improvement of an established simulated patient program. Innov Pharm. 2018;9(2):1.

Research Opportunities and Knowledge Translation: Saying "Yes" to Simulation Research for the Care of Older Adults

8

Eve Purdy, Savannah Forrester, and Victoria Brazil

Key Messages

1. It is perfectly acceptable to say "no" to doing research but sometimes saying "yes" is extremely rewarding.
2. Research needs to fill a critical gap; identifying that gap is the most important step in the process.
3. We must respect the complexity of (1) the care of older adults and (2) simulation in the questions we ask and studies we design.
4. Find a diverse team who can help with the design and conduct of high-quality research.
5. All simulation practitioners do not need to be researchers, but we all need to be scholarly in our approach to practice.

Introduction

Greater use of simulation for the care of older adults has been paralleled by an upsurge in related research publications, as demonstrated in Fig. 8.1. The purpose of this chapter is not to comprehensively summarise this diverse and growing field. Rather, it is to explore key principles related to embarking on research. Using a series of hypothetical vignettes about a fictional doctor, Dr. Jasmine Rai, we offer a framework for scholarly contributions in simulation for the care of older adults. Drawing on existing literature, we will explore when to say "no" to research and what to consider when saying "yes". Specifically, whether to position your study as (1) research *about* simulation for the care of older adults or (2) clinical or health service research about care of older adults *using* simulation as a tool or test bed. Throughout the chapter, we will highlight opportunities related to topics, methods, and partners for both approaches.

Vignette Part 1: Jasmine and Jonathan

Dr. Jasmine Rai is an emergency physician and simulation facilitator working in a tertiary care centre, Great Pines Hospital. She is the emergency department (ED) lead for simulation. In this role, she is involved in both quality improvement and education. Currently, the department has prioritised advancing care for older adults—Including improvements to clinical services and older adult emergency medicine education. The care of older adults ED lead, Dr. Jonathan Webber, sees Jasmine in the tearoom one afternoon and casually asks whether they might be able to collaborate on some research using simulation.

- If you were Jasmine, what questions would you have?
- What are the opportunities? What are the risks?
- How would you respond?

E. Purdy (✉)
Faculty of Health Sciences and Medicine, Bond University, Robina, QLD, Australia

Emergency Department, Gold Coast Hospital and Health Service, Gold Coast, QLD, Australia
e-mail: eve.purdy@health.qld.gov.au

S. Forrester
Department of Emergency Medicine, University of British Columbia, Victoria, BC, Canada

V. Brazil
Faculty of Health Sciences and Medicine, Bond University, Robina, QLD, Australia

Simulation Service, Gold Coast Hospital and Health Service, Gold Coast, QLD, Australia
e-mail: vbrazil@bond.edu.au

C. M. Smith et al. (eds.), *Comprehensive Healthcare Simulation: Geriatric Simulation*, Comprehensive Healthcare Simulation,
https://doi.org/10.1007/978-3-031-65742-9_8

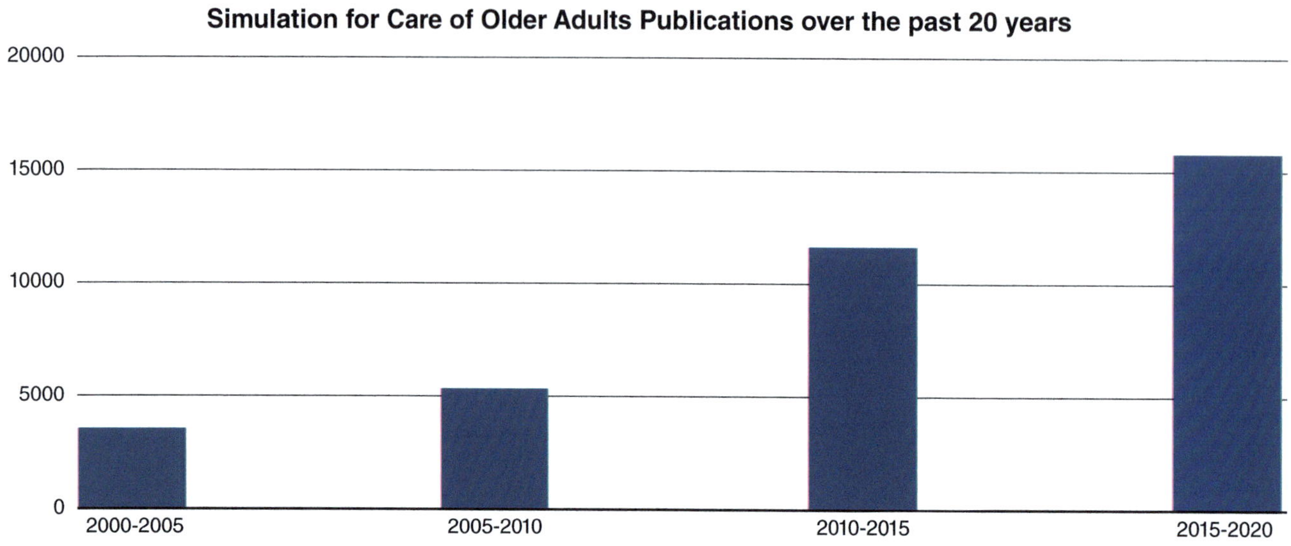

Fig. 8.1 "Geriatrics AND Simulation" in Google scholar in 5 years intervals

Saying "No" to Research

The conversation between Jasmine and Jonathan is a common one. Well-intentioned educators often have a desire to integrate simulation into their curricula but can inappropriately link that desire with the need to produce research outputs. Delivering simulation and researching simulation are different endeavours that should not be conflated. The desire to link the two are multifactorial (and largely beyond the scope of this chapter) but may be related to funding models which disproportionately reward research in the form of grants and university promotion structures [1]. Awareness and mitigation of the inherent desire to publish are necessary to avoid becoming involved in projects that are not worth the time and energy, while providing limited contribution to the field. It is entirely acceptable to conduct good simulation without researching it.

The literature is saturated with descriptions of simulation events and programmes related to the care of older adults that are analysed using limited presurvey/postsurvey designs. More studies along these lines, while attractively simple to conduct, are unlikely to meaningfully advance the understanding of either simulation or the care of older adults. Given the maturing nature of the field, research contributions need to go beyond "we did this" and "learners liked it". Research that uses simulation as a tool, or that is about simulation design, must be directly linked to relevant questions that address well-appraised gaps. The identification of specific research questions is the most important rate-limiting step in getting research off the ground. Challenges that arise related to meaningful question identification are an appropriate reason to say "no" to participating in research.

Conducting high-quality research takes time, effort, energy, commitment, and skill—above what it takes to coordinate the simulation programme itself. Just because Jasmine is an excellent simulation facilitator does not mean that she will succeed at, or enjoy, being, a simulation researcher. The required capabilities overlap but also necessitate unique strengths (Fig. 8.2). Issues related to these practical considerations are another excellent reason to say "no" to research.

Vignette Part 2A: Saying "No" to Research

Jasmine and Jonathan meet to discuss a potential collaboration. Jonathan outlines that he is interested in repurposing one of the preexisting weekly simulation sessions to focus on emergency medicine for older adults. He thinks this aligns well with the department's goals to improve care of older adults. He suggests that studying the impact would be "pretty easy"—They can do surveys before and after the session comparing confidence in caring for older patients and measure learners' thoughts about simulation as a modality. He has a few ideas for cases that he has put into the standard simulation templates and is excited to get going.

Jasmine listens carefully. She is keen on the idea of simulations for care of older adults and thinks that the programme would fit well into the already existing schedule. In fact, they would be able to start next month. She is happy to mentor Jonathan through this process and could cofacilitate with him. However, she

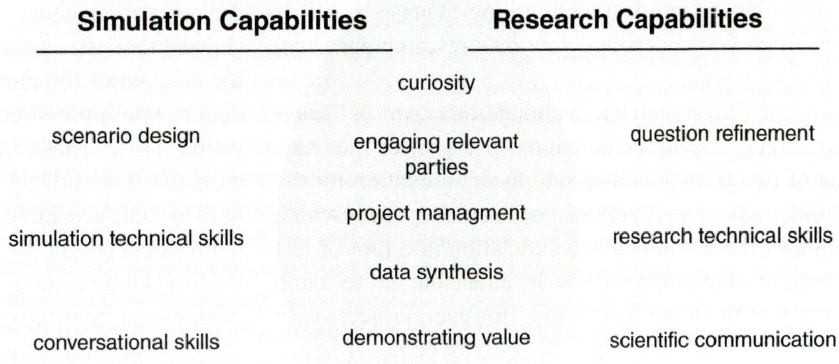

Fig. 8.2 Capabilities necessary for simulation and research

is sceptical of the research component he describes. The question is unclear and does not fill any significant gaps in the field. Furthermore, she already has two research projects ongoing and does not feel that she will have the time to commit to a third. She offers to help him design the monthly ED simulation programme for care of older adults, including a local evaluation process, but declines to be involved in research of the programme. She introduces him to some nonresearch outputs like blog posts and simulation case sharing databases that may be suitable for sharing some of their work.

- What enables you to, or prevents you, from saying "no" in similar situations?
- How do you decide what projects to take on?
- What is your current capability and bandwidth for research?

Saying "Yes" to Research

Though saying "no" to research is often the right choice; saying "yes" can be extremely rewarding too. There are special moments—like the one below between Jasmine and Jonathan—when the intersection of passion, skill, and opportunity can lead to something incredible. The chance to generate new knowledge and shape future practice can be invigorating.

Vignette Part 2B: Saying "Yes" to Research

Jasmine and Jonathan meet to discuss a potential collaboration.... [a different conversation takes place]

Jasmine listens carefully. Jonathan seems to be very enthusiastic and has several ideas about using simulation. It seems that he is interested in using it as a tool to research specific ED processes related to care of the older adult and he also has ideas about how to employ it for education. The research questions are not quite clear yet, but she thinks there is potential for meaningful work. She has just finished her masters and is keen to apply her research skills. She thinks this presents the perfect opportunity—It is a departmental priority and Jonathan mentioned that it may come with some additional funding for research support. She tells Jonathan that she will think about potential avenues for research based on what he has described and will spend some time thinking about approaches. They plan to meet up in a week's time to discuss further.

An important next step when saying "yes" to research is reflecting on your research paradigm. Research paradigms are scaffolded by understanding of reality (ontology), thoughts about how knowledge is created (epistemology), and decisions about how to explore reality and knowledge (methodology) [2]. The paradigm you are operating in impacts the research questions you are likely to ask and the way you will choose to answer them.

Table 8.1 outlines three common research paradigms. The paradigm then drives critical decisions throughout the research process: creating questions and objectives, choosing methods, analysing data, and writing manuscripts. It is imperative that you understand your own research paradigm and that of your team.

Saying "yes" to research as a simulation expert or "*simulationist*" likely means participating in a project that falls into one of two areas: (1) research *about* simulation for the care of older adults or (2) clinical or health service research about care of older adults *using* simulation as a tool or test bed. Each of these approaches is amenable to research through any of the three paradigms. However, projects with pragmatic or constructivist approaches may be better suited to exploring the complexity that is common to both care of older adults and learning through simulation. Context is increasingly recognised as critical to the success of quality improvement and educational interventions [14, 15]. Movement away from a positivist research paradigm may be uncomfortable given that those in the healthcare field are often predisposed and enculturated to this worldview. Reflecting on and shifting paradigms, when appropriate, can be a powerful first step at the beginning of your research journey.

When conducting research about simulation for the care of older adults, it is also important to think about who else might join your team or act as advisors. The answer to this question will depend on the nature of the questions and methodologies chosen, but natural collaborators may include education researchers, social scientists, consumers, or patient advocates older simulated participants are perfectly positioned to engage with as research partners because they likely have relevant consumer experience and also significant insight into the world of simulation. Looking for support beyond traditional medical research circles may be especially helpful when operating outside of the positivist paradigm.

Researching Simulation for Care of Older Adults: Understanding What Works, in What Context, and Why

Many studies, usually with a positivist research paradigm, have been conducted and show that simulation "works" as an educational intervention. Recent systematic and scoping reviews highlight that simulation results in enhanced clinical geriatric knowledge, improved interpersonal skills, increased confidence, and high degrees of satisfaction for learners [16, 17]. Most studies in these reviews are quasiexperimental and include prepost surveys, have short periods of time from intervention to measurement of impact, and vary in the inclusion of meaningful comparator groups. As examples, Fisher and Walker demonstrated that medical students who participate in simulations for care of older adults have better knowledge and more positive perceptions compared to those who did not participate in the simulation [18]; and Bradway et al. showed that after an interprofessional simulation workshop for the care of the older adult, participants felt more confident in interprofessional communication immediately afterwards [19]. These results, and many others, are not particularly surprising. Though helpful for legitimising the field in some academic circles, they are not much more informative than gestalt. We are left wanting more. This want has led to a call by certain researchers for better designed, larger, randomised controlled trials to provide more quantitative "proof" that simulation works [16]. We argue that this positivist focus on proof is the wrong future direction for most research in simulation of care of older adults.

More interesting and helpful questions are related to what works but extending to consider for what objectives, for who, in what context, and why. Realist evaluation is an example of a structured framework to approach such questions [20]. For example, were the simulations run by Fisher and Walker more effective than less costly workshops on the same topic or more effective than convenient asynchronous learning tools? Or how does the interprofessional session from Bradway et al. fit into broader learning and experiences related to interprofessionalism within the participants' contexts? These questions do not focus on proving that simulation "works" rather they allow for a deeper exploration of important contextual factors that affect impact.

We can learn from some research groups who are approaching research in a way that incorporates and acknowledges complexity. For example, Braude et al., seemingly operating from a pragmatic research paradigm, first used quantitative measures to see if their simulation programme was associated with learning and then applied qualitative methods to explore what specifically led to that learning [12]. They demonstrated that learning occurred and that the learning was likely due to the extensive curriculum mapping phase of their design process. Participants felt that the simulation programme covered gaps not addressed by teaching elsewhere in the programme. This is helpful because the initial temptation would be to take the Braude et al.'s simulation programme and apply it just as it is described at other sites. But instead, their nuanced exploration of what worked showed that the local curriculum mapping process was the key component of success. Curriculum mapping allowed simulation design to meet the needs of the local educational context and lead to the positive learning outcomes. Because of the research approach chosen, readers can learn to apply the process that led to success (curriculum mapping), instead of simply using the final product (the simulation exercise)—which in a different context may not be as effective. This example reflects the type of useful knowledge that can be

Table 8.1 The three common research paradigms with examples from the simulation for the care of older adults literature

Paradigm	Ontology	Epistemology	Methodology	Methods	Examples from the simulation for care of older adults literature
Positivism	There is a single reality	Reality can be directly measured. The goal should be to do so precisely and reliably	Experimental research	Usually quantitative:	Wen A, Wong L, Ma C, Arndt R, Katz AR, Richardson K, et al. An interprofessional team simulation exercise about a complex geriatric patient. Gerontology Geriatrics Educ. 2019;40(1):16–29. [3]
			Surveys	– Sampling	Torkshavand G, Khatiban M, Soltanian AR. Simulation-based learning to enhance students' knowledge and skills in educating older patients. Nurse Educ Pract. 2020;42:102678. [4]
				– Surveys	Gellis ZD, Kim E, Hadley D, Packel L, Poon C, Forciea MA, et al. Evaluation of interprofessional health care team communication simulation in geriatric palliative care. Gerontology Geriatrics Educ. 2019;40(1):30–42. [5]
				– Statistical analyses	Chen AMH, Kiersma ME, Yehle KS, Plake KS. Impact of the Geriatric Medication Game® on nursing students' empathy and attitudes toward older adults. Nurs Educ Today. 2015;35(1):38–43. [6]
					Fernández-Gutiérrez M, Bas-Sarmiento P, Pino-Chinchilla H del, Poza-Méndez M, Marín-Paz AJ. Effectiveness of a multimodal intervention and the simulation flow to improve empathy and attitudes towards older adults in nursing students: A crossover randomised controlled trial. Nurse Educ Pract. 2022;64:103430. [7]
					Arrogante O, Velarde-García JF, Blázquez-González P, Moro-Tejedor MN. The effects of high-fidelity simulation training on empathy and attitudes toward older people among undergraduate nursing students: A quasi-experimental study. Nurse Educ Pract. 2022;64:103441. [8]
Constructivism/ interpretivism	There is not a single, measurable, reality—rather, reality is constructed by individuals and groups	Reality is interpreted. It is discovered through people and context	Ethnography	Usually qualitative:	Lunde L, Moen A, Jakobsen RB, Møller B, Rosvold EO, Brænd AM. A preliminary simulation-based qualitative study of healthcare students' experiences of interprofessional primary care scenarios. Adv Simul. 2022;7(1):9. [9]
			Grounded theory	– Interviews	Perot JG, Jarzebowski W, Lafuente-Lafuente C, Crozet C, Belmin J. Aging-simulation experience: impact on health professionals' social representations. Bmc Geriatr. 2020;20(1):14. [10]
			Phenomenological	– Participant observation	Lee DA, Maxwell CA, Miller S. "This Is Me!" Perceptions of Older Adult Simulated Participants in an Aging and Injury Simulation Experience. J Trauma Nurs. 2021;28(1):10–20. [11]
			Action research	– Case studies	
				– Document review	
				– Thematic analysis	
Pragmatism	Truth is constantly negotiated. There may be an objective truth that exists beyond human experience, but human experience cannot be separated from reality	Reality may be measured and shaped through people and context	Mixed-methods	Combination of the above depending on the question—also more likely to include usability testing, rapid cycle testing, prototyping	Braude P, Reedy G, Dasgupta D, Dimmock V, Jaye P, Birns J. Evaluation of a simulation training programme for geriatric medicine. Age Ageing. 2015;44(4):677–82. [12]
			Action research User-based design		Weldon SM, Kneebone R, Bello F. Collaborative healthcare remodelling through sequential simulation: a patient and front-line staff perspective. Bmj Simul Technology Enhanc Learn. 2016;2(3):78. [13]

There are other research paradigms such as post-positivism, critical, subjectivism, post-structuralist, and feminist

Table 8.2 Examples of possible directions for future research at different phases of the simulation

Phase of simulation	Possible directions for future research
Preparation/program development	– Understanding barriers to implementing programmatic approaches to translational simulation for care of older adults
	– Needs analysis for faculty development specifically for simulation for care of older adults
Design	– Approaches to and impacts of partnering with consumers in design process
	– Impacts of learner designed simulations
	– Risks/benefits of disability simulations
	– Equity, diversity, inclusion in simulation design
Delivery	– Virtual reality as a simulation delivery tool
	– Impacts of the use of masks and moulage
	– Simulated participant faculty development
Debriefing	– Impacts of incorporating consumers in debriefs
	– Approaches to incorporating equity, diversity, and inclusion in debriefing
Evaluation	– Demonstrating return on investment
	– Overcoming barriers to simulation (financial, time, faculty development)

uncovered using a pragmatic research and realist evaluation approach.

Curiosity about complex issues of simulation design, delivery, debriefing, and evaluation—when matched with methodologies that respect that complexity—will be most likely to meaningfully advance the field of simulation for care of the older adult. Table 8.2 provides examples of possible directions for future research at different phases of the simulation.

Vignette Part 3a: Undertaking Research About Simulation for Care of Older Adults

Jasmine and Jonathan meet a week later to further discuss ideas for a research project. Both have spent time looking through the literature, and there appears to be an opportunity to research how healthcare consumers and their families can shape the design, delivery, and debriefing of simulations for care for older adults. They are both very excited about this topic. They feel that an action research methodology that involves consumers and their families, participants, simulation faculty, and simulated patients will likely be the best approach. Specific methods may include surveys, focus groups, and interviews, but they recognise that they will need additional expertise to help mentor them through this unique approach. They decide to start a collaborative working document to formalise their current research questions and ideas up to this point.

- What are the next best steps for Jasmine and Jonathan?
- Who else do you think they should ask to join their team at this stage?
- At your institution, where would you go for guidance?

Simulation as a Testbed: Using Simulation as a Tool to Conduct Research About the Care of the Older Adults

Simulationists like Jasmine may also find themselves involved in research, not about simulation itself, but rather focused on clinical problems that use simulation as a tool in their investigative process. The simulated environment can be an efficient and convenient place to study real-world problems. Simulation can offer an opportunity to research a diverse array of questions related to policies, protocols, processes, and environments. It can also be used to explore healthcare provider and consumer perspectives.

The opportunity to research and test clinical approaches and environments through simulation is likely underutilised in the care of older adults. Translational simulation—simulation specifically designed to meet the needs of health services—is a field in its infancy [21, 22]. However, a few examples do exist. For example, computer-based simulations have been used to research interventions related to bed capacity and patient flow in acute care geriatric units [23]. Another team effectively demonstrated the use of simulation to develop and refine a clinician decision support system (CDSS) to improve pain management for older patients in the ED [24]. In this study, providers cared for patients in a simulated environment, which included the use of a simulated electronic health record, then answered questions about the usability and functionality of the CDSS. Through five iterations of usability testing and refinement, the usability of the tool improved significantly. Another group simulated primary care encounters, to research the acceptability and usability of remote presence robots [25]. As translational simulation becomes more common and supported both institutionally and financially, it will become a more widely accepted testbed for clinician researchers and quality improvement groups to engage with. Simulation experts may look for more diverse opportunities to collaborate with clinical research colleagues in this regard.

The simulated environment also offers the opportunity to learn more about provider and consumer perspectives. Simulation can concentrate experiences or encounters over a short time. As such, it can be an efficient and effective way to learn more about a given issue. For example, Fisher et al., using an interpretivist approach, conducted a series of simulation sessions specifically related to the identification of elder abuse [26]. Though conducted with medical students, the research was not about the medical students' learning outcomes specifically—rather it focused on understanding the barriers to identifying elder abuse. Using content analysis of field notes and a transcript of the debriefing, the research team was able to identify six themes that better inform the clinical community's understanding of the barriers that exist in the identification of elder abuse. These themes might inform future clinical and educational programmes. In another example, using sequential simulations, researchers engaged with a diverse array of practitioners and patients to explore perspectives about integrated care models spanning general practice, community health, and social care [13]. This research, seemingly conducted through a pragmatic research paradigm, generated practical knowledge about perspectives that contributed directly to healthcare remodeling in the local context. Simulation researchers can be excellent partners for those in health policy, quality improvement, or clinical care looking to better understand providers and the patients they care for.

Vignette Part 3b: Doing Clinical Research That Uses Simulation as a Tool

Jasmine and Jonathan meet a week later to further discuss ideas for a research project. Jonathan is part of a large national working group that is developing a new tool for the detection of delirium. The group is particularly interested in comparing the usability of the new tool to already existing tools and understanding if there are any refinements that would be helpful for delivery for the providers using it. Jonathan had mentioned simulation as a potential option for this step of the process. The working group was enthused by that prospect. Jasmine and Jonathan decide that this collaboration might be a great opportunity to link their two portfolios.

- What are the next best steps for jasmine and Jonathan?
- Who else do you think they should contact at this stage?
- Where would you go for guidance?

Alternatives to Research: Scholarship Related to Simulation for the Care of Older Adults

While research is easily recognisable as scholarship, there are other activities that meet the standards for scholarly activity (i.e. they have clear goals, adequate preparation, appropriate methods, significant results, effective presentation, and reflective critique) [27]. Boyer proposes that the scholarship of discovery (research) is joined by scholarship of integration, of application, or of teaching in meeting these standards [28]. In practice, this supports simulationists disseminating their work through more diverse methods, including digital platforms (e.g. Simulcast), resource repositories (e.g. EM Sim Cases), conference presentations, and evaluation reports [29, 30]. Social media based scholarship has emerged as a legitimate educational activity for health profession education, and criteria for quality in these contributions have been developed [31].

Conclusion

This chapter serves as a basic introduction to simulation facilitators interested in research but is certainly not a comprehensive guide. There are numerous issues essential to the research process that are not covered here including ethics, funding, and details of different approaches to methods and analysis. We encourage you to reach out to others with experience when deciding to embark on research through either of the lenses discussed in this chapter. An excellent further resource for those hoping to learn more is "Healthcare Simulation Research: A Practical Guide".

While we strongly believe that it is perfectly acceptable to say "no" to being involved in research, we also know that "saying yes" can be the beginning of an exciting and rewarding journey.

References

1. Schimanski LA, Alperin JP. The evaluation of scholarship in academic promotion and tenure processes: past, present, and future. F1000Res. 2018;7:1605.
2. Bunniss S, Kelly DR. Research paradigms in medical education research. Med Educ. 2010;44(4):358–66.
3. Wen A, Wong L, Ma C, Arndt R, Katz AR, Richardson K, et al. An interprofessional team simulation exercise about a complex geriatric patient. Gerontol Geriatr Educ. 2019;40(1):16–29.
4. Torkshavand G, Khatiban M, Soltanian AR. Simulation-based learning to enhance students' knowledge and skills in educating older patients. Nurse Educ Pract. 2020;42:102678.
5. Gellis ZD, Kim E, Hadley D, Packel L, Poon C, Forciea MA, et al. Evaluation of interprofessional health care team communication simulation in geriatric palliative care. Gerontology Geriatrics Educ. 2019;40(1):30–42.

6. Chen AMH, Kiersma ME, Yehle KS, Plake KS. Impact of the Geriatric Medication Game® on nursing students' empathy and attitudes toward older adults. Nurs Educ Today. 2015;35(1):38–43.
7. Fernández-Gutiérrez M, Bas-Sarmiento P, del Pino-Chinchilla H, Poza-Méndez M, Marín-Paz AJ. Effectiveness of a multimodal intervention and the simulation flow to improve empathy and attitudes towards older adults in nursing students: a crossover randomised controlled trial. Nurse Educ Pract. 2022;64:103430.
8. Arrogante O, Velarde-García JF, Blázquez-González P, Moro-Tejedor MN. The effects of high-fidelity simulation training on empathy and attitudes toward older people among undergraduate nursing students: a quasi-experimental study. Nurse Educ Pract. 2022;64:103441.
9. Lunde L, Moen A, Jakobsen RB, Møller B, Rosvold EO, Brænd AM. A preliminary simulation-based qualitative study of healthcare students' experiences of interprofessional primary care scenarios. Adv Simul. 2022;7(1):9.
10. Perot JG, Jarzebowski W, Lafuente-Lafuente C, Crozet C, Belmin J. Aging-simulation experience: impact on health professionals' social representations. BMC Geriatr. 2020;20(1):14.
11. Lee DA, Maxwell CA, Miller S. "This Is Me!" perceptions of older adult simulated participants in an aging and injury simulation experience. J Trauma Nurs. 2021;28(1):10–20.
12. Braude P, Reedy G, Dasgupta D, Dimmock V, Jaye P, Birns J. Evaluation of a simulation training programme for geriatric medicine. Age Ageing. 2015;44(4):677–82.
13. Weldon SM, Kneebone R, Bello F. Collaborative healthcare remodelling through sequential simulation: a patient and front-line staff perspective. BMJ Simul Technology Enhanc Learn. 2016;2(3):78.
14. Dixon-Woods M. The problem of context in quality improvement. In: Jonathan, editor. Perspectives on context. London: The Health Foundation; 2014. p. 88–101. https://www.health.org.uk/publications/perspectives-on-context.
15. Ward B, Diug B. Prioritising and reflecting on context in medical education. Med Educ. 2022;56(1):20–2.
16. Siew AL, Wong JW, Chan EY. Effectiveness of simulated patients in geriatric education: a scoping review. Nurs Educ Today. 2021;100:104856.
17. Plakiotis C. Clinical simulation training in geriatric medicine: a review of the evidence and lessons for training of psychiatry of old age. Adv Exp Med Biol. 2017;987:161–75.
18. Fisher JM, Walker RW. A new age approach to an age old problem: using simulation to teach geriatric medicine to medical students. Age Ageing. 2014;43(3):424–8.
19. Bradway C, Cotter VT, Darrah NJ, Gibbs VD, Hadley D, Kim EH, et al. An interprofessional education simulation workshop: health professions learning palliative care communication. J Nurs Educ. 2018;57(8):493–7.
20. Graham AC, McAleer S. An overview of realist evaluation for simulation-based education. Adv Simul. 2018;3(1):13.
21. Brazil V. Translational simulation: not 'where?' but 'why?' A functional view of in situ simulation. Adv Simul. 2017;2(1):i2.
22. Nickson CP, Petrosoniak A, Barwick S, Brazil V. Translational simulation: from description to action. Adv Simul. 2021;6(1):6.
23. Franck T, Bercelli P, Aloui S, Augusto V. A generic framework to analyze and improve patient pathways within a healthcare network using process mining and discrete-event simulation. 2020 Winter Simulation Conference (WSC), Orlando, FL, USA. p. 968–79.
24. Genes N, Kim M, Thum F, Rivera L, Beato R, Song C, et al. Usability evaluation of a clinical decision support system for geriatric ED pain treatment. Appl Clin Inform. 2016;07(01):128–42.
25. Vermeersch P, Sampsel DD, Kleman C. Acceptability and usability of a telepresence robot for geriatric primary care: a pilot. Geriatr Nurs. 2015;36(3):234–8.
26. Fisher JM, Rudd MP, Walker RW, Stewart J. Training tomorrow's doctors to safeguard the patients of today: using medical student simulation training to explore barriers to recognition of elder abuse. J Am Geriatr Soc. 2016;64(1):168–73.
27. Glassick C, Huber MT, Maeroff IG. Scholarship assessed: evaluation of the professoriate [Internet]. Wiley Publishing; 1997. https://www.wiley.com/en-us/Scholarship+Assessed%3A+-Evaluation+of+the+Professoriate-p-9780787910914.
28. Boyer E. Scholarship reconsidered: priorities of the professoriate. Princeton: The Carnegie Foundation for the Advancement of Teaching; 1990.
29. Brazil V, Symon B, Spurr J, Stokes-Parish J. Simulcast—a high fidelity podcast [Internet]. 2023. http://simulationpodcast.com.
30. Baylis J, Heyd C, Canners K. EM Sim cases [Internet]. 2022. https://emsimcases.com/leadership-team/.
31. Sherbino J, Arora VM, Melle EV, Rogers R, Frank JR, Holmboe ES. Criteria for social media-based scholarship in health professions education. Postgrad Med J. 2015;91(1080):551.

Part III

Implementation

9 Building and Enhancing a Simulated Participant Program with and for Older Adults

Cate Nicholas

Key Points

1. The ASPE SOBP Domain 4—Program Management—provides a framework to successfully add SPs over 60 to your program.
2. A well-thought-out articulate vision and mission statement are the foundation upon which to build your strategic plan.
3. SP educators need to develop additional expertise in how the normal aging process relates to work as an SP, characteristics of successful older workers, and how to create an age diverse and inclusive workplace.
4. Policies and procedures should support the addition of SPs 60 and over.

Introduction

In this chapter, guidance is offered on approaches to build or enhance an SP program with older adults. Selected principles from the ASPE SOBP in Domain 4—Program Management—are used to frame the process [1]. Published in 2017 as a living document, these standards are intended to support SP educators in all facets of safe and effective SP methodology. The standards are largely based on evidence drawn from adult SP programs and may need further consideration for older adults. First, I demonstrate how to create or revise your program's mission/vison statement, and then I will describe what you need to know when adding older adult SPs to the workplace, writing or revising your policies and procedures, how to support older adult SPs, and how to implement an ongoing quality improvement process. Examples are used to illustrate each step. Throughout the chapter, older SPs refer to older adults as SPs. Additional resources are provided at the end of the chapter.

C. Nicholas (✉)
Clinical Simulation Laboratory, University of Vermont, Burlington, VT, USA
e-mail: cate.nicholas@med.uvm.edu

ASPE SOBP Domain 4: Program Management

Principle 4.1 Purpose

A strategic planning process allows you to understand where you are, where you want to go, and how to get there [2]. A clear vision and mission statement are the first step in developing a strategy.

Create or revisit your *vision statement***.** A vision statement is a broad inspirational statement meant to demonstrate what you hope to accomplish in the next 3 to 5 years.

> Sample vision: SP methodology will prepare healthcare professionals to provide inclusive and equitable patient-centered care for those 60 and over.

Develop a *mission statement* which is more specific and describes the goals of the program. Mission statements focus on what we want to do and how we will achieve these goals.

> Sample mission: Create a diverse and inclusive multigenerational workplace to recruit, train, support, and retain people aged 60 and over into an existing SP program adhering to the ASPE SOBP values of professionalism, quality, collaboration, accountability, and safety to meet the healthcare needs of an aging population and the education of all healthcare students and professionals.

While you can create the vision and or mission statement yourself, consider engaging a range of relevant parties such as your advisory committee, SP educators, faculty, and younger and older SPs. Engaging the voices of those working day to day with learners and faculty will expand your thinking and at the same time help focus your message. See the resources section below for approaches to writing vision statements.

C. M. Smith et al. (eds.), *Comprehensive Healthcare Simulation: Geriatric Simulation*, Comprehensive Healthcare Simulation,
https://doi.org/10.1007/978-3-031-65742-9_9

Table 9.1 An example of a SWOT analysis for an older SP program

Strengths	Weaknesses
35% of current SPs 60 and over	Long checklists
They can recruit other SPs	Cases require extensive memorization
Flexible work schedule	Long hours
Opportunities	*Threats*
More people retiring and looking for part time meaningful work	Hiring freezes HR policies

SWOT Analysis

While a carefully crafted vision and mission statement will guide the next steps, knowing the internal **s**trengths and **w**eakness and understanding the external **o**pportunities and **t**hreats (SWOT) to your program will inform your strategy. Since the 1960s, an approach with the mnemonic—SWOT—has been used in management practice. A SWOT analysis is often most productive done as a brainstorming session where participants are encouraged to think without interruption [3] (Table 9.1).

Now that you have a better understanding of where your program stands, the next step is to develop a strategic action plan.

Strategic Action Plan

> A good strategy is not the product of hours of careful research and modeling that leads to an inevitable and almost perfect conclusion. Instead, it's the result of a simple and quite rough-and-ready process of thinking through what it would take to achieve what you want and then assessing whether it's realistic to try. [4]

Creating an action plan is a multistep process:

1. Identify SMART goals and objectives (see below).
2. Link plan to the goals and objectives:
   (a) Identify steps to reach the goals and objectives.
   (b) Assign process owners.
   (c) Create a timeline and milestones.
   (d) Identify resources needed.
   (e) Create measures to evaluate signs of success.

SMART Goals and Objectives

Much like objectives used when creating educational activities, goals/objectives should be SMART (specific, measurable, achievable, relevant) and have a timeline [5].

Example SMART objective linked to the vision and mission. Over the next 2 years, we will increase recruitment and retention for SPs 60 years and over by 25%.

Table 9.2 Example of an action plan

	Step 1	Step 2	Step 3
	Identify SPs in program 60+	Review and address current SP program policies and procedures to identify barriers for recruitment, hiring, retaining, training, and portrayal	Remove barriers and open opportunities to hire and retain SPs over 60
Process owner	Program administrator	Program administrator	Program Director with Human Resources (HR)
Resources needed	HR records	Policies and procedures	Time Institutional will
Signs of success	Accurate count	Complete review	HR support hiring and retention of SPs over 60
Completion date	1 month	1 month	2 months

Now create an action plan linked to each objective. Each step includes who is responsible, what resources are needed, and the timeline and benchmarks of success (Table 9.2).

SP educators will be most effective when they are well versed in all aspects of SP methodology. In this case, the expertise needed is how to work with people aged 60 and over and incorporate them into a multigenerational workplace. Let us start with learning how the normal aging process relates to work as an SP, characteristics of successful older workers, and how to create an age diverse and inclusive workplace.

Principle 4.2 Expertise

> Given the growing coexistence of multiple generations in workplaces, it is imperative to understand how organizations can maximize benefits that can be derived from age diversity at work. p. 119 [6]

Normal Aging Processes

Understanding normal aging [6, 7] is essential and can influence your SP policies and procedures. Of course, some older adults will experience all of these changes, some will have just some changes, and others will not have any of these changes.

1. Biological Aging.
   (a) External changes: Changes to hair, nails, and skin may affect who you can engage and for which role.

   (b) Sensory changes: Changes to taste, smell, sight, and hearing may affect ability to participate in certain scenarios. For example, hearing loss may be an issue in hearing announcements, hearing the learner, hearing instructions, etc.
   (c) Organ system changes: Changes to the cardiovascular, pulmonary, musculoskeletal, gastrointestinal, and urinary systems may impact what cases they can portray, for example:
      (i) Moving may become more painful and require more support getting up and down from an exam table.
      (ii) Repetitive exams may be more painful or tiring and may require a limit on the numbers of encounters in any one session.
      (iii) The need to urinate more frequently may also create a need for more frequent breaks or more time between stations.
2. Psychological aging: Changes to memory, learning, cognition, personality, and coping can also affect participation or require modifications to scenarios. Learning details of SPs cases and checklists may become more challenging and anxiety producing. Building in cognitive aids or simplifying cases can be of help. It is important to understand that there may be a decline in the older SPs speed of information processing.
3. Social aging: Changes in roles and relationships (e.g., becoming grandparents, moving from employed to retired, loss of friends and family, etc.) shape the meaning of aging which can be a positive or negative experience. These changing roles can make it easier or more difficult to commit to work or specific roles. Be sure to check in frequently and remind SPs to let you know if their situation has changed (e.g., the person who used to drive is no longer there, children have asked for help with childcare needs, etc.)

Characteristics of Successful Older Workers

Fraser et al. [8] gathered data from 16 adults with an average age of 67 who were participating in regular paid employment using demographic surveys and semistructured interviews. They shared the positive and negative aspects of working and the reason they want to keep working. Understanding these elements will help with advertising, recruitment, training, and retention.

Positive Aspects of Working

- Appreciative attitude toward work and life
- Attention to detail
- Fewer distractions
- Good work ethic
- Life and work experience
- Loyalty
- Wisdom

Negative Aspects of Working

- Less endurance and less stamina
- Physical limitations
- Poor health
- Poor motivation
- Resistance to change

Why Older People Want to Work

- Additional income
- Belonging to a supportive workplace
- Having a purpose
- Improved physical and emotional health
- Keeping sharp
- Making a difference
- Social connections
- Using skills built over a lifetime

As we develop expertise in working with age diversity in the workplace, consider what the SP program staff and SPs might need in training to assure that older SPs are welcomed and treated fairly (see Chaps. 3, 4, 5, 6, 10, 11, 12, and 14).

With a better understanding of where your program stands and of working with people over 60, it is time to edit or create *Policies and Proce*dures that will help older SPs be successful in your program and for you to meet your goals.

Principle 4.3 Policies and Procedures

Gliva-McConvey et al. [9] provide a guide for creating policies and procedures for SP programs, and Smith et al. [10] provide a framework for working with older SPs from which to build your policies and procedures. Information included in policies and procedures can include but are not limited to information for SPs about what an SP does and how they will be trained, expectations of the work, compensation, logistics, etc. When expanding or developing a new SP program for older adult SPs, the policies and procedures should reference information specific to older SPs as outlined above. See the resources section below for examples of policies and procedures from other SP programs.

Principle 4.4 Records Management

For this principle, there are no additional considerations for working with older adults.

Principle 4.5 Team Management

Team management includes assuring SP psychological, physical, and environmental safety and recruiting a diverse cohort of SPs. Learning what older SPs tell us about the value of working and some of the challenges they face can guide your program [11–13]. To better understand the experience of SPs 60 and over at the University of Vermont SP program, SPs who were 60 and over were invited to participate in focus groups. Four focus groups of 5 SPs ($n = 20$) were conducted by the Director of the Program. The SPs have worked between 2 and 26 years with an average of 9 years.

When asked why they became and continue to work as an SP, they identified two major reasons:

1. Personal Benefit
   (a) Becoming a better healthcare consumer for themselves and their family
   (b) Flexible in-person and remote schedules
   (c) Interesting work
   (d) Keeping current on developing social norms
   (e) Meeting new people and creating a community with people they would have never met otherwise
   (f) Learning new things and keeping old skills sharp
   (g) Working with the best and brightest students who are motivated, focused, and engaged
2. Sense of Purpose
   (a) Becoming visible and appreciated for their experience in a culture that does not always value aging
   (b) Feeling appreciated and valued by the SP program and the learners
   (c) Giving back by using their life and healthcare experiences to improve patient care now and in the future

SP Voice

"It is a blast! I love the teaching component, working with motivated students."
"My life is balanced because of this work."
"I have direction and a focus.
Easy to decline if you don't have a focus."

When asked about challenges of the work, three main points were identified:

1. Generational difference with social norms (antiracism and gender affirming care clinical skills)
2. Issues related to normal aging:
   (a) Memory can be a challenge and a source of anxiety
   (b) Mental and physical limitations which make sitting or moving position difficult and may limit the number of hours they can work
   (c) Need more time within the sessions to learn their role, to portray their role in the scenario and additional preparation time between learners, completing the checklists or rating forms, and to prepare for feedback
   (d) Early and late work hours
      (i) Long commute
      (ii) Parking can be a challenge—long walk to the program
      (iii) Driving at night
3. Navigating technology:
   (a) New programs like ZOOM
   (b) Multiple passwords

SP Voices

"Social concepts- like pronouns usage-gender- have to wrap head around these changes and understand and work on my own identify and honoring others."
"You know old age hits you one day suddenly you are old. Sitting or moving position can be difficult. I would prefer not to do a whole day."

When asked what an SP program could do to help them work if they choose to, several suggestions were made:

1. Combine SP's own social and medical history when possible, so there is not as much to memorize.
2. Be consistent in how material is presented.
3. Create older person specific cases (e.g., facing death, fear of death, and loneliness), and also allow work on cases not specifically about older people's health (e.g., in the role of a grandparent).
4. Give SPs a clearer understanding of what the students are learning and their trajectory.
5. Keep remote working options.
6. Keep payment at a level that recognizes them for the level of work they are doing.
7. Maintain leadership and faculty who are supportive.
8. More long-range scheduling to better plan other activities/vacations better—6 months out if possible.
9. More technical assistance.
10. More time to prepare and more time during sessions.
11. Creating a workplace environment that is welcoming.

SP Voices

"Ask our opinion, recognize our value and lived experience and how you bring that into education and help learners see us and value us."

> "Keep remote options- Nice to not have to go in and lie on table. Removes challenges of physical disabilities and transportation."

Creating a Diverse and Age-Inclusive Workplace

> An age-inclusive workplace "connects each employee to the organization; encourages collaboration, flexibility and fairness and leverages diversity through the organizations so that all individuals can participate and contribute to their full potential". p. 5 [14]

Some ways your program can commit to creating an age inclusive workplace include the following:

- See if age is included in your organization's equity, diversity, and inclusion statements and strategies.
- Provide training in an age-inclusive workplace for staff and other SPs.
- Review Human Resource (HR) and program materials to make sure the language includes and invites people 60 and over to apply [15]. Table 9.3 provides examples.
- Highlight the following benefits of SP work when advertising for older SPs:
  - Flexible work schedules
  - Working from home—remote options

Table 9.3 Examples of phrases to use in age inclusive HR documents

Say this	Not that
Entry level with salary range	Recent college graduate
List specific skills and required proficiency level	Digital native Tech savvy
Agile creative thinker	Fresh
Adaptable	Young
Education level	Graduation year
List values, benefits, and DEI policies	Cultural fit
Productive	Go getter
Highly engaged	High energy
At least *x* years of experience	No more than *x* years of experience

- Create peer mentoring process so younger and older SPs can work together on projects.
- Use your institution's social media to share the work your organization is doing to create an age-inclusive workforce. Update your programs' web and social media presence to use images and text that showcase older SPs and feature profiles of those SPs.

Recruiting older adults to the workforce may require different sources than those used for other SPs. Potential sources include the following:

1. Job websites that focus on older people
2. Seniors' centers
3. Houses of worship
4. Advocacy groups supporting older adults

Use resources in your local setting to consider options (see resources section below).

Principle 4.6 Quality Management

Now that you have a better understanding of SPs 60 and over, you can integrate what you have learned into a quality management process. Smith et al. [10] provide a three-phase framework for working with SPs 60 and over. You can use this framework to organize the data you need to gather to assess if you are meeting your goals of adding and supporting older SPs to your program. See Table 9.4 for an example.

Closing

As the patient population ages, SP methodology can be on the front lines to effectively educate and train healthcare professionals in the management of patients 60 and over. Careful consideration in creating and supporting a more age diverse SP workforce with specific organizational practices described in this chapter can help prepare your program to meet the complex needs of older adults.

Table 9.4 Three-phrase framework for quality management

Pre-simulation	Simulation	Post-simulation
1. Successful hiring and retention of SPs over 60	1. Program staff present to address any issues that may arise	1. De-roling post simulation
2. SPs	2. Area is scanned for fall risks	2. Specific feedback of portrayal and assessment is provided
• Co-create cases based on their lived experience	3. Real-time support for technology is provided	3. SP/SPE professional development needs are identified
• Use their own social and medical history if appropriate	4. One SP is scheduled for the am shift and another for the pm shift	4. SP feedback to improve program management is sought
3. Number of checklist items or feedback points are manageable	5. Breaks are incorporated	5. Mentors (regardless of age) are provided to train and support older SPs
4. Recruitment for cases- considers physical, psychological, or other factors		

Resources

Standards

Association of Standardized Patient Educators (ASPE) Standards of Best Practice (SOBP). https://advancesinsimulation.biomedcentral.com/articles/10.1186/s41077-017-0043-4 [Accessed July 24, 2023]

Approaches to Writing Vision Statements

Sinek S. *Start with Why*. 1st ed. New York: Portfolio; 2009. https://thecompassforsbc.org/how-to-guide/how-develop-mission-statement [Accessed July 24, 2023]

Examples of Policies and Procedures from SP Programs

https://steps.wvu.edu/media/14794/sp-policies-2016.pdf [Accessed July 24, 2023]

https://medicine.okstate.edu/site-files/documents/academics/sim-center/sp-handbook-2021.pdf [Accessed July 24, 2023]

Examples of Websites for Recruitment of Older Adults

- American Association of Retired Persons: https://jobs.aarp.org/ [Accessed July 25, 2023]
- Flex Jobs: https://www.flexjobs.com/ [Accessed July 25, 2023]
- Seniors4Hire: https://www.seniors4hire.org/ [Accessed July 25, 2023]
- Workforce5: https://www.workforce50.com/ [Accessed July 25, 2023]
- Older Workers Australia: https://olderworkers.com.au/ [Accessed July 25, 2023]
- Indeed – Senior Citizens: https://au.indeed.com/Senior-Citizens-jobs?vjk=058e8785fa282fdf [Accessed July 25, 2023]

Examples of an Organization Supporting for or Advocating for Older Adults

International Federation of Ageing: https://ifa.ngo/driving-our-agenda/ [Accessed July 25, 2023]

References

1. Lewis KL, Bohnert CA, Gammon WL, Hölzer H, Lyman L, Smith C, Thompson TM, Wallace A, Gliva-McConvey G. The association of standardized patient educators (ASPE) standards of best practice (SOBP). Adv Simul. 2017;2(1):1–8.
2. 5 steps of the strategic planning process. https://www.lucidchart.com/blog/5-steps-of-the-strategic-planning-process. Accessed 21 Dec 2022.
3. Section 14. SWOT analysis: strengths, weaknesses, opportunities, and threats. https://ctb.ku.edu/en/table-of-contents/assessment/assessing-community-needs-and-resources/swot-analysis/main. Accessed 21 Dec 2022.
4. Martin R. The big lie of strategic planning. Harvard Business Review. Jan–Feb 2014. https://hbr.org/2014/01/the-big-lie-of-strategic-planning. Accessed 21 Dec 2022.
5. Setting goals and developing specific, measurable, achievable, relevant, and time-bound objectives SAMHSA native connections. https://www.samhsa.gov/sites/default/files/nc-smart-goals-fact-sheet.pdf. Accessed 21 Dec 2022.
6. Wang M, Fang Y. Age diversity in the workplace: facilitating opportunities with organizational practices. Public Policy Aging Rep. 2020;30(3):119–23.
7. Chalise HN. Aging: basic concept. Am J Biomed Sci Res. 2019;1(1):8–10.
8. Fraser L, McKenna K, Turpin M, Allen S, Liddle J. Older workers: an exploration of the benefits, barriers, and adaptations for older people in the workforce. Work. 2009;33(3):261–72.
9. Gliva-McConvey G, Nicholas CF, Clark L, editors. Comprehensive healthcare simulation: implementing best practices in standardized patient methodology. Cham: Springer International Publishing; 2020.
10. Smith CM, Sokoloff LG, Alsaba N. Collaborative framework for working with older simulated participants (SP). BMJ Simul Technol Enhanc Learn. 2021;7(2):112–5.
11. Schelgel C, Smith CM. "Please let me know when I do not realize it myself": a qualitative analysis of senior simulated patients' experiences. Adv Simul. 2019;4(1):1–1.
12. Smith CM, Sokoloff LG, Gallucci CE. 'It's like a shot in the arm': evaluating the experiences of older simulated participants in structured virtual meetings during COVID-19. Int J Healthc Simul. 2021;1(1):33–40.
13. Thompson J, Tiplady S, Hutchinson A, Cook G, Harrington B. Older people's views and experiences of engagement in standardized patient simulation. BMJ Simul Technol Enhanc Learn. 2017;3:154–8.
14. Government-wide diversity and inclusion strategic plan 2011. https://www.opm.gov/policy-data-oversight/diversity-equity-inclusion-and-accessibility/reports/governmentwidedistrategic-plan.pdf. Accessed 21 Dec 2022.
15. Say This, Not That: A Manager's Guide to Hiring https://employerportal.aarp.org/age-inclusive-workforce/follow-age-inclusive-recruitment-practices/guide-say-this-not-that

Working with Volunteer Older Adult Simulated Participants

10

Lisa Guttman Sokoloff, Cathy M. Smith, Anne Bellot, and Sheng-Po Kao

Key Messages

1. Working with older adult SP volunteers can be a rich and meaningful experience, beneficial both to the volunteers and the organization.
2. Developing an ongoing volunteer SP program is resource intensive, requiring the same attention to all aspects of SP methodology as are needed for a program with paid SPs. However, the cost/benefit ratio is well worth the commitment of resources.
3. Understanding the benefits and challenges that older adults identify related to volunteering as SPs can help SP educators maximize the involvement of these SPs.
4. Leveraging institutional resources (e.g., a Volunteer Services department) can support the recruitment and screening of new SPs.
5. Onboarding, training, and ongoing support of older adult volunteer SPs is necessary.
6. Acknowledging and showing appreciation for the contributions of your older adult volunteer SPs are examples of how to support them.

L. G. Sokoloff (✉)
Faculty of Applied Health and Community Studies, Sheridan College, Brampton, ON, Canada

Department of Speech Pathology, Temerty Faculty of Medicine, University of Toronto, Toronto, ON, Canada
e-mail: lisa.sokoloff@sheridancollege.ca

C. M. Smith
Baycrest Academy for Research and Education, Baycrest Centre for Geriatric Care, Toronto, ON, Canada
e-mail: CSmith4@baycrest.org

A. Bellot
NorSimS, University of Caen Normandy, Caen University Hospital, Caen, France
e-mail: bellot-a@chu-caen.fr

S.-P. Kao
Center for Humanities in Medicine, Buddhist Hualien Tzu Chi General Hospital, Tzu Chi University, Hualien, Taiwan
e-mail: spkao@tzuchi.com.tw

Vignette

For the last 2 years, you have managed a simulation program in an institution that supports healthcare professionals and students. You mainly work with manikins and run your program according to recommended practices. A recent review of the institutional training curriculum identified the care of older adults as a priority, specifically related to the development of interpersonal and behavioral skills. Clinical educators identified that they would like to create simulations that engage older adult SPs to promote better care. The head of your department has expressed strong support for working with older adult SPs. The only barrier is that there is not enough money to fund an SP program where the SPs are paid. You are wondering about the feasibility of engaging older adults as volunteer SPs. Where do you begin?

Background

Although there is much information reported about why older adults volunteer, there are few reports specifically related to working with older adult volunteers as SPs. Therefore, we begin by exploring both reasons why older adults volunteer and what is known about working with volunteer SPs in general and then present what is known about older adult volunteer SPs.

Why Do Older Adults Volunteer?

Older adults volunteer for many reasons. The literature has multiple examples of positive rationale for older adults to volunteer including altruism, making a difference, cognitive benefits, and social benefits [1–4]. Bradley [5] suggests that motivation for older adult volunteering can be divided into three categories: enhanced sense of purpose, personal growth, and continued productivity.

C. M. Smith et al. (eds.), *Comprehensive Healthcare Simulation: Geriatric Simulation*, Comprehensive Healthcare Simulation,
https://doi.org/10.1007/978-3-031-65742-9_10

Mak [6] utilized data from the "Understanding Society: UK Household Longitudinal study" [7] to investigate whether older adults receive benefits from volunteering. Their analysis found that in general, volunteers had lower levels of mental distress and better health-related quality of life and that the differences were even more prominent in the older population (Baby Boomers and adults born before 1945). They also noted that volunteering promotes the development of new social networks and roles and group identity for older adults. These are benefits that older volunteers may gain through volunteering while younger people may do so through work, schooling, or family activities.

In a review of the US Health and Retirement Study—2014 Wave [8], Lim et al. [9] noted that volunteering is integral in shaping late-life friendships. Their review also found a positive association between the number of hours spent volunteering and the number of close friends, along with the quality and contact frequency of those friendships. This was found to be of greater benefit to older women than older men, although the older men still benefited.

With the population of older adults continuing to grow exponentially, Devany postulated that after retirement, people could conceivably still live one-third of their lives, allowing much time for volunteering [2].

These reasons why older adults volunteer highlight why they are ideal candidates to volunteer in SP programs.

Volunteer SPs: Who Are They?

Volunteer SPs are well people who donate their time and who are carefully trained to portray someone else, such as a patient, client, family member, or health professional. Volunteer SPs can be *real* patients who portray themselves with their illness experience and donate their time [10]. However, for the purposes of this chapter, we focus on volunteer SPs who are **well** people; they are playing a role other than themselves. Volunteer SPs work in many contexts [11–15]. The backgrounds of volunteer SPs may include faculty or staff, alumni, retired clinicians, actors, community members, and learners [16–19]. There is variation in how volunteer SPs are supported in their work and there are no published standards for working with volunteer SPs.

Benefits to an Organization Working with Volunteer SPs

The rationale for working with volunteers is often financial [12, 16, 18, 20]. Paid SPs may be perceived as being too expensive. Volunteers are sometimes seen as being more available (especially if they are retired), and students perceive them as sometimes being friendlier than paid SPs [21]. Volunteers with content expertise (e.g., retired nurses portraying nurses) are sometimes perceived by learners as being more authentic, both in their role portrayal and feedback, and therefore more engaging [16, 22]. In addition, in educational settings, those with content expertise and experience (e.g., practicing nurses) are described as needing less training or support as they are able to distinguish levels of understanding in students and so can adjust their portrayals accordingly and assess what learners are doing more accurately than a SP without clinical knowledge [23].

Benefits to Volunteer SPs Working with Programs

Volunteer SPs identify many benefits, including filling a vocational void after retirement, gaining satisfaction from helping the next generation of learners, feeling useful through contributing, being provided with learning opportunities (including finding out more about how to manage their own health and navigate the healthcare system), receiving stimulation from the social experience, and finding a peer group [15, 17, 24–27]. Both their physical health and cognitive functions, recognized as major factors that contribute to healthy aging, can also improve. These findings are in close alignment with findings from various general studies related to the benefits of volunteering, particularly related to retired older adult volunteers [4, 28–30].

Challenges for Organizations Working with Volunteer SPs

Challenges in working with volunteer SPs include perceptions that they are less committed than paid SPs [24] and that they may have changing levels of interest and availability [22]. Difficulties may ensue because they do not want to be held to program standards [24] and may not be able to sustain interest and commitment over the long term [18]. Those who have clinical content knowledge may fill gaps in or move into the role of being an instructor rather than a simulated participant [11].

Challenges for Volunteer SPs Working with Programs

SP volunteers identify challenges such as the time commitment, feeling too much responsibility, worrying that they will fail, having anxiety about not being prepared properly, being concerned about their ability to remember details, and having the stamina to participate and overall health concerns [4, 25]. Worrying about a lack of formal performance training or the ability to portray more advanced roles (e.g., those with heightened affects or complicated histories) may discourage volunteer SPs from participating [18]. The literature about volunteering in general also suggests that volunteers will quit if their motivations are not satisfied and if they do not feel supported and/or appreciated [28].

Recommended Practices for Working with Older Adult Volunteers

Sellon, in a 2014 review of the literature, identifies seven recommended practices for engaging with older adult volunteers, including personal invitation, role flexibility, stipends, social interaction, support from staff, meaningfulness, and recognition [31]. She goes onto note that "identifying and utilizing the strengths of individuals and communities and volunteer goal setting are … additional best practices that may be particularly relevant in attracting a diverse set of older adult volunteers" (p. 421).

There are many resources available for setting up volunteer programs [32–35]. Some SP programs may be affiliated with institutions that already have volunteer departments with established recruitment and screening policies and procedures [36], offering the opportunity for partnership and leveraging of resources.

Comparing Three International Volunteer SP Programs

Now that we have provided this overview, we will describe our three simulation programs where we work with older adult volunteer SPs, all within institutions with established volunteer departments. Our programs are in Canada, France, and Taiwan. All our programs follow recommended practices in simulation [37, 38]. Table 10.1 provides an outline of important features of each program that might be helpful to consider when developing or refining a volunteer SP program. We have also provided some flow charts illustrating the infrastructure used in two of our programs (see Figs. 10.1 and 10.2).

Similarities Between the Programs

Despite being based in different countries, and developing independently of one another, our programs are remarkably similar. All three programs take an evidence-informed approach and have rigorous infrastructure, training, and research components. Each program recognizes that there are costs associated with running a volunteer SP program and have organizational support, including funding for an SP educator, even if part time. These SP educators have knowledge of SP methodology, program needs, and special considerations for older adults. A long-term commitment by the volunteers is also important and helps to establish a sense of community among the older adult SPs. We have also all found that dedicated administrative support, in addition to the SP educator, is necessary.

NorSimS SP Program

The NorSimS SP program in Caen, France, was developed in 2017 within the NorSimS simulation center. In response to requests to develop "breaking bad news" encounters for medical residents, the NorSimS team was in need of SPs. Since 2020, the roles of the SPs were progressively extended to other types of simulation such as hybrid training around obstetrical delivery procedures with midwifes, consultations in anesthetics, and emergency situations.

The NorSimS SP's ages range from 19 to 74 years old. The SPs participate in as many simulation sessions as they want. Their feedback is used to adapt training sessions and scenarios. All NorSimS SPs are volunteers in the program. They come from various backgrounds (e.g., students, workers in the healthcare system and outside of it, retirees). The older adult SPs are all retired and active. Some of them do other volunteer work as well; some take classes at the university. The recruitment of the older adult SPs is mainly done via word of mouth. Approximately 11% of the SPs are older adults. Conversations with the older adult SPs reveal their appreciation of participating in the training and assessment of future healthcare professionals.

Michèle, age 68 "I'm already a volunteer blood donor, I can as well donate some of my time for medical education."

Denise, age 71, "The health system takes care of us, we can help in medical education; …

Simulation Activities for Gerontological Education (SAGE)

The SAGE program at Baycrest in Toronto, Canada, was developed in response to a need for more face-to-face interactions and training for healthcare workers and families, specifically tailored toward person-centered care for older adults. All the SAGE SPs are over 60 years old. Besides participating in live simulations, both in person and virtually, a large part of the program includes the development of reflective videos that are embedded into eLearning modules and/or used for teaching. SAGE SPs are often codevelopers of scenarios, and they are recognized and celebrated for the wisdom, authenticity, and knowledge they bring to the team.

All SAGE SPs are volunteers, and their recruitment is coordinated by Baycrest's Volunteer Department. Many of the SPs have disclosed that they also volunteer in other areas at Baycrest and find that the work they do as SPs also enhances their other volunteer experiences by exposing them to different scenarios or ways of thinking about things. The SPs often report that they value their volunteer experiences

Table 10.1 Comparison of three International Volunteer SP programs

Country	France	Taiwan	Canada
Name of organization	NorSimS	Hualien Tzu Chi General Hospital	Baycrest Academy for Research and Education at Baycrest Centre for Geriatric Care
Title of program	NorSimS SP Program	Tzu Chi Standardized Patient Program for Medical Education	Simulation Activities for Gerontological Education (SAGE)
	https://norsims.unicaen.fr	https://hlm.tzuchi.com.tw/spcenter/	https://www.baycrest.org/Baycrest/Academic-Education-Training/Training-and-Simulation-Division/Programs
When program was established (year)	2017	2006	2015
Age range of older adult Volunteer SPs	65–75	65–81	65–95
Number of SPs	99	159	13
Number (%) older adults	11 (11%)	30 (18.8%)	13 (100%)
Gender of older adult SPs (%)	7 male, 4 female	10 male, 20 female	4 male, 9 female
Principal focus	Summative assessment—Participating in OSCE's	Summative assessment—Participating in nationwide OSCEs	Formative training and assessment focused on older adult cognition, brain health, dementia care
Learner Group	3rd, 4th, 5th and 6th year medical students, residents, healthcare students and healthcare workers	6th (final) year medical students, paramedical undergraduate students and postgraduate residents	Healthcare workers, students, community members
Staffing costs	Two SP trainers: 10 h/month: screening, training, follow up of SP's	SP trainers 8 h/month; recruiting, training, retaining SPs	Simulationist 28 h/month
	One administrator 48 h/month (takes care of all the SPs)	One administrator 40 h/week (takes care of all the SPs)	Simulation educators 28 h/month
Other associated costs	Incidental costs for props, wardrobe, moulage, refreshments, meals, parking, fees for paid SPs	Transportation Expenses Space (e.g., simulation room) Equipment (e.g., audiovisual)	Costs to make videos (e.g., videographer), incidental costs for props, wardrobe, moulage, refreshments, parking, fees for paid SPs who are hired occasionally
Volunteer SP recruitment strategy	Program is promoted via email to the "inter-age university" (an association that promotes activities in Normandy for people of any age. Although anyone can register and attend any class or activity proposed, mainly seniors and retired people are part of it), word of mouth	Program is promoted through the organization's volunteer services orientation, word of mouth from SPs in the program	Program is promoted through the organization's volunteer services orientation, word of mouth from SPs in the program
SP screening and/or orientation	15-min screening that includes an interview by two SP educators: a psychologist and a physician	SP screening is incorporated into the SP training program During "Acting technique training" and "Scenario training and dry run" sections of the training program, the SP trainers will observe and select the SPs who fit the program	60-min session that includes improvisation exercises

SP training program	3 h in one session	6 h:	3 h (held as two separate 90-min sessions)
	Interactive on-site training including an introduction to simulation, the role of the SPs in the program, our expectations, the working tools (scenarios sheets, visit of the simulation center), and exercises on playing emotions	2 h on SP professionalism (role clarity, expectation, simulation process)	Interactive training focused on: what is simulation, who are SPs, role clarity, description of expectations and processes, practice training with sample scenario
		2 h on acting technique training	
		2 h for scenario training and dry run	
Continuing development for SPs	None yet	6-h Continuing curriculum (including workshop) every 3 months (4 times/year)	Advanced training session on Giving Feedback
			During COVID—continued Zoom meetings to work on skills (e.g., mindfulness, storytelling, improvisation and use of technology as an SP)
Program research and scholarship	SPs engaged in a qualitative study on "teaching empathy to residents using simulation" [39]	SPs engaged as participants in research studies regarding their motivation for the program and opinions about the program [40–43]	SPs engaged as subjects in research and presentations regarding their lived experiences as SPs in the program [25, 26, 44–46]
Future plans	Expanding older adult SP pool to extend activities (training and OCSE sessions)	Follow up and caring for the older adult SPs	Increased online work
		Older adult SPs sharing their life stories for medical humanities curriculum	Expanding SP pool to provide more diversity
			Recording the life stories of SPs as a basis for creating characters in future scenarios

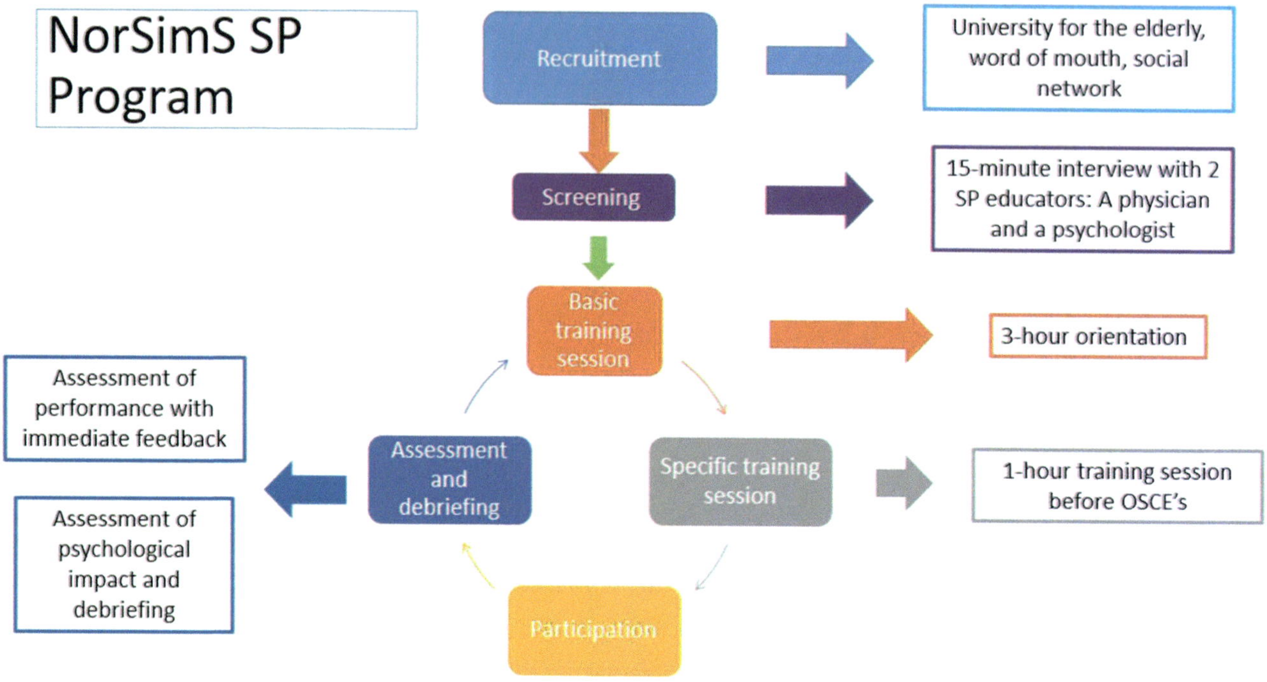

Fig. 10.1 NorSimS Volunteer SP program flow chart

greatly and that they are "getting more out of it than they are giving."

Although Baycrest is publicly funded, and SAGE membership is open to all who meet the screening criteria, Baycrest is a faith-based organization that embraces the long-standing Jewish tradition of *tikkun olam*—taking action to improve and repair the world. As volunteers, the SAGE SPs support this tradition.

Noreen, age 82 "I told myself - you can do this - it's important for people your age and future generations, they don't know what's to come and hopefully we are helping nurses. It's fun. I love it! I feel good about myself… it makes me feel important to myself."

Essie, age 87 "I love doing a little bit of acting and meeting the great people that belong to this group, and also, most of all, I feel like I'm helping. But the best thing is that I'm getting more out of it than I'm giving."

Tzu Chi Standardized Patient Program for Medical Education

The Tzu Chi SP program was developed in 2006 at the Buddhist Hualien Tzu Chi General Hospital in Eastern Taiwan and currently has 159 SPs aged from 26 to 81 years old. While the SPs come from various backgrounds, they are all volunteers of the Buddhist Tzu Chi Foundation, and all share a common goal of helping to improve the healthcare system. Members of the Buddhist Tzu Chi Foundation have a specific focus on community service and outreach, especially medical and educational service [47]. Subsequently, by volunteering their time and expertise, SPs can make a difference in the lives of future healthcare professionals and further support the values of the Buddhist Tzu Chi Foundation.

The SPs provide a unique opportunity for students to practice their clinical skills in a safe and supportive environment. The SPs participate in the national Objective Structured Clinical Examination (OSCE), which is a prerequisite for the medical licensure examination. They also support teaching activities of medical students and are involved in the training of paramedical undergraduate students and postgraduate residency. The SPs also participate in research projects that aim to improve the quality of healthcare education.

The SPs report that their physical health and cognitive functions, recognized as the major factors for healthy aging, have improved since joining the program. This is likely due to the program providing them with opportunities to stay active and engaged in their community. The SPs report the program to be a rewarding way to give back to the healthcare community.

Lin, age 69, "Given my age, the requirement of reciting the script and performing immediately has helped me a lot with my memory. In addition to acting, which requires high concentration and flexibility, we need to give students constructive feedback immediately. I will probably not have dementia in the future."

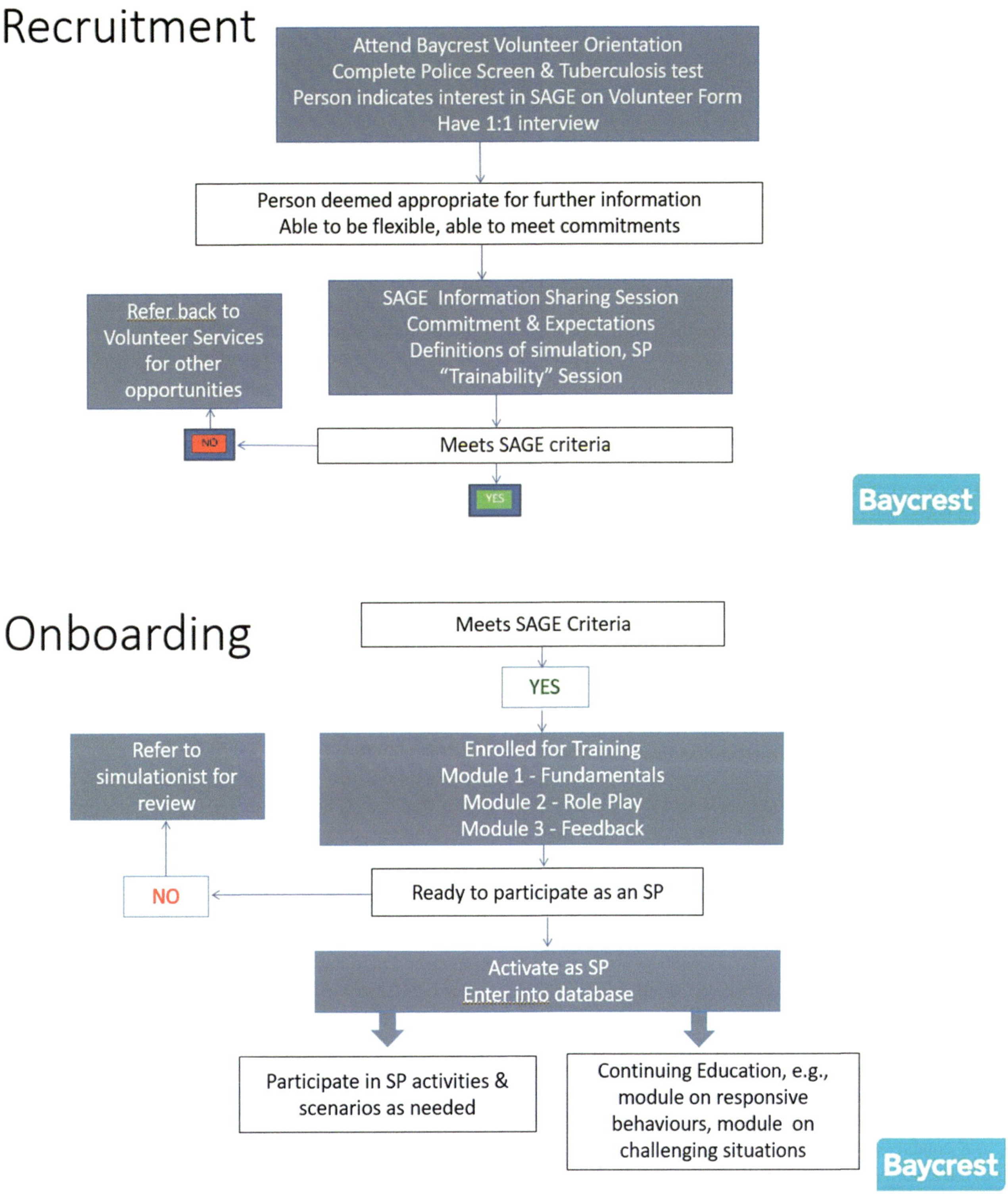

Fig. 10.2 Baycrest SAGE Volunteer SP program flow chart

Frequently Asked Questions About Volunteer SPs

In the next section, we share questions that sometimes arise when considering working with older adult volunteers, along with our responses.

Q: What is the cost to run a program if the SPs are volunteers?

Response: Despite not having to pay a salary or compensation to the volunteer SPs, there are still many associated costs. These budget items may include the salary for a trained SP educator/staff or having a hybrid model where some SPs are paid, and others are volunteers. Other costs may include administrative costs, continuing professional curriculum for SPs, honoraria, parking, and refreshments/catering for SPs. It is important to have support from organizational leadership so that they recognize there are associated direct and indirect costs.

Q: Are volunteer SPs less committed than paid SPs?

Response: Despite literature supporting the **perception** that volunteer SPs are less committed [22], there is no published evidence to support volunteer SPs being less committed than paid SPs. Paid SPs may sometimes drop out at the last minute, usually because of other potentially more lucrative work opportunities. In one of our programs, when compared with another local center, volunteer SPs had a higher attendance rate (100%) than the paid SPs at OSCEs. It is important to frame expectations about commitment and have clear communication processes in place if a volunteer SP must cancel. Our experience has been that volunteer SPs are remarkably committed and usually only cancel if they are unwell or have a family emergency. SPs in our programs tell us that they will cancel other engagements, so they can attend training or simulation sessions.

Q: By not paying volunteers, is that taking advantage of them?

Response: There are many benefits to older adults who volunteer, including possibly reducing risk of cognitive decline. Anderson et al. [4] noted that the articles they reviewed "most consistently reveal that volunteering is associated with reduced symptoms of depression, better self-reported health, fewer functional limitations, and lower mortality" (p. 1505). The authors concluded that volunteering by older adults is associated with cognitive, physical, psychosocial, and functional benefits.

In another article, it was noted that older adult volunteer SPs overwhelmingly reported that participating in education of students was rewarding and provided the chance for them to provide input to care of older adults in the health system [15].

At Baycrest, during the height of the COVID-19 pandemic, we conducted an interview-based study to explore the lived experience of older adult SPs during this time. Some SPs mentioned that being SPs improved their physical and cognitive well-being [26].

Q: Does a volunteer SP program need infrastructure or human resources management? If the SPs are volunteers, they are not employees.

Response: Regardless of whether payment is involved, structure is required. Not all volunteers can be SPs. Recruitment strategies are required to ensure that SPs fit program requirements and learners' needs. At times, both paid and volunteer SPs may be warranted.

Each of our programs has an established infrastructure (see Figs. 10.1 and 10.2) to direct orientation, recruitment, and training/development. In the SAGE program at Baycrest, in response to feedback from the older adult SPs, orientation was split into two 90-min sessions, rather than one 3-h session as the SPs felt it was too long.

Q: Since the SPs are volunteers, can anyone participate?

Response: As with paid SPs, older adult volunteer SPs must be carefully screened. Not all people are appropriate or ready for SP work, either paid or volunteer. Reasons that volunteers may not be accepted as SPs include the following:

- Personal motivations that are not congruent with the program's goals (e.g., having a personal agenda to "fix the system/learners" rather than be in service to the learners/learning objective)
- Attitudes incongruent with program standards (e.g., refusing to participate in training sessions, not following established protocols, treating others disrespectfully)
- Not meeting the required skill set for the program as identified in the orientation/recruitment phase
- Not emotionally available to take on the content of the work
- Inability to meet the time commitments required
- Inability to participate in structured/rigorous training

If a volunteer is not able to meet the requirements of the SP program, they could be redirected to other volunteer activities.

Q: Should volunteers use their own life stories when playing a role?

Response: There are differing thoughts about this. Use of personal stories may have unanticipated complications. Details could be introduced that have the potential to trigger the SP or the learners that then takes away from the learning objectives/focus of the scenario. While we recognize that SPs will draw on some aspects of their own lived experiences when playing a role, we caution that, if SPs are enacting roles that are parallel to their own life stories (e.g., portraying someone taking care of a family member living with dementia), or that could evoke strong emotions, there are processes in place, including debriefing and deroling, that attend to their psychological safety. SPs should always have the option to withdraw from a simulation for any reason. Throughout the process, SP educators need to be vigilant in monitoring for, and supporting, this aspect of SP work. On a positive note, the lived experience of older adult SPs can add depth to a role.

Q: How much can we expect of SPs who are volunteers? Should we apply the same standards that we would for a program with paid SPs?

Response: The same simulation standards [37, 38] apply to all SPs, whether they be volunteers or paid. With careful selection, training, coaching, and ongoing support, volunteer SPs can play the same roles as a paid SP [40]. Older adult SP volunteers can act as educators and/or trainers and administrators [41–44]. There are also reports of volunteer SPs contributing to scenario development [45]. Special considerations should be acknowledged when working with older adult volunteer SPs (e.g., memory changes), and roles may need to be adapted so they fit an SP's current abilities. With aging related changes, roles and other processes may require further adaptation [46].

Q: Are volunteer SPs as effective as paid SPs?

Response: There is no agreement or strong evidence whether volunteer SPs are more or less effective than paid SPs. While several studies describe characteristics of effective SPs, the volunteer status does not appear to be a significant variable [10, 11, 16, 18, 48–50]. As is the case when working with all SPs, it is important to know the abilities of the older volunteer SPs you work with, to attend to their needs and changes they may undergo as they age, and to adapt as required. Volunteer SPs work across a broad spectrum of activities, including OSCEs [39, 43].

Summary/Conclusions

In this chapter, we introduced three older adult volunteer SP programs. We highlighted both the benefits and challenges of working with older adult volunteer SPs and reviewed some evidence that informs the creation of a positive and meaningful experience for the volunteers, the learners, and the organizations. We also addressed some frequently asked questions about volunteer SPs. We encourage SP educators to consider working with older adult volunteer SPs and strongly recommend creating and applying a program structure that follows best practices.

References

1. Taghian M, D'Souza C, Polonsky M. A study of older Australians' volunteering and quality of life: empirical evidence and policy implications. J Nonprofit Publ Sect Market. 2012;24(2):101–22.
2. Devaney C, Kearns N, Fives A, Canavan J, Lyons R, Eaton P. Recruiting and retaining older adult volunteers: implications for practice. J Nonprofit Publ Sect Market. 2015;27(4):331–50.
3. Greenfield EA, Marks NF. Formal volunteering as a protective factor for older adults' psychological well-being. J Gerontol Ser B Psychol Sci Soc Sci. 2004;59(5):S258–S64.
4. Anderson ND, Damianakis T, Kröger E, Wagner LM, Dawson DR, Binns MA, et al. The benefits associated with volunteering among seniors: a critical review and recommendations for future research. Psychol Bull. 2014;140(6):1505–33.
5. Bradley DB. A reason to rise each morning: the meaning of volunteering in the lives of older adults. Generations. 1999;23(4):45–50.
6. Mak HWK. Why do older generations benefit more from volunteering? [Internet]. University of Essex, UK: UK Data Service, Economic and Social Research Council; 25 Feb 2022. https://blog.ukdataservice.ac.uk/older-generations-volunteering-benefits/.
7. University of Essex Institute for Social and Economic Research. Understanding Society, 9th release. [Internet]. Essex: UK Data Service; 2023. https://doi.org/10.5255/UKDA-Series-2000053.
8. The Health and Retirement Study—2014 wave [Internet]. Ann Arbor: The Regents of the University of Michigan; 2014. https://hrs.isr.umich.edu/about.
9. Lim E, Peng C, Burr J. Volunteering and friendship in later life: does gender moderate the relationship? Innov Aging. 2020;4(Suppl 1):416.
10. Cleland JA, Abe K, Rethans JJ. The use of simulated patients in medical education: AMEE Guide No 42.1. Med Teach. 2009;31(6):477–86.
11. Smithson J, Bellingan M, Glass B, Mills J. Standardized patients in pharmacy education: an integrative literature review. Curr Pharm Teach Learn. 2015;7(6):851–63.
12. Blickendorf JM, Adkins EJ, Boulger C, Bahner DP. Trained simulated ultrasound patients medical students as models, learners, and teachers. J Ultrasound Med. 2014;33(1):35–8.
13. Ghate D, Bodnarchuk B, Sanders S, Deokule S, Kedar S. The ability of healthy volunteers to simulate a neurologic field defect on automated perimetry. Ophthalmology. 2014;121(3):759–62.
14. King MA, Ott J. Actors needed: clinical faculty get the call. Nurse Educ. 2012;37(3):105–7.
15. Hackel JM, Roberts TME. The effectiveness of an educational project using older adult volunteers for training primary care nurse practitioners in geriatric assessment. J Nurs Educ Pract. 2020;10(3) https://doi.org/10.5430/jnep.v10n3p51.
16. Mavis B, Turner J, Lovell K, Wagner D. Developments: faculty, students, and actors as standardized patients: expanding opportunities for performance assessment. Teach Learn Med. 2006;18(2):130–6.
17. Carlton KH. Community and alumni Volunteers enhancing simulation fidelity and quality across curriculum: lab coordination and management perspective. Clin Simul Nurs. 2012;8(8):e396–7.
18. Nestel D, Calandra A, Elliott RA. Using volunteer simulated patients in development of pre-registration pharmacists: learning from the experience. Pharm Educ. 2007;7(1):35–42.
19. Nestel D, Tierney T. Role-play for medical students learning about communication: guidelines for maximising benefits. BMC Med Educ. 2007;7:3.
20. Jones J, Staub J, Seymore A, Scott LA. Securing the second front: achieving first receiver safety and security through competency-based tools. Prehosp Disaster Med. 2014;29(6):643–7.
21. Clever SL, Dudas RA, Solomon BS, Yeh HC, Levine D, Bertram A, et al. Medical student and faculty perceptions of volunteer outpatients versus simulated patients in communication skills training. Acad Med. 2011;86(11):1437–42.
22. Sanko JS, Shekhter I. Using embedded simulated persons (aka "confederates"). In: Maxworthy J, Epps C, Okuda Y, Mancini M, Palaganas J, editors. Defining excellence in simulation programs. 2nd ed. Philadelphia: Lippincott Williams & Wilkins; 2022. p. 825–37.
23. Bokken L, Rethans JJ, Van Heurn L, Duvivier R, Scherpbier A, Van Der Vleuten C. Students' views on the use of real patients and simulated patients in undergraduate medical education. Acad Med. 2009;84(7):958–63.

24. Heine N, Ferguson D. Management of standardized patient programs. In: Maxworthy J, Epps C, Okuda Y, Mancini M, Palaganas J, editors. Defining excellence in simulation programs. 2nd ed. Philadelphia: Lippincott Williams & Wilkins; 2022. p. 317–404.
25. Schelgel C, Smith CM. "Please let me know when I do not realize it myself": a qualitative analysis of senior simulated patients' experiences. Adv Simul. 2019;4(1):18.
26. Smith CM, Sokoloff LG, Gallucci CE. 'It's like a shot in the arm': evaluating the experiences of older simulated participants in structured virtual meetings during COVID-19. Int J Healthc Simul. 2021;1(1):33–40.
27. Crittenden J, Thompson K. Motivations and experiences of older adult volunteers in a telehealth nursing simulation activity. Innov Aging. 2021;5(Suppl 1):945.
28. Morrow-Howell N, Mui AC. Elderly volunteers: reasons for initiating and terminating service. J Gerontol Soc Work. 1989;13(3-4):21–34.
29. Morrow-Howell N, Hinterlong J, Rozario PA, Tang F. Effects of volunteering on the well-being of older adults. J Gerontol Ser B Psychol Sci Soc Sci. 2003;58(3):S137–S45.
30. Fischer LR, Schaffer KB. Older volunteers: a guide to research and practice. Newbury Park: Sage; 1993.
31. Sellon AM. Recruiting and retaining older adults in volunteer programs: best practices and next steps. Ageing Int. 2014;39:421–37.
32. Engaging volunteers: older adults [Internet]. Ottawa: Volunteer Canada; 2020. https://volunteer.ca/index.php?MenuItemID=342.
33. Volunteer management [Internet]. Caledon: Older Adult Centres' Association of Ontario; 2023.
34. CivicPlus. How to start a volunteer program in your community [2022 Updates] [Internet]. Manhattan: CivicPlus; 2023. https://www.civicplus.com/blog/pr/how-to-create-an-effective-volunteer-program.
35. Braverman J. Tapping into strengths of our older volunteer [Internet]. St. Paul: Minnesota Alliance for Volunteer Advancement; 2020. https://www.mavanetwork.org/content.aspx?page_id=5&club_id=286912&item_id=59999
36. Becoming a Volunteer [Internet]. Toronto: Baycrest; 2023. https://www.baycrest.org/Baycrest-Pages/Get-Involved/Volunteer/Becoming-a-Volunteer.
37. Lewis KL, Bohnert CA, Gammon WL, Hölzer H, Lyman L, Smith C, et al. The association of standardized patient educators (ASPE) Standards of Best Practice (SOBP). Adv Simul. 2017;2(1):10.
38. INACSL Standards Committee. Healthcare simulation standards of best practice™. Clin Simul Nurs. 2021;58:1–66.
39. Bellot A, Albert C, Ristovski M, Dolley P, Guillois B. Création d'un groupe de patients simulés bénévoles: un atout pour la formation et l'évaluation à l'heure de la réforme du deuxième cycle des études médicales en France. Pédagogie Médicale. 2023;24:97–102.
40. Kao S-P, Chen T-Y, Hsieh M-L. Effectiveness of a training program on the role recognition and case portrayal of standardized patients. Tzu-Chi Med J. 2018;30(1):37.
41. Chien T-C, Lin M-R, Lin C-T, Lee C-J, Hsieh M-L, Hsieh M-C. The effects of medical education from religious mission—examples of model "good teachings, as well as good mentors". 醫學教育. 2017;21(1):43–8.
42. Kao S-P, Tseng P-H, Chiang J-P, Chentao P-Y, Liu M-L, Hsieh M-L. Feasibility of veteran standardized patients as trainers of standardized patients. 醫學教育. 2020;24(2):86–92.
43. Kao S-P, Wang L-Y, Tseng P-H, Hsieh M-C, Chu S-Y. Feasibility of using standardized patients as examiners in an objective structured clinical examination (OSCE) of medical students. 醫學教育. 2021;25(1):8–15.
44. Smith CD, Sokoloff LP. SAGE documentary: red carpet event 2021 [Video Film]. Toronto, ON; 2021 [38:26 minutes]. https://www.youtube.com/watch?v=vshH6_9gzc8.
45. Smith C, Poerschke K, Bernick L, Kramer B, Meyer R, Adams M. Ruth's story: co-creating inclusive, authentic and engaging scenarios with simulated participants (SPs). Toronto: SimExpo; 2022.
46. Smith CM, Sokoloff LG, Alsaba N. Collaborative framework for working with older simulated participants (SP). BMJ Simul Technol Enhanc Learn. 2021;7(2):112.
47. Tzu Chi [Internet]. Hualien: Buddhist Compassion Relief Tzu Chi Foundation; 2023. https://www.tzuchi.org.tw/en/Hualien.
48. Gallimore C, George AK, Brown MC. Pharmacy students' preferences for various types of simulated patients. Am J Pharm Educ. 2008;72(1):04.
49. Collins J, Harden R. AMEE Medical Education Guide No. 13: real patients, simulated patients and simulators in clinical examinations. Med Teach. 1998;20(6):508–21.
50. Murphy S, Imam B, MacIntyre DL. Standardized patients versus volunteer patients for physical therapy students' interviewing practice: a pilot study. Physiother Can. 2015;67(4):378–84.

Embedding Simulation for the Care of Older Adults into Programs

11

Lou Clark, Holly Gerzina, and Tamara Owens

Key Messages

1. Use a model when initiating a geriatric simulation curriculum; consider the *Human Simulation Ethics & Best Practices Curriculum Design Model*. This model encourages readers to apply an ethical lens and best practices of SP methodology to prioritize safety for older adult SPs.
2. Embrace an iterative approach to safety in geriatric simulation curriculum design.
3. Include, value, and learn from the lived experiences of older adult SPs as relevant to the geriatric curriculum development process.
4. Understand that a collaborative approach by a geriatric curriculum development team that has inclusive membership with clearly noted roles and responsibilities will produce a higher quality simulation to benefit learners and ultimately older adult patients.
5. Use the *Checklist for Designing New Geriatric Simulation Curriculum* for guidance.

Overview

Embedding geriatric simulation into health professions' curriculum is imperative for the welfare and dignity of older adults as patients and people. To best support curricular efforts, educators must be prepared to collaborate with key partners, including SP Educators (SPEs) and other simulation professionals, clinician educators, geriatric specialists, and the older adult simulated participants/patients (SPs) who bring their lived experiences to the process.

This chapter provides practical advice on how to design and operationalize a simulation curriculum for health professions' learners that focuses on the care of older adults. The practical advice is anchored in our new *Human Simulation Ethics & Best Practices Curriculum Design Model* introduced in this chapter and the Collaborative Framework for working with older adult simulated participants (SPs) [1]. Our model contextualizes the traditional approach to simulation curriculum design within an ethical lens, applying best practices of SP methodology. Additionally, we take readers through a newly expanded seven-step framework for human simulation curriculum design [2], highlight older adult SP voices via narrative reflections, and feature a new, three-phase (pre-, real-time, and post-simulation) checklist for those designing, implementing, and evaluating geriatric curriculum with older adult SPs. Our goal is that these tools support readers in using best practices when embedding simulation for the care of older adults into their curriculum to prioritize safety for all involved, including the older adult SPs who bring this curriculum to life.

Introduction and Background

> I have found my work as an SP to be among the most meaningful work I have ever done. I am gratified to know I am helping students learn to be better communicators and practitioners, as well as helping their future patients receive better care… In my 14 years working here, I have moved from playing middle-aged roles to more senior ones. As the population itself ages, medical professionals who can provide geriatric care will be in great need. It is my privilege to allow them to practice on me for the betterment of healthcare provided to my peers as these students move forward in their careers.—Sid

SPs, including Sid, represent a growing international population of older adults in our simulation programs and in our

L. Clark (✉)
M Simulation, University of Minnesota, Minneapolis, MN, USA
e-mail: louclark@umn.edu

H. Gerzina
Wasson Center and Interprofessional Education Services, Northeast Ohio Medical University, Rootstown, OH, USA
e-mail: hgerzina@neomed.edu

T. Owens
Simulation and Clinical Skills Center, Interprofessional Education Committee, Howard University, Washington, DC, USA
e-mail: tlowens@howard.edu

C. M. Smith et al. (eds.), *Comprehensive Healthcare Simulation: Geriatric Simulation*, Comprehensive Healthcare Simulation,
https://doi.org/10.1007/978-3-031-65742-9_11

communities. Globally, people are living longer—well into their sixties and beyond. The World Health Organization states "By 2030, 1 in 6 people in the world will be aged 60 years or over" [3]. The growth in older adults is outpacing the health professionals specifically trained to treat this population. Predictions show that the medical field will experience a healthcare worker shortage, as a disproportionate number of physicians will retire in the next 10 years. The Association of American Medical Colleges' research indicates that by 2034, the United States will be short anywhere from 37,800 to 124,000 physicians [4]. This anticipated shortfall, in addition to adults living longer, provides a necessary opportunity to expand health professions' education curriculum.

In this chapter, we introduce the *Human Simulation Ethics & Best Practices Curriculum Design Model* (Fig. 11.1) and apply it to the design and implementation of geriatric simulation education curriculum for health profession students. This model prioritizes a new lens for this curricular work with SPs, grounded in the Healthcare Simulation Code of Ethics [5] and the Association of SP Educator (ASPE) Standards of Best Practices [6].

We intend for this conceptual model to expand the traditional logistical approach to human simulation curriculum design to one informed first by ethics as applied to human simulation and followed by best practices of SP methodology. As we guide you through the seven steps for curriculum design—(1) establish rationale, (2) build development team, (3) perform needs assessment, (4) develop case including learning objectives and case piloting/testing process, (5) recruit and train older adult SPs calibrating abilities and support resources informed by the pilot, (6) implement simulation, and (7) evaluate and gather feedback—our goal is to inspire readers to apply an ethical lens toward prioritizing safety for SPs. Safety—as a value and a practice—is the first of the five core domains of the ASPE Standards of Best Practices [6], which all collaborators should adopt when working with all SPs. This begins with considering SPs and their safety in each curriculum design step, because SPs literally bring the curriculum to life. If they do not feel confident and safe in doing so, the curriculum will suffer, as may the SPs themselves. Applying the tenets of this model tracked through each curriculum design step will support readers to create coherence, sequence, continuity, and integration

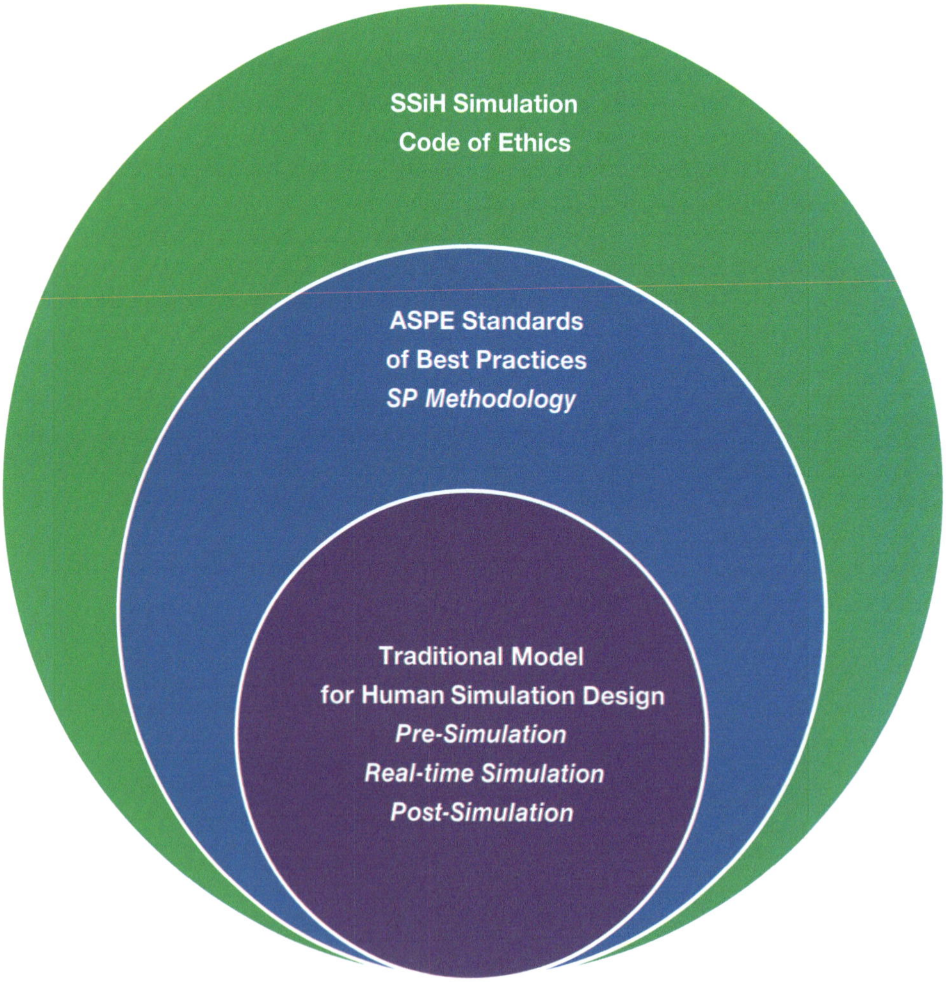

Fig. 11.1 Human simulation ethics & best practices curriculum design model

for the design and implementation of geriatric simulation education events [2] while necessarily prioritizing the safety of older adult SPs [7].

Checklist for Designing New Geriatric Simulation Curriculum

The following checklist for healthcare educators can be used when designing and implementing geriatric simulations with older adult SPs. During each of the three phases—pre-simulation, during, and post-simulation—considerations are proposed to enhance the differing cognitive, physical, and sensory abilities that may occur with older adult SPs. The *Checklist for Designing New Geriatric Simulation Curriculum* (Table 11.1) focuses on the three phases critical for optimal geriatric simulation curriculum design and delivery. These phases, as emphasized throughout the chapter, are framed with an ethical lens and with best practices of SP methodology as guiding principles.

Table 11.1 Checklist for designing new geriatric simulation curriculum

Seven-step curriculum design framework & associated tasks	Responsible key partner(s)	Ethics & SP methodology best practices questions & checks
Phase I: Pre-simulation *Time: 6–8 months before event*		
Establish **Rationale**:		
• Is this geriatric simulation needed in the curriculum?	• Curriculum expert(s) or course director.	• Consider the fact that older adult SPs will bring this curriculum to life if implemented. What initial concerns come to mind for older adult SP safety when doing this?
• How does it support learners to achieve curricular goals?	• This should be in collaboration with SPE input.	
Build **Development Team**:		
• What expertise is needed, and who is needed to design this curriculum?	• Curriculum expert(s) or course director. • SPE. • Older adult SPs. • Assessment expert (if applicable).	• Is the team diverse and inclusive of older adult perspectives, including SP perspectives since they will bring this curriculum to life?
Perform **Resource Needs Assessment**:		
• What resources (e.g. financial, human, time) are needed to design and implement this curriculum?	• Curriculum expert or course director. • Director of Simulation Program & SPE, (if not same person).	• How will utilizing these resources further geriatric curriculum and care? • How might expanding the simulation curriculum impact all involved (e.g. benefits, bandwidth)?
Develop **Case:**		
• SP Case Development is optimal as a collaborative and inclusive process. We recommend to have-at minimum-team members listed in the middle column.	• Curriculum expert(s) or course director.	• Did you include SPEs?
Tasks in this section below are underlined and include: Create Learning Objectives, Co-Author New Geriatric SP Case, Pilot New Geriatric SP Case, and Calibrate Abilities of Older Adult SPs and Resources Needed to Support Them.	• In collaboration with SPE. The SPE provides insight and expertise on applying best practices of SP Methodology to the Case Development process. • In collaboration with older adult SPs.	• Did you include older adult SP voices? • How did I approach inclusivity if SPEs and/or SPs are not available (e.g. community volunteers, individuals outside of the experts)?
Create ***Learning Objectives:***		
• Write learning objectives prior to co-authoring the SP case or proceeding with any further development work.	• Same development team members as listed above for *Develop* **Case**	• Is simulation the best methodology to achieve the learning objectives?*
• Learning objectives should be actionable items that trainees can achieve through engaging in the simulation.		• Are the objectives best achieved through human simulation, and specifically with a case designed to be portrayed by older adult SPs?*
• Each learning objective should be observable and measureable.		** If the answer to either of the above questions is "No", stop designing this simulation and advise your team as to why this is not the best approach. This will save resources including time and funds.*
• Write your learning objectives beginning with an action verb, (hint—this is a learning objective that begins with an action verb)!		

(continued)

Table 11.1 (continued)

Seven-step curriculum design framework & associated tasks	Responsible key partner(s)	Ethics & SP methodology best practices questions & checks
Co-Author ***New Geriatric SP Case:***		
• Include input and lived experiences from older adult SPs.	• Same development team members as listed above for *Develop* **Case**.	• How did I encourage and facilitate participation in the SP case development process from all development team members? (This includes practicalities like technology and font size, in addition to fostering inclusive spaces for all to express their thoughts and suggestions openly.
Pilot ***New Geriatric SP Case:***		
• Allows key partners to assess feasibility for older adult SPs, including any issues related to mobility, memory, vision, and hearing.	• Curricular expert/course director.	• How did the pilot simulation allow the learner(s) to achieve (or not achieve) the learning objectives created by the development team?
• It is also important to assess mental and emotional well-being when older adult SPs portray patients with age-related illnesses and issues.	• This should be in collaboration with SPE, and with input from lived experiences from older adult SPs.	• What worked well in terms of implementation for the older adult SP(s)?
	• SPs provide constructive feedback immediately after pilot encounter(s).	• What-if any-physical, emotional, cognitive challenges did the older adult SP(s) experience when bringing the simulation to life?
	• A debrief with all parties should immediately follow the pilot run.	
Calibrate **Abilities** *of Older Adult SPs and* **Resources** *Needed to Support Them:*		
Remember: calibrate, not underestimate!	• Ideally by SPE.	• What-if any-changes must occur for simulation implementation plan to ensure learning objectives may be achieved without compromising the physical, emotional, or cognitive well-being of the older adult SPs?
	• By other educator if SPE is not available.	
	• Learning from the pilot test run, SPEs should plan for needed time and other resources to support older adult SPs on the day of the geriatric simulation.	
Recruit & Train **SPs:**		
• Share case topic with older adult SPs and send SP case in advance, so they make an informed decision about whether or not to participate.	• Ideally led by SPE.	• How did I approach recruiting older adult SPs for from an ethical approach; assess comfort with age-related case material?
• At the start of the training, let the older adult SPs know that it is ok to excuse themselves at any point.	• Led by another educator if SPE is not available.	• How will I navigate any age-related feelings an older adult SP might experience in training that may manifest when working in simulated learner encounters?
• Set a moderate pace, taking care not to rush and build in assessment checks to confirm older adult SPs understand the material being presented.	• With active participation from older adult SPs.	• What training methods did I use to verify older adult SPs understood material without being patronizing to them?
• Include time to debrief the older adult SPs at the end of the training to check-in regarding their well-being.	• Course director and/or subject matter experts participate as needed.	• How did I prepare older adult SPs to provide verbal and/or written feedback to learners especially if they felt triggered in an encounter?
Phase 2: Real-time simulation		
Time: TDB based on timing of Phase 1 & number of learners		
Implement **Simulation**		
	• Simulation Operations team (e.g. space, technology, logistics).	• How did preparations in Phase 1 of this curriculum design process support the team in implementing the geriatric simulation prioritizing and upholding safety for all participants including the older adult SPs?
	• Curriculum experts orient, observe, and debrief learners; note that simulation professionals may collaborate on any/all of these tasks.	
	• Older adult SPs directly supported by SPEs.	

(continued)

Table 11.1 (continued)

Seven-step curriculum design framework & associated tasks	Responsible key partner(s)	Ethics & SP methodology best practices questions & checks
Phase 3: Post-simulation		
Time: TDB based on timing of Phase 2 & number of learners		
Conduct **Evaluation & Feedback**		
	• Learners evaluate the simulation ideally immediately following it.	• How was safety prioritized and upheld for both learners and older adult SPs participating in the geriatric simulation event?
	• Older adult SPs should evaluate their experience of both the SP training process and of participating in the simulation event itself; SPs should also participate in a facilitated debrief session with the SPE or another simulation team professional prior to departing from the geriatric simulation event as part of a well-being check.	• How did the simulation support learners to achieve, (or not) the learning objectives on caring for older adults?
	• Development team members should evaluate their experiences working independently and together, ideally having a post-simulation debrief session within the week following the event.	• What should the development team change for next time to improve the event?
	• Relevant feedback disseminated to learners including written feedback from the patient perspective authored by the older adult SPs.	• How did the participation of older adult SPs including their shared lived experiences benefit learners in this geriatric simulation event?

Phase 1: Pre-simulation

The pre-simulation phase includes five steps of the framework: (1) establishing the rationale, (2) building the development team, (3) performing a resources needs assessment, (4) developing the case, and (5) recruiting and training SPs.

Establish Rationale

The first step in the framework is to state the rationale for embedding geriatric simulation education events into your program's health professions' curriculum. As noted above, there will be a shortage of healthcare professionals trained to care for older adult populations in the next decade. Therefore, simulation education events may introduce learners to geriatric medicine/care of older adults, who may not have previously considered the specialty. Additionally, the rationale to use simulation as opposed to a lecture or observation is that students prefer an active approach to acquiring knowledge [8].

Importantly, geriatric simulation curriculum may reflect an interprofessional (IPE) or care team approach, namely, when providers from two or more health professions care for older adult patients in collaboration with one another. Simulation events designed for IPE learning teams enable healthcare trainees to practice associated core competencies critical for successful team-based care, including practicing team-based communication and fulfilling designated roles and responsibilities as part of the team [9]. This is needed as older adults are living longer with increasing rates of chronic conditions ideally managed by healthcare teams versus providers operating independently from one another.

Build Development Team

The second framework step is to build the development team of experts to design the simulation curriculum. Assembling an inclusive team will greatly assist with the curriculum development and integration. Course directors and curricular experts must be prepared to collaborate with key partners, which includes SP educators and other simulation professionals, clinician educators from various healthcare professions, and geriatric specialists. SPEs will be key partners in the process, so it is helpful to understand their role, which is defined as "those who work to develop expertise in SP methodology and are responsible for training and/or administering SP based simulation" [6]. As noted in the previous section, SPs offer critical voices on the development team because they bring lived experiences as older adults to this process.

For an IPE simulation program, key partners may include relevant faculty in medicine, nursing, social work, dentistry, nutrition and dietetics, occupational therapy, pharmacy, physical therapy, exercise science, paramedics, and other disciplines. Importantly, a geriatric IPE simulated encounter will optimally represent many health professions, even those not available to participate in the training. Patient progress notes can be provided for any profession with pertinent healthcare knowledge. SPEs, staff, and SPs collaborate with curricular experts from applicable professions to design and implement the simulation. When applying best practices, designing a simulation education event is an iterative team process and an inclusive one.

Through their lived experiences, older adult SPs hold the potential to be valuable collaborators in developing robust geriatric simulation education design. Taking an ethical lens to this process necessitates that we consider older adult SPs as curricular experts along with healthcare faculty and other key partners. This is because—as older adults themselves—they best understand emotional, physical, and psychological safety needs when bringing geriatric curriculum to life. While authentic and realistic scenarios can support learners' perspectives on engaging and preserving the welfare and dignity of older adults as patients and people, this should not come at the expense of older adult SPs [7].

Actively including older adult SP voices in curriculum design holds the power to improve the authenticity of the simulation while simultaneously attending to safety concerns. For example, while simulated scenarios about dementia and falls may be excellent learning experiences for healthcare trainees, including SP voices in the development process can foster agency in advance of the SPs portraying these vulnerable patients. At minimum, including older adult SP voices in this process may serve to acknowledge that the simulated scenarios they portray may be challenging for them—even if they themselves are not experiencing the actual illnesses. Beyond an acknowledgment, including older SP adults as collaborators may prevent or mitigate triggering negative feelings they may encounter due to any lived experiences—their own or a loved ones—with these health issues. In this way, older adult SPs are ethically and actively valued as vital contributors in the geriatric curriculum design process from the beginning, heightening the positive outcomes for learners. As older adult SP Sid notes, she is aware that SP work is critical as our global population ages. Including voices like Sid's in the curriculum design process may heighten positive outcomes for healthcare trainees while also prioritizing and attending to older adult SP safety concerns and needs.

In the reflection below, SP Rhea demonstrates the power of curriculum design when it is inclusive. Her perspective as the spouse in this scenario highlights how the patient's condition influences the whole family:

> I've participated as a 'spouse' whose husband had a stroke with resultant aphasia. This included two sessions, three months apart. It was a wonderful opportunity for students to interact with a family member over an extended period of time, particularly as the husband's status changed over the first 90 days after the stroke. As the spouse, I became increasingly concerned about how I was going to manage taking care of my husband. I enjoyed this case because it simulated common family issues and not just patient issues.—Rhea

Rhea's reflection ends by touching on the power of a geriatric simulation curriculum to include family member caregivers and loved ones in addition to patient care issues. In this way, educators may listen to and incorporate humanistic and social elements into writing simulation cases while learning directly from older adult SPs as to what is logistically feasible for them emotionally, mentally, and physically [1]. Chances are that without SP input, educators who are not older adults may inadvertently over- or underestimate the abilities of the SPs.

Perform Resources Needs Assessment

The third of the seven-step framework is to perform a needs assessment to identify existing and needed resources for your geriatric simulation event. Numerous resources already exist for the general design and operation of human simulation curriculum, and educators should use these as a foundation to develop and implement SP education events for the care of older adults. Key resources for SP case development, SP training, and SP methodology include the following:

- The Association of SP Educators (ASPE) website at https://www.aspeducators.org/ [10]
- The ASPE Case Development template found on the ASPE website [10]
- The ASPE Standards of Best Practices publication found on the ASPE website [6]
- The book *Comprehensive Healthcare Simulation: Implementing Best Practices in Standardized Patient Methodology* [11]
- The book *Defining Excellence in Simulation Programs*, Chap. 3 Standardized Patients [2]

The above resources will provide practical guidance and "how to" approaches on best practices for designing and implementing human simulation curriculum with SPs.

Next, the development team should examine other resources such as their SP pool, training time, staff support, and budget. First, investigate the most important and accessible resources you have which are the older adult SPs working with your program. It is recommended to directly invite older adult SPs to participate in the needs assessment process. This will save time later as involving older adult SPs from the beginning allows for feedback as to whether the vision for the geriatric curriculum is feasible for them to implement. It is better to do this early on rather than invest time and resources into developing curriculum that is not feasible. In addition, there is great joy in working with SPs and appreciating the unique backgrounds and experience that they bring to the work. This may also be helpful—and even inspiring—when designing geriatric simulation curriculum.

Interestingly, for an IPE SP case, the older adult patient and an older adult caregiver may both be present as simulated patient and simulated participant when presenting to the IPE healthcare team. To clarify, this case would require two SPs—one as the simulated patient while the second SP as a spouse, sibling, or adult child. If resources are not available and it becomes cost prohibitive to have both a simulated patient and a simulated participant, the development team may choose to write the case for one SP who shares knowledge about the other role. For example, an adult child could share their concerns about the patient, or the patient could share that their adult child has concerns about them. Additionally, having one to two SPs simultaneously interviewed by multiple health professions learners can streamline event logistics, provide the opportunity to cost share across programs with limited resources, and align the goals and objectives of the development team for each profession's roles and responsibilities as well as for team competencies in a geriatric curriculum.

The curriculum development team should also assess the unique training needs for a geriatric simulation. Older adults often enjoy fellowshipping and sharing lived experiences. It is optimal to create an SP training agenda that is flexible and includes open discussion time. It is best for SPEs not to rush the rich discussions that often add to how the older adult SPs process and internalize their role in the simulation. In addition, it is important to understand the technological acumen needed for older adult SPs to participate so that you can address the technology needs for an onsite or online simulation. Technology is just one example of how underestimating the abilities of older adult SPs may have unwanted influence on curricular programming. While some older adult SPs struggle with technological advances, many are adept at navigating this terrain—as we witnessed in the pandemic.

A key to the success of older adult SPs working successfully with technology is support. This may include a tech-savvy proctor, staff, SPE, or faculty facilitator on the simulation event day. However, prior to the actual training event, this support often begins with the SPE conducting a technology assessment as part of SP training. In the pandemic, SPEs at the first author's workplace routinely performed technology assessments with all SPs working remotely. They found that the older adult SPs were motivated to master the technology needed to work. While some older adult SPs did not need additional coaching, others did need further coaching. A key takeaway from this experience is that it is critical not to underestimate additional time that may be required for older adult SPs to learn new information or skills.

The development team must also assess the need for staff support essential for implementation of the geriatric simulation education event. As stated earlier, it is important to include the SPE as an expert on the development team as the professional versed in best practices of human simulation/SP methodology. SPEs are experts in coaching SPs to portray older adult patients in ways that provide students with opportunities to achieve the case learning objectives. This requires that SPEs intentionally coach older adults on case content details, on how to provide constructive verbal feedback, and on nuances of any needed technology. Lesser-resourced programs with fewer staff may experience challenges in providing this type of 1:1 coaching support.

Lastly, included in the needs assessment is the budget. The budget should reflect all issues discussed in this chapter. The development team should itemize all costs for an optimal simulation. Budget program considerations depend on varying resources. Specific line items in this budget should include (but are not limited to) pay/compensation for older adult SPs to complete both a training session and the simulation event(s), space rental (if applicable), any associated equipment costs, audiovisual recording costs, consultancy costs (if applicable), and disposable items (paper drapes, table paper, tissues, etc.).

Another key item to discuss in relation to the budget is time for older adult SPs to provide feedback to learners immediately following simulated patient-provider encounters. Older adult SPs may have a different perspective of the interaction that allows them to provide authentic feedback based on their age and lived experience. When students hear their experiences through constructive verbal feedback sessions, this provides them opportunities to respond with compassionate communication. SP Linda shares an example:

> It is gratifying to portray a caregiver of an elderly partner or the grandmother of a dying child as I know these situations are common and health professionals need to be comfortable with them. The students really appreciate the practice and feedback from us as SPs.—Linda

As SP Linda emphasizes, learners appreciate verbal feedback from SPs, which is likely because they receive a gauge on their performance in real time. SP verbal feedback to learners may be especially helpful if the faculty-to-student ratio is large. In this way, SPs may act in the role of faculty extenders, especially if they are trained to provide focused feedback that reinforces the learning objectives.

Develop the Case

After conducting a needs assessment to determine whether any simulation event is truly required to achieve curricular or professional goals, the next step is to develop the case. This should always begin by creating learning objectives on which to base the simulation curriculum. The development team should use a collaborative approach in which curricular experts work side by side with SPEs. The learning objectives should state what the students should be able to do or perform following the simulation. This "establishes measurable learning objectives" [2], meaning raters can assess whether learners are able to achieve each learning objective. To create the learning objectives for a geriatric simulation, the development team must revisit the rationale for the educational event and align the simulation objectives with the overall health professions program objectives.

Once the team creates learning objectives, the next part of this process is to co-author a draft of the new case. It is critical to involve the voices of older adult SPs in this process so that they may contribute lived experience; they will be the ones bringing this curriculum to life with their own bodies, so they will be the ones most apt to identify safety concerns. Additionally, oftentimes the development team includes mostly or only clinicians, and so it is important to include older adult SPs who do not possess clinical knowledge. This is because their lived experiences, perspectives on healthcare, and associated concerns and worries are most reflective of the majority of the patient population, namely, those who do not possess formal clinical training or knowledge.

Following completion of an advanced draft of the new case, the development team should pilot or test the new case. This is to determine if revisions are needed to optimize the case for the intended learner group so that the development team can ensure that the learners may achieve the newly created learning objectives. When piloting a new geriatric case, it is important to recruit an older adult SP who is comfortable with improvising, as this is often needed in the pilot process. This SP should be comfortable providing feedback about the case and willing to replay the case with different variations as needed. Additionally, the team will need to identify an individual willing to act as the learner. Ideally, this is a person who is similar to the learner group but slightly more experienced—perhaps already having been at the time point in the curriculum for which this case is indicated. For example, it often works to have a fourth-year medical student helping to pilot cases intended for earlier placement in the medical school curriculum. As the team tries different variations of the case, it is important to pause and reflect on what is working and what needs revising. During this process, it is critical to actively solicit feedback from the older adult SP, to maximize their contributory potential. Actively soliciting the perspective of the older adult SPs in the case piloting process will ensure a smoother, more efficient, and more effective new case from this point forward. This is critical, as resources, including time and funding, are often limited as the team moves closer to implementation.

Recruit and Train Older Adult SPs

Given that there is ample and relevant content on this topic covered in other chapters of this book (see Chaps. 4, 6, and 9 for further information), we will not spend much time on this topic here. The most critical component to emphasize in this chapter is that any needs or concerns identified by older adult SPs as part of the case piloting process should be identified and accounted for in advance of and during any subsequent SP training sessions. This will help ensure that older adult SPs recruited to portray new cases receive needed support, including ample time and resources, in order to participate fully and successfully in the SP training process. SPEs should lead the SP training session with other key partners, including faculty, participating as needed. Most importantly, SPEs and any other key partners must regard an SP's physical, psychological, and emotional safety as paramount during SP training in addition to the simulation event itself.

Phase 2: Real-Time Simulation

The sixth step of the seven-step framework is to create a plan for the real-time implementation of the new geriatric simulation. During the needs assessment step, the development team should determine where in the health professions' curriculum the geriatric simulation event would be embedded. This information will inform the implementation plan.

Implement Simulation

Based on this timeline, the SPE (implementation lead) and other simulation professionals should meet to discuss the event and devise the implementation plan. The plan should include the following:

- Simulation activity setup time allocation
- Simulation activity start and end timing
- SP arrival time
- Plan for backup/understudy SP in case an SP unexpectedly cannot attend this event (critical as this often happens with SPs of any age)
- SP orientation timing and content (often led by the SPE)
- Learner orientation timing and content (which may be led by subject matter expert or another member of the simulation team)
- Student/SP encounter timing
- Student post encounter activity (writeup, reflection, etc.) time length
- Logistics for SP assessment of learners (if needed)
- SP constructive verbal feedback to learners (if indicated as activity component)
- Learner debriefing session with faculty, which often includes a simulation professional facilitating
- SP debriefing session
- Transition time between SP encounters and other event components (e.g. debriefing)

- Breaks (recommended for all, including the older adult SPs)
- Simulation activity breakdown time allocation

The simulation team should consider the number of learners for the event to determine the number of iterations of encounters needed. This usually depends on available spaces for individual SP-learner encounters. Once the implementation plan for the simulation is developed, we recommend that it is distributed to the team for clear communication during the real-time simulation.

Phase 3: Post-simulation

The final step for embedding older adult simulation into programs and curriculum is to evaluate and measure success of the new simulation case implemented based on iterative feedback from all key partners.

Evaluation and Feedback

Many simulation center teams gather partial information from universal evaluation forms used for simulation events within their centers. These forms often ask for the level of learner as well as any related clinical experiences. Evaluation questions to consider include those about learning success, knowledge gains, workshop organization, and effectiveness of teaching—as well as change in attitude of teamwork and communication. Importantly, we recommend asking a question pertaining to the learning impact of this new case as one that involved the learner working with an older adult SP. Additionally, if the event involved an interprofessional training experience, one may ask about intent to practice collaboratively soon [12]. Curricular experts and faculty facilitators may provide anecdotal feedback regarding organization of workshop, challenges with learners, and challenges with technology.

Similarly, SPs can provide general feedback regarding training, active role portrayal, and feedback sessions to students as well as team members. Older adult SPs may provide feedback on the feasibility of their participation in the simulation regarding any physical, emotional, or cognitive challenges they may have experienced during the simulation. [See Chap. 7 for further information on program evaluation.] It is of the utmost importance that SPEs debrief the SPs just as curricular experts debrief learners. For SPEs, the SPs are also learners, and it is critical that they depart from the workplace feeling heard and seen especially in the event of any triggering encounters (for age-related or other reasons).

Summary

I started my work as an SP over 15 years ago to show gratitude to a Geriatric Clinic that was helping care for my parents, and the residents had participated with SPs. I'm so appreciative that not only did I give back for my parents, I am still involved as an SP, and now as a more senior SP and a Baby Boomer! I'm interacting with the students, helping them with their communication and physical skills to reduce patient risk in a clinical and hospital setting. And now, helping with geriatric education for me and other Baby Boomers is so rewarding! I'm also seeing more different ethnicities involved in the SP program and I'm pleased to still be involved assisting preparing the students for their future patients!—Elaine

Our aim in this chapter was to provide a starting point on which simulation educators and other key partners can build geriatric simulation curriculum together. Critical to this process is working ethically and safely with older adult SPs who value this work and put their trust and bodies literally in our hands. It is our job to uphold that trust while collaborating with them to advance healthcare sciences training that will ensure optimal care for our ever-increasing population of older adults.

Acknowledgments Profound thanks to the talented older adult SPs who work as part of the M Simulation SP Program at the University of Minnesota, who provided the narrative reflections that are included in this chapter.

References

1. Smith CM, Sokoloff LG, Alsaba N. Collaborative framework for working with older simulated participants (SP). BMJ Simul Technol Enhanc Learn. 2021;7(2):112.
2. Owens T, Gliva G. Standardized patients. In: Palaganas J, Maxworthy J, Epps C, Mancini M, editors. Defining excellence in simulation programs. Philadelphia: Wolters Kluwer; 2014. p. 199–212.
3. World Health Organization. Aging and health. 2023. https://www.who.int/news-room/fact-sheets/detail/ageing-and-health.
4. Association of American Medical Colleges. AAMC report reinforces mounting physician shortage. 2021.
5. Park CS, Murphy TF. The Code of Ethics Working Group. Healthcare simulation code of ethics [Internet]. https://www.ssih.org/SSH-Resources/Code-of-Ethics. Accessed 3 Mar 2023.
6. Lewis KL, Bohnert CA, Gammon WL, Hölzer H, Lyman L, Smith C, Thompson TM, Wallace A, Gliva-McConvey G. The association of standardized patient educators (ASPE) standards of best practice (SOBP). Adv Simul. 2017;2(1):1–8.
7. Clark L, Woll A, Owens TL, Shropshire D, Kiser B, Gephardt G, Park CS. SP safety, autonomy and healthcare simulation practice in the COVID-19 era. BMJ Simul Technol Enhanc Learn. 2021;7(5):450.
8. Reime MH, Johnsgaard T, Kvam FI, et al. Learning by viewing versus learning by doing: a comparative study of observer and participant experiences during an interprofessional simulation training. J Interprof Care. 2017;31:51–8.

9. Interprofessional Education Collaborative. https://www.ipecollaborative.org/ipec-core-competencies. Accessed 27 Mar 2023.
10. Association of SP Educators. https://www.aspeducators.org/. Accessed 31 Jan 2023.
11. Gliva-McConvey G, Nicholas CF, Clark L, editors. Comprehensive healthcare simulation: implementing best practices in standardized patient methodology. Cham: Springer; 2020.
12. Berger S, Mahler C, Krug K, Szecsenyi J, Schultz J. Evaluation of interprofessional education: lessons learned through the development and implementation of an interprofessional seminar on team communication for undergraduate health care students in Heidelberg—a project report. GMS J Med Educ. 2016;33(2):Doc22. https://doi.org/10.3205/zma001021.

Faculty Reflections: Supporting Older Adult Simulated Participants in Giving Feedback

12

Carol Fleishman and Tanya Tierney

Key Messages

1. Feedback from the SP's perspective provides valuable insight for the learner about how the patient felt during the interaction.
2. Older adult SPs' diverse life experiences may translate into wisdom that can enhance the feedback they offer and bridge the age gap between learner and SP.
3. Older adult SPs may have physical, cognitive, or sensory changes that result in the need for specific training or support during the session.
4. Each older adult SP's needs will be different and may shift with time, so regular one-to-one conversations are important.

Introduction

One of the key benefits of using simulation is the opportunity for learners to receive feedback from multiple perspectives. This may include others involved in the simulation (simulated participants {SP} and peers) as well as those observing the simulation (facilitator and peers). Each perspective brings different insights for the learners. Even though the facilitator is likely to bring valuable, subject-specific knowledge, as an observer, their perspective may differ from those who were immersed in the simulation.

In particular, the SP, as a participant of the simulation, has a unique viewpoint. While observers of the simulation (facilitator and peers) can provide feedback about behaviours and demonstration of learner's skills, only the SP has a felt sense of the impact of those behaviours and skills on the person the SP was portraying. When the feedback from the SP captures these nuances, it can have profound impact on the learner in understanding how their behaviour effects the people with whom they are interacting.

Feedback can take both verbal and written forms and may be structured differently depending on the purpose of the simulation (e.g., formative vs. summative, dyadic consultation vs. a group activity, conversation only vs. physical exam vs. hybrid simulation vs. high fidelity simulation). This chapter focusses more on feedback offered in the context of a simulated consultation; however, these principles can be applied in other contexts.

Table 12.1 summarises some general guidelines for SP feedback. On the right-hand side, we included some description and considerations when working with SPs. We kept this detail brief (as more detailed guidelines for the delivery of feedback in general can be found elsewhere). Our intention is to highlight areas that may invite additional attention when working with older adult SPs. Some of the points raised in Table 12.1 are elaborated on later in the chapter.

C. Fleishman (✉)
Johns Hopkins Medicine Simulation Center, Johns Hopkins Medicine, Baltimore, MD, USA
e-mail: cfleish2@jhmi.edu

T. Tierney
Lee Kong Chian School of Medicine, Nanyang Technological University, Singapore, Singapore
e-mail: tanyatierney@ntu.edu.sg

C. M. Smith et al. (eds.), *Comprehensive Healthcare Simulation: Geriatric Simulation*, Comprehensive Healthcare Simulation,
https://doi.org/10.1007/978-3-031-65742-9_12

Table 12.1 Feedback guidelines

Guideline	Some thoughts
Offered at the right time	Usually soon after the event, after a brief pause for participants to collect their thoughts.
Provides balance	Addresses both what the learner is doing well (and is encouraged to retain) and what was done less well, with suggestions for improvement (for self-reflection). A structured model (e.g. Pendleton [1]) can provide a format for SPs to follow.
Describes SPs' experience of the event	SPs have the unique perspective of knowing what it felt like to be directly engaged with the learner. When SPs express how the patient felt, their feedback can prompt the learner to have a better understanding of patients.
Describes behaviours, not personal characteristics	It is important to focus on what the learner did (behaviours) and avoid reference to personal characteristics (as these cannot be changed).
Takes the feelings of the learner into account	If not carefully worded and feels like criticism, feedback can be met with resistance or cause distress to learners.
Has a familiar structure	SPs often find it helpful to have a "template" to phrase their feedback, e.g. "When you …, I felt…". This can help them remember to include the behaviour of the learner and their feelings in their feedback.
Connected with learning outcomes as provided by faculty	Having the feedback focussed on the learning outcomes of the activity allows for a more effective discussion for achieving the educational goals of the curriculum.

Opportunities and Challenges

An older adult SP brings a wealth of complex and interrelated life experiences, which can enhance or detract from the effectiveness of their feedback. One aspect of these experiences is their health as an older person. A younger learner may struggle to imagine what it may be like to grow older. Learners need to understand the impact of illness for all patients, but with older adult patients who may have multiple medical conditions on top of the natural process of aging, it can provide more for the learner to appreciate. If applicable to the learning outcomes, this complexity of health issues can be discussed by the SP during feedback, providing the learner with their perspective about how the learner interacted with the patient, assisting them in bridging the age gap when working with older adult patients.

Secondly, they bring professional experiences. While some older adult SPs may have engaged in SP work for a long time, others may take up SP work later in life. People who move into SP work after retiring from other careers may bring diverse transferable skills to the SP community. Some may have worked in healthcare or education and can directly apply their knowledge to their delivery of feedback. Understanding some principles of education and/or the culture of healthcare can allow the SP to word their feedback in ways that align with medical education theory. Those with experience in the corporate sector may also bring relevant transferable skills that underpin their feedback delivery. On the other hand, awareness of changes in workplace culture and theory over time is needed. Workplaces, education, and healthcare have moved towards more person-centred practices (including feedback delivery), so SPs who have a long history in the workplace may benefit from support to align their approaches with current practice.

For SPs who retired from a healthcare setting and chose to contribute to medical education, their understanding of healthcare can be valuable as they understand what is expected of learners. They can frame their feedback with this understanding in mind. On the other hand, SPs with a history of working in healthcare may need to put aside their own preconceptions as their healthcare experience may differ from the learner's context. In addition, there may be difficulty in setting aside the clinical lens to ensure the feedback they provide is from a patient perspective.

Thirdly, the wording and tone used by SPs in their feedback may also be shaped by their personal life experiences. They may be parents or even grandparents, and their own parental relationships may influence their interactions with learners (e.g., if the learner is of similar age to their own children). The SP may come across as nurturing in the delivery of their feedback, which can create a helpful learning environment. On the other hand, strong feelings about how a younger person should act could result in the SP coming across as more "paternalistic," so care should be taken to manage this. Some older adult SPs may be parents to healthcare professionals and this perspective can also influence their feedback. They may bring a level of empathy for clinicians that can enhance their feedback. Conversely, some may need to take care not to compare each learner with their own family member who works in a clinical setting.

Older adult SPs are also likely to have had more interactions as recipients of healthcare; in fact, many are inspired to start working as an SP by their own experiences as patients or caregivers. While some are inspired by positive experiences, it is unfortunate that a significant number choose to explore SP work after negative experiences in healthcare and may feel motivated to "improve the system". Whichever the motivation, it is important for the feedback process to allow the SP to focus on what happened in the current simulation and on their feedback to the learner(s) involved. Any residual feelings about their own interactions with healthcare need to be put aside, so it does not influence the feedback to the learner.

Summarising, there is a complex interconnection of life experiences that older adult SPs bring to their feedback: health, professional, and family life. They have a unique lens through which they see their experiences of portraying older adults who are interacting with learners.

Impact of Aging on SPs

The natural process of aging results in changes that may impact the ability of SPs to provide feedback. For example, SPs may experience decline in working memory, cognitive function, or comfort with technology [2].

The ability to give detailed, learner-centred feedback requires the SP to recall in detail what happened during the interaction. During the roleplay, the SP needs to pay attention to their portrayal while also taking mental note of what is happening between the patient and the learner to provide feedback later. These parallel processes require close attention and can take a lot of "bandwidth". If the SP is experiencing any decline in working memory or cognitive function due to increasing age, this process becomes more difficult. If more attention is needed to remember the details of the scenario and manage the portrayal, the "bandwidth" left to pay attention and inform the feedback can be reduced, and hence SPs may start to struggle with providing detailed and nuanced feedback. To ensure enough "bandwidth" is left to take note of what is happening and inform feedback, the SP may need to spend more time preparing for the scenario and practising feedback specific to the learning outcomes. The more instinctive the portrayal is, the easier it becomes for the SP to balance their attention between the two processes.

It is worth considering the session flow to allow time and space for preparing feedback. For example, it is a good practice to have a brief pause after the simulation/role-play for the participants (learners and SPs) and observers to gather their thoughts. During this time, the SP can de-role and prepare their feedback. Most SPs find it helpful to write a few notes to help the structure their verbal feedback. This may be on a designated written feedback form, or it may simply be unstructured notes for their own reference. If resources are available, the older adult SPs could have a partner who is observing and who can take notes and assist the SP in preparing their feedback.

The mental space given in the session for verbal feedback is important. If a facilitator is involved while feedback is being offered, they may need to give a little more time, so the older adult SP does not feel rushed. If the SP's feedback is brief or lacks a required component, the facilitator's prompts can be helpful. For example, if SPs are encouraged to link how the learner's behaviour impacted the emotions of the patient, a facilitator can encourage elaboration, as presented in Table 12.2.

Table 12.2 Facilitator prompts for improving SP feedback

Example 1
SP "It was good that you said you could see it was hard for me when I told you my daughter was leaving home."
Facilitator "Yes, I thought that was a helpful empathic statement. Could you tell Robert a little more about how you felt when he said that?"
SP "Since my husband died, it has been just me and my daughter at home. With her going to university I worry about how I will cope. Robert, when you acknowledged how hard that is for me, I really felt heard and supported. It meant a lot to me that you realised that managing my illness while living alone is going to be a challenge."
Example 2
SP "I felt really comfortable sharing my worries with you."
Facilitator "That's lovely. Could you explain to Grace what she did that helped you to feel comfortable?"
SP "Oh yes. I think it was the way you softened your tone of voice when you saw I was worried. You pulled your chair in a little closer and gave space and time for me to explain what I was worried about."

The additional scaffolding provided by the facilitators in the examples contained in Table 12.2 can help the SP structure their feedback and offer enough detail to the learners about their performance.

When the session involves written feedback, some older adult SPs may need adaptations to enhance accessibility. Older adult SPs may prefer using pen and paper over electronic technology. If pen and paper is used, the environment needs to be considered. For example, is there a place to store the paper during the encounter and easily accessed when needed, and a table or surface to use while completing the paper? Physical changes with age may make it uncomfortable to write in a less ergonomically setup environment. If SPs have any decline in their visual acuity, another way that may assist them is to increase the font size of the document being used.

With increasing use of digital platforms, however, written feedback may be captured on electronic devices rather than on paper. Older adult SPs may be less familiar with using digital platforms and need more support [3]. In addition, the COVID-19 pandemic has driven a shift towards fully remote sessions. Despite the return to in-person sessions, telemedicine remains a significant feature of medicine, and as such a proportion of sessions still take place online. It is worth noting here that if the SP finds providing written feedback by digital means more difficult, it may also be true that support is harder to access in remote sessions. The example case study shown in Box 12.1 highlights why older adult SPs, who are more likely to need support with technology, may find providing written feedback during a remote session more challenging.

Box 12.1 Technical Challenges with Documenting Feedback: Case Study

At one medical school, the written feedback form used during communication skills teaching is delivered via a digital platform. The platform can be accessed via an iPhone or iPad app, or a web browser. During in-person teaching sessions, SPs are issued iPads. The app is already downloaded, open, and the role-account user is logged in. The correct form is bookmarked under "favourites," so it is immediately obvious which form to complete. During the session, if an SP has difficulties, they can ask for assistance from the facilitator or even from the learner (e.g. if the SP cannot find the learner's name on the list). In addition, administrators who are overseeing the session are on-hand to help with technical difficulties.

During the COVID-19 pandemic, all communication skills teaching was online using Zoom. To participate in the sessions, SPs needed to have the appropriate technology to participate (a device to access Zoom with good internet access, plus a second device to access the feedback form). The SPs needed to download the app on their own device and be able to follow the instructions to locate the appropriate form, identify the learner, and be able to complete the feedback form while at home. Support was provided via WhatsApp. The need to manage the technology from home with less support created significant difficulty for many older adult SPs.

Training and Support

These opportunities and challenges can be kept in mind when planning training and support for older adult SPs. For example, preserving additional time for self-introductions at the beginning of a group training allows for diverse life experiences to emerge. This can be insightful for the SP educator and for the SPs. As well as the immediate benefit of community building, skillful facilitation can also highlight how each SP's context brings wisdom to the feedback they can offer. Keeping the schedule more spacious in general is a good practice when working with older people. This allows more time for on-topic discussions, as well as community building during the breaks. Additional time during training is also helpful for reviewing and practising aspects of the case content and digital platforms older adult SPs may find more difficult.

Some older adult SPs who work for multiple programs, or for different projects within a program, may find they are needing to learn a variety of feedback protocols. SP educators should review how feedback is handled at their location and for their project just before an activity starts and, if feasible, have a summary of the protocol on the feedback form.

And lastly, it is important not to generalise or make assumptions. Each SP will bring different strengths and weaknesses, so taking time to understand what additional training and/or support each SP requires is important. These conversations should take place periodically, as additional difficulties may emerge or increase with time, as SPs age.

Closing

In this chapter, we explored the opportunities and challenges for older adult SPs providing feedback to learners. We highlighted points to consider when planning training and support for older adult SPs providing feedback.

References

1. Pendleton D, et al. Implementation of the approach to teaching and learning. In: The new consultation: developing doctor-patient communication. Oxford: Oxford Academic; 2003. p. 120–9. https://doi.org/10.1093/med/9780192632883.003.0011.
2. Smith CM, Sokoloff LG, Alsaba N. Collaborative framework for working with older simulated participants (SP). BMJ Simul Technol Enhanc Learn. 2020;7(2):112–5. https://doi.org/10.1136/bmjstel-2020-000613.
3. Czaja SJ, Charness N, Rogers WA, Sharit J. Factors predicting the use of technology: findings from the Center for Research and Education on Aging and Technology Enhancement (CREATE). Psychol Aging. 2006;21(2):333–52.

13 Innovations in Older Adult Simulated Participant Methodology

Lisa Guttman Sokoloff, Jordan Holmes, and Lisa Krinsky

Key Messages

1. Technology is a good way to introduce innovation in simulation. Using technology can enhance knowledge transfer and reach a wider audience.
2. Behavioural skills can be addressed in unique ways (e.g. VR, embedded interactive reflective videos) that promote everyone's safety and allow learners to experience situations they may not otherwise encounter; this is especially relevant when training deescalation of behaviours seen in people living with dementia that could be dangerous for SPs or learners to practise in person. Potentially sensitive topics can also be addressed through these simulation modalities.
3. Filming interactive reflective videos allows for consideration of older adult SPs' needs (e.g. breaks between takes, filming in short chunks to reduce cognitive or physical load).
4. Collaboration and partnership are invaluable when being innovative; each person/group can bring their specialised knowledge to the table.
5. When selecting new simulation methods and technologies, careful attention must be paid to aligning the learning objectives with the capabilities and strengths of the methods.

L. G. Sokoloff (✉)
Faculty of Applied Health and Community Studies, Sheridan College, Brampton, ON, Canada

Department of Speech Pathology, Temerty Faculty of Medicine, University of Toronto, Toronto, ON, Canada
e-mail: lisa.sokoloff@sheridancollege.ca

J. Holmes
Centre for Teaching Support & Innovation, University of Toronto, Toronto, ON, Canada
e-mail: jordan.holmes@utoronto.ca

L. Krinsky
LGBTQIA+ Aging Project, The Fenway Institute, Boston, MA, USA
e-mail: LKrinsky@fenwayhealth.org

Introduction

Simulation itself can be considered "innovative" or "non-traditional" especially in healthcare education [1] despite introduction of mannikins for CPR practice in over 60 years ago [2]. The use of technology, mannikins and live interactions to practice skills is constantly growing and developing. Simulation innovations tend to parallel advances in technology such as wearable simulators or hybrid simulation [3], augmented, virtual and mixed reality (AR/VR/MR) [4], three-dimensional printers [5], etc. Simulation educators, however, should still use best practices, standards and guiding principles [6, 7] to choose which form or modality of simulation, if any, is most appropriate for their situation and not just choose something because it is "cool" or "cutting edge".

This chapter will introduce different and innovative modes and methods for simulation related to the care of older adults through two examples of innovative simulation modalities—virtual reality (VR) and embedded interactive reflective videos—that allow learners to experience scenarios and situations they might not otherwise encounter.

In caring for older adults, there are often times when situations arise that are uncomfortable, unfamiliar and/or dangerous. This may include caring for someone against whom you have bias (conscious or unconscious) because of their sexual orientation or gender identity based on your own personal beliefs and/or lack of exposure to this group. It may also include working with a client who has dementia or other mental health issues that can result in aggressive behaviours. By using VR or embedded interactive reflective videos that are carefully crafted to highlight specific topics, learners can be exposed to scenarios in a way that is both physically and psychologically safe. Another benefit of utilising technology is that it allows for greater spread and scalability.

C. M. Smith et al. (eds.), *Comprehensive Healthcare Simulation: Geriatric Simulation*, Comprehensive Healthcare Simulation,
https://doi.org/10.1007/978-3-031-65742-9_13

Case Examples

Embedded Interactive Reflective Videos

The LGBTQIA+ Aging Project, a program of the Fenway Institute at Fenway Health in Boston, MA, USA, works towards equity, inclusion and community for lesbian, gay, bisexual, transgender, queer/questioning, intersex and asexual older adults, ensuring that they can age with the dignity and respect they deserve. (Note: language regarding sexual orientation and gender identity continues to evolve and varies widely. The LGBT Aging Project became the LGBTQIA+ Aging Project in 2021 after the production of their training module; for the purpose of this chapter, we will use LGBTQ.)

In 2019, the Aging Project developed *LGBT Aging in Massachusetts*, a 1-hour interactive online eLearning module to fulfil Massachusetts' first in the nation legislation mandating that the state's network of elder care providers complete LGBTQ cultural competency training. Massachusetts' elder care network is broad and includes community-based services, in-home care, residential settings (assisted living, long-term care) and more. This training ensures that regardless of where an older adult lives in Massachusetts, they have access to providers with a basic foundation of knowledge regarding LGBTQ older adults.

LGBTQ Case Scenarios

LGBT Aging in Massachusetts is comprised of didactic learning about sexual orientation and gender identity and expression, understanding of LGBTQ history, stigma and resilience, best practices for individuals and organisations and next steps. Case scenarios included throughout the eLearning module are based on real situations encountered by LGBTQ older adults and caregivers.

Themes of the Scenarios

- Home care: A gay man reporting to a case manager about homophobic verbal abuse from his home care worker
- Senior Centre: A lesbian coming out to a senior Centre staff member
- Nursing home: Nursing home staff preparing to welcome their first transgender patient
- Interview questions: Staff asking sexual orientation and gender identity questions of older adults as part of the demographic questions in their standard assessment
- Personal beliefs: Home health aides navigating their personal beliefs and professional standards of care
- Home visit: Authentic ways to be LGBTQ inclusive during a home visit
- Assisted living: Using welcoming and inclusive language when LGBTQ people seek assisted living communities
- Adult day health: Inclusive language and meaningful conversations in adult day health settings

The overarching goals of the training, regardless of elder care setting, were to educate learners about the challenges faced by LGBTQ older adults, build empathy and present examples of varied approaches across elder care settings. Early on, it was recognised that having carefully scripted video simulations of these scenarios and embedding them in the eLearning module would model varied interactions and allow learners to reflect on their practice and responses. However, the Aging Project team had never worked with SPs before and had not developed videos. Collaboration with the Volunteer SP program at Baycrest, a geriatric health system in Toronto, Canada, gave them access to Simulationists who were skilled in scenario writing and development of interactive reflective videos as well as working with older adult SPs. The value of interactive video simulations compared with noninteractive videos of simulations has been highlighted especially since the COVID pandemic. Musa et al. [8] noted that interactive videos promoted students' learning and were perceived to be more authentic than noninteractive video simulations.

Each scenario had an initial short video of the situation, followed by two or three possible response option videos. The response options included those identified as "not a good response" and some reasons why. For example, not addressing issues directly, not being empathic to the LGBTQ older adult, or putting one's personal feelings ahead of their professional role when engaging with the LGBTQ older adult. Those identified as "a good response" were explained as clear, direct and responsive to the LGBTQ older adults or elder care workers with whom they engaged. In the case of the third option, it was identified as having some positive qualities but not fully addressing all issues raised in the scenario. For every option selected, learners were provided with some education regarding why their choice was not a good response, somewhat acceptable, or a good response.

Engaging and training older adult simulated participants (SPs) to play these roles in a realistic and meaningful way included sharing information with them about the work of the LGBTQIA+ Aging Project, the intention of the eLearning module and the true stories upon which the scenarios were based. The SPs who participated in this project are part of a group of older adult volunteer SPs who are trained to use improvisation and storytelling in their simulations. The SPs noted that hearing the original stories from the Aging Project staff directly helped them to better understand their roles. The SPs were diverse across race, ethnicity and sexual orientation, features that were incorporated into the scenarios as well.

Two scenarios in particular that incorporated SP identities into the case scenarios raised concerns around authenticity, respectful representation and psychological safety of the SPs. The following examples demonstrate how we modified our processes to ensure respect and psychological safety.

Recognising that a large population of Massachusetts' home health aides are women of colour raised in cultures that are not affirming of the LGBTQ community, the case scenario that featured two home health aides addressed that issue directly. It was written specifically with the intention to create a scenario that might resonate for some home health aides and offered a model of navigating one's personal beliefs along with fulfilling their obligation to meet professional standards of care for their clients. With this intention, both SPs cast in this scenario are women of colour. One of the SPs featured in the video is a staff nurse at the healthcare facility where the videos were filmed. Initially, she was reluctant to participate in the role of the homophobic home health aide because she was concerned that if her colleagues saw the video, they would assume she was espousing her own personal beliefs, rather than playing a role. Everyone producing the video wanted to relieve the SP's concerns; once she understood that the audience for the eLearning module was in Massachusetts, and not anywhere near her workplace, she agreed to play the role and support the learning objective illustrating how to balance personal beliefs and professional obligations.

The case scenario that illustrated the experience of a transgender person being admitted to a nursing home and the staff reluctance to provide assistance with bathing was intended to address the staff person's personal discomfort with their new resident and the best way for them to fulfil their professional obligation to care for that resident. It was important that we represented the transgender community authentically in this scenario; however, we were unable to find an older SP from the transgender community to play the new resident. Rather than having a cisgender SP play the role of the transgender resident, we rewrote the scenario to be a discussion between the reluctant staff person and her supervisor about how best to care for transgender residents, instead of between the staff person and transgender resident directly. This modification enabled us to still meet the overall learning objective of addressing how best to care for and interact with transgender residents.

Although the situations highlighted in both examples of providing care to older adults are relevant to SPs of any age, they were included as a reminder of the importance of psychological safety and respect of all participants.

Using embedded interactive reflective videos throughout the online learning modules allows learners to see an illustration of a learning concept as well as consider their own responses to the case scenarios. This can be particularly helpful with topics that may be unfamiliar or make the learner uncomfortable, for example, directly asking an older adult their sexual orientation or gender identity. The multiple response options offered were scripted so that some were egregiously "not good" responses—reassuring learners' self-confidence while they learn and practice new skills ("well even I know not to say *that*...even if I'm not sure what I should say").

These videos also support impactful training of large audiences. In this case, the Massachusetts elder care network, comprised of community-based care managers, staff at senior centres, adult day health centres, long-term care providers, home health aides and more, were estimated at about 200,000 providers across the state. In compliance with state law, all those providers were required to complete the 1-hour eLearning training by June 30, 2022. Any new staff hired after that date must complete the training module within 9 months of hire. The online eLearning module with these embedded videos has been so well received that organisations are recommending training for other staff not just those mandated by state requirement. The use of technology easily enabled the wide spread of this eLearning module.

As is frequently the case, it is the stories in the case scenarios, and the way the SPs conveyed the impact of those "good" and "not good" responses, that give the video simulations the greatest impact and are best remembered by learners. Anecdotal comments from learners include "Seemed so realistic", "Great to hear exact language, what someone might say to be welcoming as well as how to apologise if they have not been" and that the videos are the "best part of training" with the "greatest impact".

Virtual Reality for Deescalation of Responsive Behaviours

Providing experiential opportunities for formal and informal caregivers of persons with dementia (PWD) to develop skills that maximise safe, compassionate care is a key priority in healthcare. For several years, the simulation team at the Michener Institute has collaborated with clinical educators to develop conventional in-person simulation sessions for nurses and other healthcare providers who encounter PWD with responsive behaviours. We are proud of the work we have done here to better prepare caregivers to respond to difficult and potentially dangerous situations.

However, in these sessions, we found that conventional simulation can have significant limitations that limit their effectiveness. First, the full expression of patient behaviours must be limited to ensure that both learners and simulated participants (SPs) are not physically harmed. Our team often had to tell the SP to "pull back" their affect and behaviour so as not to put anyone at risk, even in situations where such escalation would have been clinically authentic. We found that this often compromised the authenticity of the simulations and limited the effectiveness of training, as learners were not able to fully experience management of complex behaviours that risked progressing to physical threat.

Second, learners in conventional simulations do not have the opportunity to fully experience the perspective of the patient, which we believe limits the potential for development of empathy and compassionate care. While we always value and hold an essential place for the perspective of the SP during debriefing, what if we could go further? What if we could see through the eyes of the patient? Could this give learners a more visceral insight into the patient experience?

Similarly, in conventional simulations, educators and observing learners do not have the opportunity to truly "be in the shoes" of the learner in the hot seat. During debriefing, we often ask them to describe what they were seeing or paying attention to. What if we could see for ourselves?

To attempt to address the limitations of conventional simulation in the deescalation, we collaborated with the Ottawa Hospital Research Institute (OHRI) to develop a headset-mounted display (HMD)-based VR platform where simulations were delivered in a risk-free environment that fully leverages opportunities for deescalation training, situational awareness and perspective-taking.

We collaborated with subject matter experts at Baycrest, a geriatric health centre in Toronto that specialises in care of older adults, to refine the VR platform and simulation scenario to maximise opportunities for effective education for formal and informal caregivers.

Learners had the opportunity to don the VR headset and enter a virtual clinical space where they encountered a person with dementia, portrayed by a human SP (also wearing a VR headset). Communication and interaction happened naturally, in real time. The objective for the learner was to manage the responsive behaviours of the person with dementia. Simulation educators and observing learners were able to view the perspective of the SP, the caregiver, or take a "fly on the wall" view (see Fig. 13.1).

While a formal mixed-methods research study regarding the efficacy of this platform is still underway, we see great potential in VR as a medium through which to teach deescalation skills. In particular, our team has observed that VR allows for the safe incorporation of the environment in deescalation scenarios, such as when the SP choses to use an IV pole or a chair

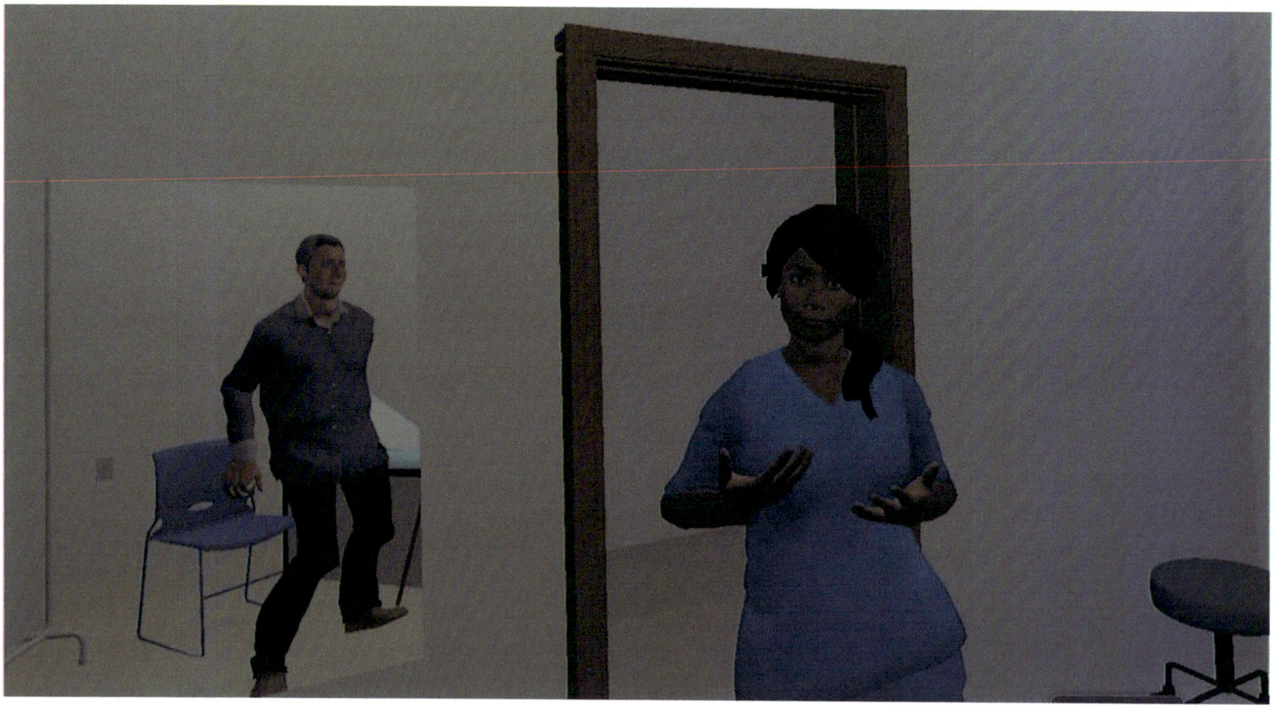

Fig. 13.1 VR de-escalation of responsive behaviours using the platform developed by OHRI, Michener, and Baycrest

to threaten or attempt to harm the caregiver. Escalating to this degree was not possible during our in-person simulations and allows for us to explore the boundaries of deescalation versus calling a code white (an emergency response for a violent person). However, we also learned that VR is in its relative infancy, and there are some current limitations to its potential:

- While the technology has come down in price, cost of entry remains a barrier
- Nonverbal communication is currently very rudimentary—this could affect the "toolkit" that learners have available to leverage when using verbal deescalation techniques and applying situational awareness skills
- More so than even conventional simulation, learners must be orientated to the technology: for first-timers, VR takes time to master the basic movement controls
- Some users experience "cyber sickness" (dizziness, nausea, headaches), especially if using the headset for too long [9, 10]—this is of particular concern for SPs who conduct multiple patient portrayals in a session

Regardless, we believe that VR technology will continue to improve and deliver on its potential to transform our perspectives of what is possible to do in simulation.

However, it is important to note that our work with VR-based simulation is also challenging the ways that we think about and hold ourselves accountable to principles of inclusion, diversity, equity and accessibility (IDEA). When we first devised the VR solution for deescalation of responsive behaviours, one of our practical goals was to leverage the avatar format of VR to be able to have a young SP represent an older person with dementia. Our rationale was that when engaging in deescalation scenarios with older adult SPs in conventional face-to-face simulations, we often observed that the scenarios could be quite physically and emotionally taxing for the SP. With VR, we could have a younger SP present as a geriatric avatar, so as to "relieve" the older SP from the exhausting nature of the simulations. Our simulation team has since had second thoughts about the implications of an unreflexive application of this practice, as we face the very real possibility of using avatars as a surface-level engagement with IDEA principles (e.g. artificial representations of Black, indigenous, people of colour, various populations with disabilities, older adults, etc.). This could further marginalise SPs from equity-deserving groups by excluding them from the education process, causing a form of "epistemic injustice". Picketts and colleagues [11] make the argument that SPs should represent the communities we serve and should contribute to case writing and portrayals whenever possible [11]. We echo this call to action, and our own work in VR has provided us with a new perspective on the ethical conduct of simulation.

Summary

In this chapter, we used two examples of technology-based innovative approaches to simulation, one each for VR and embedded interactive reflective videos. Despite being nontraditional, they both still followed the best practices and standards related to simulation. The expected outcome is to encourage others to think "outside the box" especially when training behavioural skills such as communication and deescalation and appropriate use of terminology. Thinking of different ways to utilise simulation may be beneficial in situations where sensitive or potentially dangerous topics are being addressed. We encourage those working in simulation to think of creative and unique ways to deliver learning opportunities and to partner with others who have skills and knowledge in diverse areas.

References

1. Issenberg SB, Scalese RJ. Simulation in health care education. Perspect Biol Med. 2008;51(1):31–46. https://doi.org/10.1353/pbm.2008.0004.
2. Loke S. The face of CPR. BMJ. 2020;371:m3899. https://doi.org/10.1136/bmj.m3899.
3. Brown WJ, Reid C. Implementing a cost effective and configurable hybrid simulation platform in healthcare education, using wearable and web-based technologies. Smart Learn Environ. 2022;9:20. https://doi.org/10.1186/s40561-022-00201-1.
4. Viglialoro RM, Condino S, Turini G, Carbone M, Ferrari V, Gesi M. Augmented reality, mixed reality, and hybrid approach in healthcare simulation: a systematic review. Appl Sci. 2021;11:2338. https://doi.org/10.3390/app11052338.
5. Micallef J, Broekhuyse A, Vuyyuru S, et al. Application of 3D printing in training health care providers; the development of diverse facial overlays for simulation-based medical training. Cureus. 2022;14(7):e26637. https://doi.org/10.7759/cureus.26637.
6. Lewis KL, Bohnert CA, Gammon WL, et al. The Association of Standardized Patient Educators (ASPE) Standards of Best Practice (SOBP). Adv Simul. 2017;2:10. https://doi.org/10.1186/s41077-017-0043-4.
7. INACSL Standards Committee. Onward and upward: introducing the healthcare simulation standards of best practice™. Clin Simul Nurs. 2021;58:1–4. https://doi.org/10.1016/j.ecns.2021.08.006.
8. Musa D, Gonzalez L, Penney H, Daher S. Interactive video simulation for remote healthcare learning. Front Surg. 2021;8:1–16. https://doi.org/10.3389/fsurg.2021.713119.
9. Weech S, Kenny S, Barnett-Cowan M. Presence and cybersickness in virtual reality are negatively related: a review. Front Psychol. 2019;10:158. https://doi.org/10.3389/fpsyg.2019.00158.
10. Yildirim C. Cybersickness during VR gaming undermines game enjoyment: a mediation model. Displays. 2019;59:35–43. https://doi.org/10.1016/j.displa.2019.07.002.
11. Picketts L, Warren MD, Bohnert C. Diversity and inclusion in simulation: addressing ethical and psychological safety concerns when working with simulated participants. BMJ Simul Technol Enhanc Learn. 2021;7(6):590–9. https://doi.org/10.1136/bmjstel-2020-000853.

Creative Development Opportunities for Older Adult Simulated Participants

14

Cathy M. Smith, Tim Dotson, Jamie Pitt, and Tanya Tierney

Key Messages

1. Many older adults are highly motivated to learn new things.
2. Older adult SPs benefit from regular ongoing creative development opportunities.
3. Specific SP skills and competencies such as active listening, being in the moment, and empathy are enhanced by creative development activities.
4. SP educators and SPs can apply these activities when preparing for specific roles.
5. Opportunities for leadership growth, peer mentorship, and intergenerational collaboration can be promoted by drawing on the expertise of SPs to develop and lead these activities.
6. Facilitators need to be able to adapt activities to possible age-related changes and attend to both the physical and psychological safety of the older adult SPs.

Vignette

You are managing an SP program that is part of the educational unit attached to a hospital. You started this program about 5 years ago. Some of the SPs are older adults, aged between 60 and 90 years. These SPs are all highly engaged and committed. Although they are experienced and valued members of your team, you only work with them sporadically, as the sessions they are involved in typically happen only a few times a year. Some of them have expressed a desire to be more involved in the program or wonder why they are not being contacted. You would like to engage with them more consistently. You have also noticed that some of them are experiencing cognitive, sensory, and/or physical changes between the times that they work at your program. You would like to find opportunities to support them in maintaining, adapting, and further developing their SP skills.

Introduction

Older adults can derive immense value from their involvement as SPs, including feeling a sense of purpose, making a meaningful contribution, building cohesive group connections, enhancing their skills and competence, and appreciating the opportunity to have fun and learn new things [1–5]. These findings align with broader research about what motivates older adults to learn, volunteer, or continue working [6, 7].

However, older adult SPs can become discouraged and even distressed if they are not regularly engaged [1]. They may even think they have been let go from an SP program for substandard performance without receiving any feedback, even when this is not the case [1]. They further identify that they can experience anxiety as an SP related to cognitive, sensory, and physical challenges of ageing [1, 4, 5].

It can be challenging for SP educators to engage with older adult SPs on a regular basis, especially if their programs are underresourced or if their program/curriculum does not require many older adult SPs for scenarios. Depending on the program, the roles that older adult SPs portray may be infrequently scheduled. In some contexts, the challenge of connecting has been magnified since the COVID-19 pandemic, including the need to adapt to new ways of working such as shifting from in-person to virtual

C. M. Smith (✉)
Baycrest Academy for Research and Education, Baycrest Centre for Geriatric Care, Toronto, ON, Canada
e-mail: CSmith4@baycrest.org

T. Dotson · J. Pitt
University of Tennessee Health Science Center, Center for Healthcare Improvement and Patient Simulation (CHIPS), Memphis, TN, USA
e-mail: tdotson5@uthsc.edu; jpitt6@uthsc.edu

T. Tierney
Lee Kong Chian School of Medicine, Nanyang Technological University, Singapore, Singapore
e-mail: tanyatierney@ntu.edu.sg

C. M. Smith et al. (eds.), *Comprehensive Healthcare Simulation: Geriatric Simulation*, Comprehensive Healthcare Simulation,
https://doi.org/10.1007/978-3-031-65742-9_14

sessions. Some older adults may lack the resources, ability, or confidence to work with technology [8, 9]. If sessions are being delivered in person, older adult SPs may not feel safe to attend (e.g., related to risks of being exposed to infectious diseases such as COVID-19) [10].

Despite these challenges, older adult SPs want opportunities to maintain current abilities and to further develop as SPs [1].They identity active listening, empathy, and being in the moment as important SP skills they can derive from creative development activities [1, 2].

Applications

We present some applications of development opportunities for older adult SPs—drawn from the fields of improvisation, the expressive arts, and mindfulness—that have been shown to be beneficial for older adults in general. For each application, we provide a brief overview and rationale as well as some specific activities for SP educators to try in their specific context. An underlying assumption is that the facilitators of these development sessions need to be able to adapt activities to possible age-related changes and attend to both the physical and psychological safety of the older adult SPs [8].

Improvisation

What Is it?

While modern improvisational theater involves a troupe of players performing short unscripted scenes based on games selected for them by a host or audience, it has its roots in sixteenth-century Commedia dell' arte [11]. Games include audience suggestions that are unknown to the players until right before a game is performed and a set of rules for what the players can or cannot do in the game. Viola Spolin (1906–1994) and Paul Sills (1927–2008) created many of the techniques used today. Spolin invented "Theater Games" while teaching dramatics to children and recent immigrants. Traditional teaching methods were ineffective in crossing divisions of culture and language, but when lessons became a game, her students incorporated the ideas organically. Spolin noted: "The games emerged out of necessity. I didn't sit at home and dream them up. When I had a problem, I made up a game. Then another problem came up, I just made up a new game" [12, para. 5]. Through these games, Spolin aimed for spontaneity and truthfulness rather than comedy [13].

Why Do It?

Improvisation is a perfect solution for meeting the unique creative development needs of older adult SPs. Involvement in improvisation can have a positive effect on their physical and mental health as well as on their cognitive function and social engagement, regardless of their ability [14, 15]. Improvisation creates a flexible but structured environment for varying abilities. Improvisation games do not require the participants to prepare anything or to have contextual knowledge. Anyone can participate, regardless of age, background, skill level, or physical/cognitive status.

The first two principles of improvisation are "yes" and "yes, and…" [16]. These principles support accepting the contribution of another and building on it. Games can have a liberating effect, allowing for spontaneous group performance rather than a focus on one individual. Playing games can give a sense of control from opt-in participation, progress, and belonging because everyone plays by the same rules to reach a common goal. Improvisation can be ideal for older adult SPs who might be nervous about performing or who are experiencing some memory loss, as it prepares them for the unexpected. Improvisation enlists cognitive functions, encourages narrative development, and relies on consensus-building [17].

How Do You Do It?

Improvisation "requires an environment in which experiencing can take place, a person free to experience, and an activity that brings about spontaneity" [18, p. 4]. Fostering a psychologically safe space is important. The ASPE SOBP outlines some strategies that SP educators can use to foster psychological safety when working with SPs [19]. One way is to state or post the Basic Assumption™, a concept developed at the Center for Medical Simulation, Boston, that was derived from research in previous fields such as psychology [20]. The Basic Assumption™ states: "We believe that everyone participating is intelligent, capable, cares about doing their best, and wants to improve" [21].

Introduce Fundamental Improvisational Principles

- Say "yes" to whatever is proposed.
- Say "and" then add on to what was proposed.
- Make statements (avoid questions).
- Accept "mistakes" as opportunities.

Fu [22] offers examples of how these principles could be applied to an improvisation game called "Story Swap" (see Table 14.1).

SP Educator Tips for Facilitating Improvisation Activities (in General)

- Explain games using simple directions.
- Model first: demonstrate activities.
- Use familiar words, for example, imagine, pretend, and observe; What did you notice? Experience? Think? Feel?
- Pacing: run a relaxed but focused game.

Table 14.1 Applying principles of improvisation to an improvisation game

Description of improvisation game called "Story Swap"		
• SPs sit in a circle. • Facilitator either asks for a volunteer or selects a SP (SP 1) to start the story. • SP 1 begins to tell a story (based on a topic selected by the facilitator or the group or related to a scenario or role). • After SP 1 has started to tell the story, the facilitator claps and shouts out "*Swap*" and either points to another SP in the group or invites other SPs to jump in and continue telling the story. • SP 2 continues the story exactly where the first SP left off until the facilitator claps and calls out "*Swap*" and the process is repeated until all SPs have had a chance to participate, if they choose. • Here is a demonstration of three ways the interaction could proceed:		
Version 1	*Version 2—Take 1*	*Version 2—Take 2*
Improvisation principles are used to build a collective story:	What might happen if improvisation principles are not used (e.g., Saying "Yes, **but**" instead of "Yes, **and**" and asking a question rather than making a statement)	Facilitator steps in and redirects the interaction so that improvisation principles are used:
SP 1: Let's have a party!	**SP 1: Let's have a party!**	*Facilitator: "Let's try that again, this time I invite you to try using 'Yes, and' then adding a statement that will build on what SP 1 said. Do you have an idea for a statement, or would you like suggestions from the team? "*
SP Educator claps their hands and shouts "Swap!"	*SP Educator claps their hands and shouts "Swap!"*	*SP 2: "Maybe I could say that we should hire a party planner."*
SP 2: Yes, and we'll have balloons!	**SP 2: Yes, but why would we have a party today?"**	*Facilitator: "Okay- let's start again, with the first line from SP 1. Time in."*
SP Educator claps their hands and shouts" Swap!"	*SP Educator* [to SP]: *"Time out."*	**SP 1: Let's have a party!**
SP 3: Yes, and we'll have a picnic in the sky!		*SP Educator claps their hands and shouts "Swap!"*
		SP 2: Yes, and maybe we should hire a party planner.
		SP Educator claps their hands and shouts "Swap!"
		SP 3: Yes, and we should invite all our friends!

Adapted from Fu B. Common ground: frameworks for teaching improvisational ability in medical education. Teaching and learning in medicine. 2019;31(3):342–55.

- Reinforce improvisation skills: listening, observing, and saying "yes" to ideas.
- Always provide a way out for SPs (e.g., they can take a time out) if you sense that they are upset or overwhelmed.
- Give positive acknowledgment using supportive words like "yes" and "thanks"; avoid evaluative words such as "excellent" or "perfect" [23].

Additional Facilitation Tips When Facilitating Improvisation with Older Adults

- Stress safety in exercising bodies and brains if there are limitations (e.g., remaining seated, not moving anything heavy).
- Whether or not SPs have cognitive or physical limitations, always permit observation, and rest.
- Use printed instructions with enlarged text.
- Use clear diction, repeating instructions; verbal repetition can aid memory and enhance understanding.
- Encourage group engagement and staying involved.
- Check in: Pause games to invite review: "Would someone please describe what we just did?"
- Follow with reflection: "What did you notice/experience?" "What were you thinking/feeling?" [23].
- Highlight applicability: "How could/does this apply to your work as an SP?

Improvisation Games

There are many examples of improvisation games. SP educators may need to adapt these games for older adult SPs, maintaining the objectives but being willing to change how to accomplish them. See Table 14.2 for some examples. The Spolin Games Online website [24] also has demonstrations on how to run the games we outline as well as many other resources.

What We Have Learned

- The degree of difficulty in games should be challenging but balanced to mitigate any potential feelings of frustration amongst group members.
- SP educators using improvisation should focus on the abilities of older adults in the group.

Table 14.2 Improvisation games

Name of game	Purpose of game	Directions for facilitating the game	Facilitator tips for working with SPs
Pass the clap	• To warm-up the group	• Have SPs stand (or sit) in a circle.	• The key to this game is for SPs to maintain eye contact and clear body language, i.e., coaching SPs to turn toward each other and to watch each other's hands.
		• Inform the SPs that they will be passing a clap to the person beside them.	• If the sender and the receiver get out of sync, ask them to slow down.
		• The facilitator identifies the SP who will start the activity.	
		• The first SP (sender) starts by turning to the SP beside them (receiver), making eye contact, and preparing to clap.	
		• The sender and the receiver try to clap at the same time without speaking.	
		• The receiver then becomes the sender and passes the clap onto the person next to them (the new receiver).	
		• Once a full rotation of the circle has been completed, the sender can reverse the direction of the clap by remaining focused on the SP who passed the clap to them and clapping back to them or keeping the same direction.	
Tell me the story	• To promote active listening	• SPs arrange themselves in a group of 3, sitting in chairs.	• Give SPs the opportunity to be both listeners and talkers; however, also allow them to stay in the role that feels most comfortable.
	• To develop focus when faced with multiple stimuli (especially if SPs must portray a role and give feedback or do a written assessment)	• One SP (the listener) sits in a middle chair with two other SPs (the talkers) sitting in chairs on either side facing them.	• Recognize the impact of possible sensory or cognitive deficits. A SP with hearing loss may not be able to hear clearly; a SP with memory issues may not be able to remember. These issues may affect their comfort in the role of listener or talker.
		• When the facilitator says "*Go*," the two SPs who are the talkers tell the middle SP (listener) a short story that they make up as they are telling it. The story can be a random topic such as "what happened on my walk today" or be specifically related to a scenario being trained. When the facilitator says "*Stop*," the speakers stop talking and the listener SP re-tells both stories with as much detail as they can remember.	• Keep the topic simple and the timing short, especially when starting so as not to overwhelm SPs.
Story swap	• To promote active listening and staying in the moment	• SPs sit in a circle.	• Remind SPs to apply the principles of "yes" and "yes and."
	• To practice the principles of "yes" and "yes, and"	• Facilitate either asks for a volunteer or selects a SP to start the story.	• Ask SPs to speak up and to make eye contact with the other SPs in the group.
	• To reinforce the notion of working as a team	• SP 1 begins to tell a story. The story can be based on a topic selected by the facilitator or the group or related to a scenario or role.	• If a SP did not hear something, assure them that they can ask for the story detail to be repeated.
		• After SP 1 has started to tell the story, the facilitator claps and shouts out "*Swap*" and either selects another SP in the group or invites other SPs to jump in and continue telling the story.	• Remind SPs that there is no right or wrong way to do this exercise.
		• SP 2 continues the story exactly where the first SP left off until the facilitator claps and calls out "*Swap*" and the process is repeated again, until all SPs have had a chance to participate.	• Offer SPs the choice of saying "*Pass*" when it's their turn to tell the story if they are not sure what to say or choose not to participate.

(continued)

Table 14.2 (continued)

Name of game	Purpose of game	Directions for facilitating the game	Facilitator tips for working with SPs
Gibberish[a]	• To encourage SPs to cultivate an emotional, physical, and psychological connection with the story of the person that they are portraying	• Ask SPs to pair up, either sitting or standing, evenly distributed throughout the space you are in.	• Placing SPs in pairs promotes psychological safety by allowing them to explore at their own pace and without feeling possible pressure to perform in front of or entertain the whole group
		• Ask one partner to tell the other partner the story of the person they are portraying using gibberish, that is, speech sounds that are not actual words in any language but that portray meaning through the sounds being made. The focus should be on how the SP is speaking rather than what they are saying. (For an example of gibberish, refer to this example: https://www.youtube.com/watch?v=EUdE0gYmBDM).	• Provide SPs with the option of sitting or standing or adjusting their bodies in a way that will make them feel physically comfortable.
		• Give SPs a set time to tell their story (e.g., a minute)—then call "*Stop*."	
		• Ask SPs to tell the same story again to their partner using actual words but trying to also capture the same vocal tones and movements that they used when they were speaking gibberish.	
		• Repeat with the second SP now telling the story in gibberish and then repeating it back using actual words.	
Mirror[a]	• To develop focus and the ability to work with a partner	• In pairs, two SP stand face-to-face.	• Encourage SPs to keep their attention entirely on their partner rather than on themselves.
		• One SP leads the movement while the other follows. After some time, the facilitator can ask the SPs to switch who is the leader and who is the follower. Ask SPs to always make themselves an exact mirror of their partner by following their partner's movements.	• Remind SPs to be aware of any physical limitations and to only move in ways that are comfortable for them and their partner.
		• Encourage SPs to start by making small movements such as with their head or arms, and then bring in other body parts as they are able to and feel comfortable doing.	• Offer SPs the opportunity to sit rather than stand if they are more physically comfortable.
One word story	• To promote being in the moment	• Have SPs sit in a group in a circle.	• Remind the group to speak clearly and to project their voices so all can hear.
	• To reinforce the power of listening and working as a team	• Facilitator initially provides the title of a story (e.g., trip to the store).	• Offer SPs the option of saying "*Pass*" in case they can't come up with a word, so they do not feel self-conscious or embarrassed.
	• To practice "yes and"	• To start, one SP says a single word to begin a story.	• Encourage all SPs to stay in the flow by listing to the story that emerges.
		• Then, sequentially, each SP contributes one word at a time to make a story.	• Point out how small contributions (e.g., adding "and" or "the") are important.
		• The story continues until it has gone around the circle a few times.	• Once you have played this game a few times, you can encourage SPs in the group to come up with the topic and for one of them to call "*The end*" themselves.
		• The facilitator gives a signal to end the exercise.	

[a]Adapted from: Spolin V. Theater games for the classroom: a teacher's handbook. Evanston: Northwestern University Press; 1986

Expressive Arts

What Is It?

Expressive arts can include visual arts, music, dance/movement, writing, and poetry. Expressive arts play an increasingly significant role in contemporary health science education, and they can be used as a way to focus on helping learners better understand themselves and others [25].

Why Do It?

Activities drawn from the expressive arts have been identified as having a wide variety of positive physical, interpersonal, social, and mental health effects for older adults, including helping them to relax, providing them with a sense of control, encouraging playfulness and a sense of humor, improving cognition, promoting self-expression, and improving communication with others [26, 27]. In the ongoing creative development of older adult SPs, expressive arts can be an innovative way to engage them, including those who may have age-related challenges. For example, making art or even viewing art causes the brain to continue to reshape, adapt, and restructure, thus expanding the potential to increase brain reserve capacity and perhaps make memorization easier [26].

How to Do It

One example is through creative writing activities that feature personal stories that have the power to illuminate a person's life, providing them with ways to use elements of their history to gain self-awareness of who they are and the richness they bring to their work as SPs. Stories can also facilitate the retrieval of experiences, resources, values, and wishes. We describe two creative writing activities for working with older adult SPs to support them in accessing their stories.

Identity Charts

Identity charts are a graphic tool that can help older adult SPs consider the many factors that shape who they are as individuals [28].

Instructions

- Take an 8.5 by 11 inch sheet of paper and turn it so it is on the horizontal plane.
- In the center of the page, ask the SP to write their name.
- Drawing lines out from their name, ask the SP to identify ways they define themselves and perhaps the labels that others use to describe them.
- Provide a blank template or brainstorm with the SP to create cues.
- Figure 14.1 illustrates how an SP, Thomas, would use these cues, to fill in his personal identity chart.

What We Have Learned

- Identity charts explore the labels that others give older adults and the labels they place on themselves.
- Completing an identity chart can foster individual and group identity by having older adult SPs reflect on their personal experiences, relationships, and connections to their community.
- It is a helpful idea to share an example of a completed identity chart before asking the older adult SPs to create their own.
- Once the identity chart is completed, have the older adult SP circle three items that are most significant in shaping their identity.
- If you plan on having SPs share their identity charts with a partner or in groups, it is important that they know in advance and are comfortable sharing any of these details.
- An identity chart can also be a useful training tool SPs can use to study and retain information about a character they may portray in a simulation scenario. Here is an example of how the identity chart can be modified with cues for a specific role a SP is portraying in a simulation scenario (see Fig. 14.2).

Biopoems

A biopoem is another helpful activity that can help older adult SPs engage in creative self-discovery [29]. Biopoems are useful tools that can assist older adult SPs to go beyond the aspects of identity that are often more obvious and familiar (such as ethnicity, gender, and age) by having them to focus on factors that mold their identity, such as life experiences, relationships, hopes, and interests.

Instructions

Select the focus of the biopoem. SPs typically write biopoems about themselves, but the poems can also be written about a character in a simulation scenario.

Select what to include in the biopoem. A biopoem typically can include the following information:

- Begins with your first name
- Adjectives that you would use to describe yourself
- Relationships in your life (e.g., friend, brother, daughter)
- Things you love (e.g., hobbies, people, things)
- Important moments
- Fears
- Accomplishments

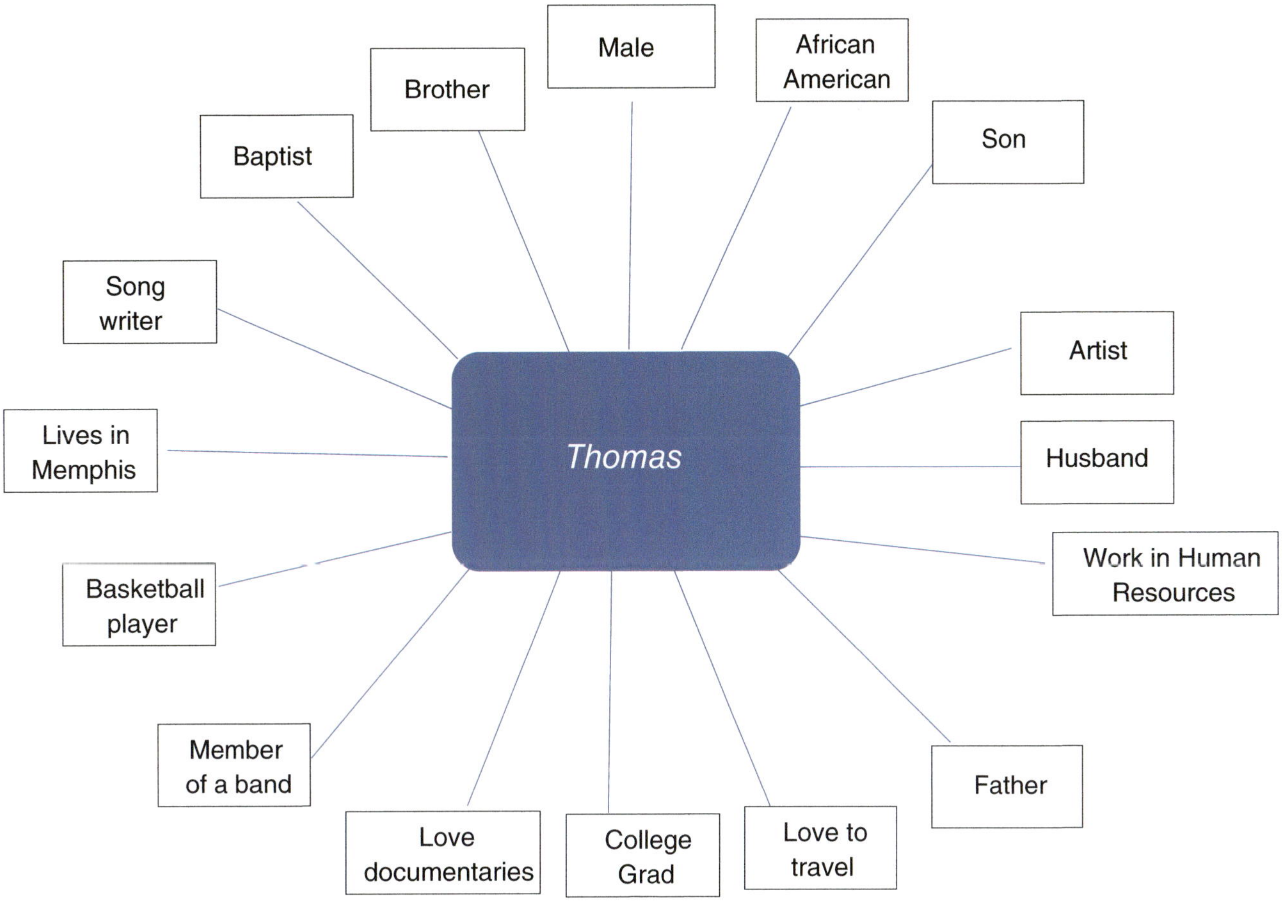

Fig. 14.1 Identity chart filled in by an SP named Thomas

- Hopes and wishes
- Home (location)
- Ends with your last name
- This format can be adapted to include other themes, such as important moments, heroes, beliefs, and special sayings or words.

What We Have Learned

- Before writing the biopoem, have older adult SPs brainstorm ideas they might include or provide some cues.
- It is helpful to provide a sample biopoem to help explain the format to the older adult SPs (see Fig. 14.3). Sharing biopoems with peers can be done in a variety of ways, such as posting the poems around the room as part of a gallery walk or sharing them with a partner or group.
- Biopoems can provide space for older adult SPs to develop enhanced self-awareness through reflecting on their life experiences, relationships, hopes, and interests.
- Creating and sharing of biopoems can strengthen relationships in a group and promote empathy and understanding for the experiences of others.
- To make the activity a psychologically safe space to explore, stress to SPs that the most important thing is an open attitude to creativity in everyday life; they do not need to be artists or have any special skills to express themselves through art making [25].

Mindfulness

What Is It?

Mindfulness can be defined as the intentional awareness that arises through paying attention, on purpose and without judgment to the unfolding experience moment to moment [30]. Mindfulness practices can take many forms, ranging from formal practices such as sitting meditation to informal practices related to bringing one's attention to whatever is being done at the moment (e.g., walking, having a conversation with someone) [31].

Why Do It?

There is an increasing body of evidence that illustrates how practicing mindfulness promotes body awareness, self-awareness, regulation of emotion, and regulation of attention [32]. Focus, concentration, flexibility, empathy, and situational awareness can be developed and enhanced

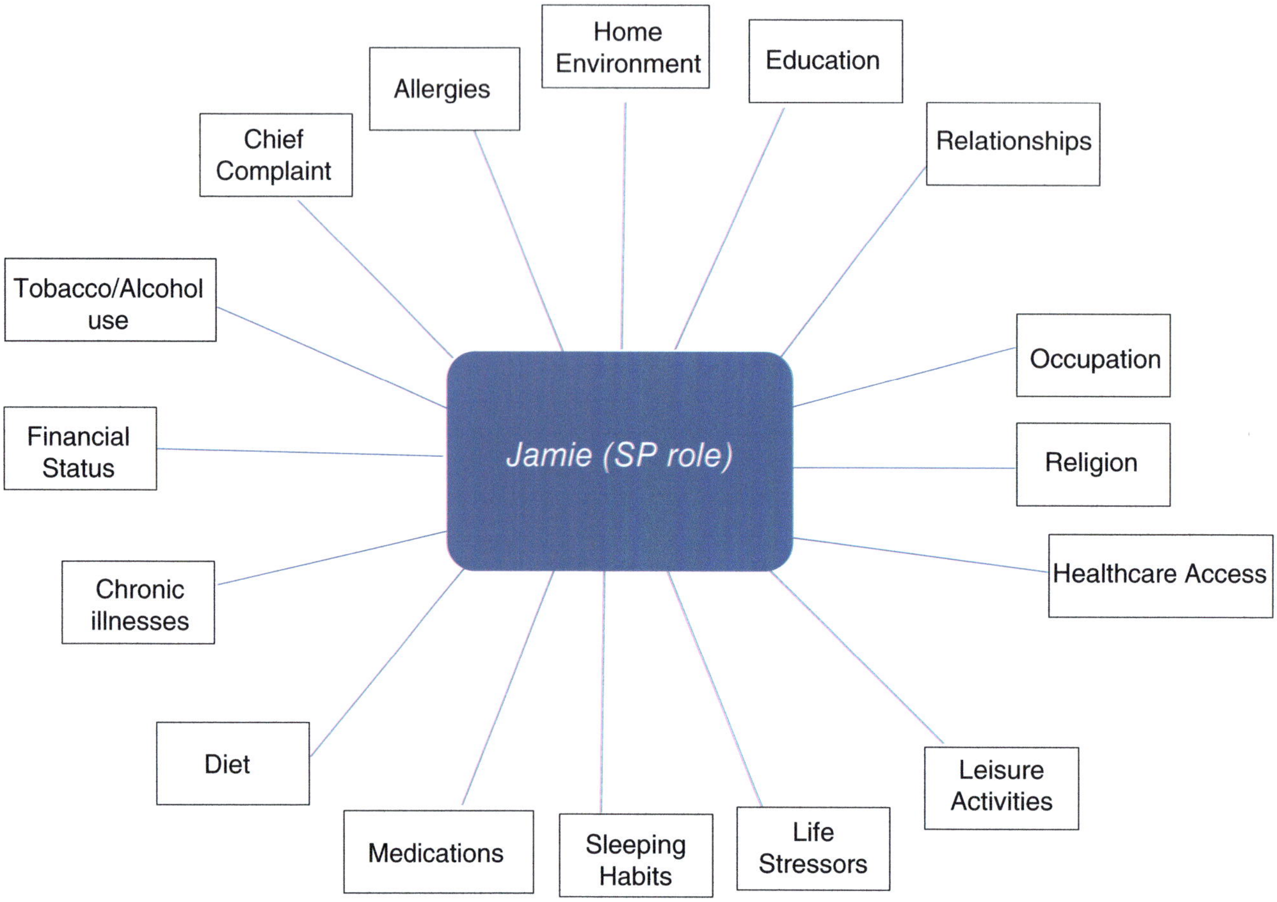

Fig. 14.2 Example of an identity chart with cues for an SP to fill in related to their portrayal of the role of Jamie

Fig. 14.3 Example of a biopoem

Tim

Funny, friendly, talented, smart

Son of Eugenia and Henry

Who loves writing, my wife, and traveling.

Who enjoys performing on stage, mentoring artists, and playing games.

Who fears disappointing love-ones, failure, and spiders.

An award-winning poet and playwright

Hoping to one day complete my book and produce a show for TV.

Lives in Memphis, Tennessee

Dotson

through mindfulness [33]. Compassion, presence, and resilience can be fostered [34]. Mindfulness has been shown to promote emotional and possibly physical well-being and increase self-awareness and promote the growth of social relationships in older adults [31, 32]. This way of being present may also facilitate older adult SPs' cognitive recall [35]. Because of these powerful benefits, mindfulness is being adopted increasingly as an educational strategy in various contexts, including health provider's education [36, 37]. There are also some reports of mindfulness being applied to SP practice, including with older adult SPs [2].

How to Do It

Considerations When Facilitating Mindfulness Practices

Psychological safety, defined as an atmosphere in which people feel comfortable participating, asking questions, opting out, and sharing their experiences without fear of negative repercussions such as judgment [38], is an important consideration for the facilitator leading a mindfulness practice. Guidelines for facilitators to keep in mind that can help to foster this kind of atmosphere include the following:

1. Let participants know that they have choices. For example, they can keep their eyes open or closed. If the practice is online, they can keep their camera on or turn it off. They can stop doing the exercise at any point or they can opt out of doing it altogether.
2. Offer participants ways to adapt the practice. This may mean inviting them to shift their posture or pause to open their eyes and take a drink of water.
3. Carefully brief and debrief these practices. In the debriefing, allow people to share their experiences without trying to fix anything. Create space for the expression of diverse experiences and the opportunity to ask questions or make comments.
4. Start with short activities, allowing participants to gradually become familiar with the practice of mindfulness and engage at their own pace.

Example of a Short Mindfulness Practice: "Follow Your Breath"

Box 14.1 contains a sample script for a short mindfulness practice to introduce SPs to this activity. The SP educator can modify the language as needed.

Box 14.1 Sample Script for "follow your breath": A Short Mindfulness Practice

As an SP, it is important that you are able to carefully listen to and respond to a learner. This short mindfulness exercise can help you to develop these skills by offering you the opportunity to develop increased awareness of what you are actually experiencing from moment-to-moment. There is no right or wrong way to do this exercise. Your experience is your experience. I will offer you options for how to do something, and you are at choice in terms of how you want to experience this exercise. If something doesn't feel comfortable, you can adjust how you are sitting. If you want to stop doing the exercise at any point, that is fine. The exercise will take under five minutes. I will be guiding you through it. Then there will be time for you to reflect on this experience within the group. Before we start, does anyone have any questions?

I invite you to settle into your chair and notice how your body is connecting with the chair. You may want to close your eyes or keep them open. If you keep them open, consider gazing softly into the distance rather than focusing on anything so you can concentrate on your experience. At any point in this exercise, you can change your posture, open your eyes, or stop doing it.

Now I invite you to notice any physical sensations, thoughts, or feelings. Is there a way you can notice them without judging them?

Now I invite you to bring your attention to your breath. Notice what happens when I ask you to do that. Breathe at your normal pace. Where do you notice your breath going as you inhale and exhale? Where are you noticing any other sensations, thoughts, or feelings? As you notice these sensations, thoughts, and feelings, the invitation is to allow them to move along as if they are floating away from you on your exhale.

Now I invite you to follow your breath for about 30 seconds. By this I mean to focus on inhaling and exhaling at a normal pace. If you notice that your attention starts to go somewhere else - for example, to plans you might have later in the day - is there a way you can notice that your mind has gone to that place, and without judgment, allow those thoughts to float along on the exhale, and invite your attention to come back to your breath. Know that this is an opportunity for you to practice mindfulness or awareness of what is happening for you from moment-to-moment. I am going to give you about 30 seconds to experience this process on your own.

[After 30 s or so] *Now, I invite you to notice any sensations, thoughts, or feelings once again. Start to wiggle your fingers and toes, gently blink your eyes and stretch if you need to and come back into the group space.*

Now I offer you the opportunity to reflect on your experience. [Note to SP educator: Questions you might ask] *What was that experience like for you? What will you take with you from this experience that you can apply to your work as an SP? Any other insights or questions?*

Applying Mindfulness to SP Role Portrayal

Once SPs have been introduced to mindfulness and have had the opportunity to practice, SP educators may want to apply a mindfulness approach to training and de-roling SPs. Here are two suggestions.

Applying Mindfulness to "Stepping into a Role"

Applying mindfulness to guiding SPs to draw awareness as to how they might step into the role of the person they are portraying can help them to embody the thoughts, feelings, and intentions of this person. Brief the SPs on the purpose of the exercise and answer any questions that they might have. Let them know that there will be an opportunity to debrief after this exercise where they can share their experiences and ask questions.

Box 14.2 contains a suggested script.

Box 14.2 Sample Script for Applying Mindfulness to "stepping into a role"

I invite you to sit in a chair and get comfortable. You may want to close your eyes or keep them open. If you keep them open, consider gazing softly into the distance rather than focusing on anything so you can concentrate on the visualization. At any point in this exercise, you can change your posture, open your eyes, or stop doing it.

I invite you to visualize the person you are portraying sitting in front of you. I am going to ask a series of questions. You can think silently about your answers, and we will discuss your responses at the end of the exercise. Notice what this person is wearing, their posture, their facial expression. What else do you notice? Any movements or behaviors, e.g., slow breathing, sighing, looking around, fidgeting? [Note to SP educator: Tailor these behaviors to the role the SP is playing and pace the questions appropriately.]

You may want to imagine yourself sitting down into this person's chair – sitting into the person you are portraying. Allow your body to take on their posture. Allow your face to take on their expression. Do you notice any sensation in this person's body – any pain, any discomfort? Where is it? What does it feel like? Do you notice any emotions that are present? What might they be? Do you notice any thoughts that are present? Is there a prevalent thought? What might that thought be? Just think it rather than say it out loud. Are there any concerns this person has? Why have they come here today?

Now I invite you to take a few breaths and come back into your own body. Breathe this person out. Feel your feet firmly on the ground. Then start to wiggle your fingers and toes, shake your hands, stretch or move if you like, have a drink of water, open your eyes, and come back into the group space.

Now I offer you the opportunity to reflect on your experience. [Note to SP educator: Questions you might ask] *What was that experience like for you? What things did you learn about the person that you are going to portray? What further questions do you have? What will you take with you from this experience? Any other insights or questions?*

De-roling Using Mindfulness

The act of de-roling can be supported by asking SPs to draw their awareness to how they have been affected by the portrayal of a role and to envision stepping out of this experience. This technique can be used by SPs in brief breaks between learners to reset and refresh before the next learner. SPs can be encouraged to visualize separating from the experience of the person they are portraying through changing their breathing or through intentional physical actions that contrast with the demeanor of the person that they portrayed. For example, suggest that they slow down their breath if they were breathing rapidly when they portrayed this person, or stand up and shake out their body if the person they were portraying was tired or closed off, or adopt a different facial expression than what they had during their role portrayal.

Example of a Mindfulness Practice for De-roling Older Adult SPs

Longer de-roling practices can be offered at the end of a simulation session before SPs leave for the day by guiding them to draw their awareness to what is happening in their body and with their breath and offering them the opportunity to release anything associated with their role portrayal (see Box 14.3).

Box 14.3 Sample Script for Applying Mindfulness to De-roling for Older Adult SPs

Let's take a few minutes now so you have the opportunity to further de-role your experience. Then you will have a chance to reflect.

I invite you to make yourself comfortable. You may want to close your eyes or keep them open. If you keep them open, consider gazing softly into the distance rather than focusing on anything so you can concentrate on your experience.

I invite you to take a few breaths and settle in. What are you noticing about your breath? If you are breathing quickly, is there a way you can slow your breathing down? What are you noticing in your body? Do you need to move or stretch or shake anything off? If you move, make sure your eyes are open and you have your balance. Is there anything else you need to leave behind?

Now I invite you to feel your feet firmly on the ground. Then start to wiggle your fingers and toes, stretch or move if you like, have a drink of water, open your eyes, and come back into the group space.

Now I offer you the opportunity to reflect on your experience. (Note to SP educator- at this point, consider moving into a debrief with the SPs of this experience and of the simulation session)

What We Have Learned

- Paying close attention to each moment can enable an older SP to be more attuned to their behavior as well as to that of the learner.
- The opportunity for older adult SPs to practice together and share their experience of practice can be an opportunity for connection and the promotion of empathy through understanding others' perspectives.
- Offer older adult SPs the choice to share their experiences in the debriefing sessions.
- There may be a variety of responses reported by older adult SPs; stress that there is no right or wrong way for them to experience mindfulness because each of them is paying attention, on purpose and without judgement, to their uniquely unfolding experience from moment-to-moment.
- Despite the perception that the purpose of mindfulness is to promote relaxation, this outcome does not always happen. Normalize for the group that it is okay to have a different response than being relaxed.
- Recognize that the mindfulness practices you present may not resonate with everyone in the group.
- During the debrief, some SPs may identify other versions of mindfulness that they practice (e.g., a walk in the woods).
- Consider making audio recordings of mindfulness practices that SPs can do on their own.

Closing

In this chapter, we have outlined the value of having ongoing creative development opportunities for older adult SPs and provided examples of some activities you might consider in your context drawn from the fields of improvisation, the expressive arts, and mindfulness. You may also find that you have those who have expertise in various fields, beyond what we have offered, both within the older adult SP group and among the larger SP pool or within your institution or community. Opportunities for leadership growth, peer mentorship, and intergenerational collaboration can be promoted by drawing on the experience of SPs in your program. Meaningful development activities for older adult SPs can create a sense of security, provide strategies for supporting them to adapt to changing abilities, acknowledge their contributions, and provide valuable opportunities for them to stay connected with a SP program.

References

1. Schelgel C, Smith CM. "Please let me know when I do not realize it myself": a qualitative analysis of senior simulated patients' experiences. Adv Simul. 2019;4(1):18.
2. Smith CM, Sokoloff LG, Gallucci CE. 'It's like a shot in the arm': evaluating the experiences of older simulated participants in structured virtual meetings during COVID-19. Int J Healthc Simul. 2021;1(1):33–40.
3. Davis K. Utilizing older adult standardized patients to enhance the education of health professional students. Age Action. 2017;32(2):1.
4. Thompson J, Tiplady S, Hutchinson A, Cook G, Harrington B. Older people's views and experiences of engagement in standardised patient simulation. BMJ Simul Technol Enhanc Learn. 2017;3(4):154–8.
5. Lee DA, Maxwell CA, Miller S. "This Is Me!" Perceptions of older adult simulated participants in an aging and injury simulation experience. J Trauma Nursing. 2021;28(1):10–20.
6. Anderson ND, Damianakis T, Kröger E, Wagner LM, Dawson DR, Binns MA, et al. The benefits associated with volunteering among seniors: a critical review and recommendations for future research. Psychol Bull. 2014;140(6):1505–33.
7. Kakulla B. Lifelong learning attracts older adults for personal growth and cognitive health [Internet]. Washington, DC: AARP Research; 2022. https://www.aarp.org/research/topics/life/info-2022/lifelong-learning-older-adults.html.
8. Smith CM, Sokoloff LG, Alsaba N. Collaborative framework for working with older simulated participants (SP). BMJ Simul Technol Enhanc Learn. 2021;7(2):112.
9. Murciano-Hueso A, Martín-García A-V, Cardoso AP. Technology and quality of life of older people in times of COVID: a qualitative study on their changed digital profile. Int J Environ Res Public Health. 2022;19(16):10459.
10. Clark L, Woll A, Owens TL, Shropshire D, Kiser B, Gephardt G, et al. SP safety, autonomy and healthcare simulation practice in the COVID-19 era. BMJ Simul Technol Enhanc Learn. 2021;7(5):450–1.
11. Kuritz P. The making of theatre history. Prentice Hall: Englewood Cliffs; 1988.
12. Folkart BA. Viola Spolin; Guru of improvisational theater methods. Los Angeles Times [Internet]. 26 Nov 1994. https://www.latimes.com/archives/la-xpm-1994-11-26-mn-1560-story.html.
13. Spolin V. Improvisation for the theatre. 2nd ed. Evanston: Northwestern University Press; 1983.
14. Cohen GD, Perlstein S, Chapline J, Kelly J, Firth KM, Simmens S. The impact of professionally conducted cultural programs on the physical health, mental health, and social functioning of older adults. Gerontologist. 2006;46(6):726–34.
15. Rajan K, Rajan R. Staying engaged: health patterns of older Americans who participate in the arts [Internet]. Washington, DC: National Endowment for the Arts; 2017. https://www.arts.gov/impact/research/publications/staying-engaged-health-patterns-older-americans-who-participate-arts.
16. Leonard K, Yorton T. Yes, and: how improvisation reverses" no, but" thinking and improves creativity and collaboration—lessons from the Second City. New York: HarperCollins; 2015.
17. Magerko B, Manzoul W, Riedl M, Baumer A, Fuller D, Luther K, et al., editors. An empirical study of cognition and theatrical improvisation. In: Proceedings of the seventh ACM conference on Creativity and cognition; 2009.
18. Spolin V. Improvisation for the theater: a handbook of teaching and directing techniques. Evanston: Northwestern University Press; 1999.
19. Lewis KL, Bohnert CA, Gammon WL, Hölzer H, Lyman L, Smith C, et al. The Association of Standardized Patient Educators (ASPE) Standards of Best Practice (SOBP). Adv Simul. 2017;2(1):10.
20. Rudolph J. What's up with the basic assumption™? [Internet]. Boston: Center for Medical Education; 2023. https://harvardmedsim.org/blog/whats-up-with-the-basic-assumption/.
21. Center for Medical Simulation. The Basic Assumption™ | Center for Medical Simulation [Internet]. Boston: Center for

Medical Simulation; 2022. https://harvardmedsim.org/resources/the-basic-assumption/.
22. Fu B. Common ground: frameworks for teaching improvisational ability in medical education. Teach Learn Med. 2019;31(3):342–55.
23. Dunford CM, Yoshizaki-Gibbons HM, Morhardt D. The Memory Ensemble: improvising connections among performance, disability, and ageing. Res Drama Educ. 2017;22(3):420–6.
24. Swartz G. Spolin Games online [Internet]. WP-Tutoring; 2018. https://spolingamesonline.org/.
25. Blomqvist L, Pitkälä K, Routasalo P. Images of loneliness: using art as an educational method in professional training. J Cont Educ Nurs. 2007;38(2):89–93.
26. Bagan B. Aging: what's art got to do with it [Internet]. Spring City: Great Valley Publishing Company; 2009. https://www.todaysgeriatricmedicine.com/news/ex_082809_03.shtml.
27. Castora-Binkley M, Noelker L, Prohaska T, Satariano W. Impact of arts participation on health outcomes for older adults. J Aging Human Arts. 2010;4(4):352–67.
28. Identity charts [Internet]. Boston: Facing History & Ourselves; 2009. https://www.facinghistory.org/resource-library.
29. Bio-poem: connecting Identity and Poetry [Internet]. Boston: Facing History and Ourselves; 2008. https://www.facinghistory.org/resource-library/bio-poem-connecting-identity-and-poetry.
30. Kabat-Zinn J. Mindfulness-based interventions in context: past, present, and future. Clin Psychol Sci Pract. 2003;10(2):144–56.
31. Mindful Staff. What is mindfulness? [Internet]. Mindful Communications & Such, PBC; 2020. https://www.mindful.org/what-is-mindfulness/.
32. Hölzel BK, Lazar SW, Gard T, Schuman-Olivier Z, Vago DR, Ott U. How does mindfulness meditation work? Proposing mechanisms of action from a conceptual and neural perspective. Perspect Psychol Sci. 2011;6(6):537–59.
33. Ince S. Positive psychology: Harnessing the power of happiness, personal strength, and mindfulness. Boston: Harvard Health Publications; 2009.
34. Cuddy A. Presence: bringing your boldest self to your biggest challenges. Hachette: Orion; 2015.
35. Sevinc G, Rusche J, Wong B, Datta T, Kaufman R, Gutz SE, et al. Mindfulness training improves cognition and strengthens intrinsic connectivity between the hippocampus and posteromedial cortex in healthy older adults. Front Aging Neurosci. 2021;13:702796.
36. Epstein R. Attending: medicine, mindfulness, and humanity. New York: Simon and Schuster; 2018.
37. Hassed C. The art of introducing mindfulness into medical and allied health curricula. Mindfulness. 2021;12(8):1909–19.
38. Turner S, Harder N. Psychological safe environment: a concept analysis. Clin Simul Nurs. 2018;18:47–55.

Part IV

Applications: Older Adult Care and Assessment

Assessing Physical Function in Older Adults

15

Target Learner Group: Second Year Medical Students

Jeanne Farnan, Shellie Williams, and Kris Slawinski

Background

This scenario is one of four formative encounters provided to second year medical students to provide practice of physical and mental assessment of the geriatric patient. Students attend a 1.5 h lecture in which key points of medical assessment of the elderly are explored. The class ($N = 90$) then breaks into cohorts of ~20–24 to rotate through four encounters in the Clinical Performance Center in groups of four. Each performs one interview and observes peers in their group perform the other three, so that all are exposed to each experience/topic. All participate in providing feedback, facilitated by a faculty preceptor observing encounters in each room.

Key Session Information

Description of the scenario	Mildred Ortiz, 66 years old, is a new patient at this clinic to establish primary care. She reports she is feeling well and that her son's worries are unrealistic. Patient will be referred to as female going forward If a male SP is recruited, the name Milton can be used in place of Mildred
Setting	Outpatient geriatric clinic, University of Chicago
Learning objectives	• Elicit patient's ADL and IADL history • Assess upper extremity function • Assess lower extremity function and gait by performing the Get-Up-And-Go Test • Describe the proper use of a cane

Adjunct materials	• Cane, incorrectly adjusted for height (too low or too tall)
	• Coin, positioned near patient on table surface
	• Documents listing steps of the Physical Function Screen, for student reference during encounter, on desktop (links provided in references and resources section):
	  • Assess home setting
	  • Determine history of falls or fear of falling
	  • Assess function: ADLs and IADLs [1, 2]
	  • Assess gait and gait device [3–5]

Participants	Learners: • One student who will perform the interview and physical function assessment • Three student observers • One faculty feedback facilitator • One SP presenting as the patient per encounter (SP performs role four times before a break. It is recommended to limit total encounters per day to eight).
Age range of SP	SP should appear to be the stated age of the role
Scenario length	15 min
Session schedule	30 min/encounter, total 2 h • 15 min for encounter • 10 min for feedback • 5 min to travel to next encounter room
Room setup	• One chair for student at desk, with its back facing the back of the room, so they cannot see observing peers and feedback facilitator • One chair for SP next to desk, facing student chair and observers at back of room • Four chairs at back of room facing SP and interviewing student, for observing students and feedback facilitator
Props	• Coin on desk or tabletop in view of student and SP • Cane, adjusted to be too tall, to be held by SP • Interviewing student and observers can have note pad to use during the session

J. Farnan
Medical School Education, Pritzker School of Medicine, University of Chicago, Chicago, IL, USA
e-mail: jfarnan@medicine.bsd.uchicago.edu

S. Williams
Faculty Physicians, University of Chicago, Chicago, IL, USA
e-mail: swillia2@medicine.bsd.uchicago.edu

K. Slawinski (✉)
SP Program and Clinical Performance Center, Pritzker School of Medicine, University of Chicago, Chicago, IL, USA

C. M. Smith et al. (eds.), *Comprehensive Healthcare Simulation: Geriatric Simulation*, Comprehensive Healthcare Simulation,
https://doi.org/10.1007/978-3-031-65742-9_15

Instructions to Learners

The following Door Chart/Student Instruction is available on the course intranet system for preparation beforehand, as well as provided to students on the day of the event.

Assessing Physical Function

Patient	Mildred Ortiz, 66-year-old retired English teacher
Setting	She is a new patient to the Outpatient Geriatric Clinic. Earlier on the phone, her son said he was worried the patient is not "getting around as well as before." Dr. Williams has asked you to introduce yourself, explain why you are there, and assess Mrs. Ortiz's physical function.
Diagnosis	Osteoarthritis
Your task	Determine living situation: Living environment, social supports

Assess physical function by:

1. ADLs and IADLs level of (I)ndependence, (A)ssistance or (D)ependence [1, 2]
2. Perform the Get-Up-And-Go, upper extremity test [3, 4]
3. Observe and instruct patient on proper use of cane [5]

Suggestions:

- No need to take a full history: just introduce yourself and begin discussion of home environment and supports.
- Use the screening guides on the desktop in the exam room.

Instructions to SPs

Short Patient Description

You are Mildred Ortiz, a 66-year-old retired English teacher.

Your Opening Statement and Perception of Why You Are Here Today

"My son is concerned that I'm not getting by as well as I used to."

If asked to elaborate: "I'm not quite sure what he is talking about. I know I've slowed down, but I think he doesn't know what it means or feels like to get old."

(Note: the responses suggested in this role are suggestions; they do not have to be delivered verbatim. However, whatever opening statement the trainer and SP determine to use should be standardized throughout all the student encounters for this case).

Your Affect

You are a cheerful, pleasant, intelligent older woman and are open to answering any questions the student may have or performing the physical exam steps.

What to Expect Today

Students will rotate through in groups of four. The first three will be seated before the interviewing student enters the room. Refrain from talking with them or the preceptor before the final student enters. The interview will last 15 min, and there will be 10 min for the feedback portion.

Let the student guide the interview. If the student gets stuck and asks for a *timeout*, do not engage in conversation or make eye contact with the students. Reengage with your student wherever they pick up the interview after receiving guidance from the preceptor.

History of Present Illness

- You have arthritis of the knees and hands, as well as mild high blood pressure, controlled with diet and doing relatively well.
- If asked, you are also beginning to have significant problems with your physical function because of increasing muscle weakness in your legs from the arthritis in your knees.
- Your son and grandson do not live nearby, and your other children (you can use actual children's names, info) live out of state. Your old neighbors have either moved away or died, and, unless you go out, which is increasingly difficult for you to do, you do not have daily contact with anyone.
- You are able to perform bathing, dressing, toileting, grooming, and feeding independently.
- You are able to organize your medications, cook, and do light housework independently.
- You have difficulty with heavy housework because of knee pain.
- You have difficulty with shopping because you do not drive and do not own a car.
- You live on your social security and a small teacher's pension, which totals $2080 a month. As a result, you have trouble paying your bills because of the costs of your food and your gas heat. If asked, your son assists you financially when needed.

Guidelines for Functional History

Students Should Ask You Questions About Your Functional Status (ADLs and IADLs)

ADLs (Activities of Daily Living)

- Do you have any problems:
  - Getting out of bed or a chair by yourself?
    - No.
  - Using the toilet by yourself?
    - No, but I did almost fall a couple times.
  - Taking a bath or shower by yourself?

    - No, I take sink baths.
  - Getting completely dressed by yourself?
    - No.
  - Controlling your urine?
    - Only if I don't get to the toilet on time.

IADLs (Instrumental Activities of Daily Living)

- Do you have any problems:
  - Preparing your own meals?
    - No.
  - Doing all your own shopping by yourself?
    - No, my son takes me most times.
  - Getting where you need to go by yourself?
    - That is a problem.
  - Using the telephone by yourself?
    - No.
  - Doing your own housekeeping by yourself?
    - I have someone come in once a week.
  - Doing your laundry yourself?
    - My helper does that.
  - Handling your own finances by yourself?
    - My son is always butting in.
  - Taking your medications by yourself?
    - No.

Home Environment

You live in a house, with two floors and a basement. There are about five exterior steps to your front porch: every time you go out, you have to climb these.

If asked, if you have any trouble with stairs inside or outside of your home:

"Lord, yes! I can hardly get upstairs sometimes because of my knees. I could do my own laundry, you know, if it weren't in the basement. And those steps up to my front porch are murderous."

Social Support

Who would be able to help you in case of an emergency?

"Well, my son and grandson would help, of course, but they live at a bit of a distance. Most of my neighbors are gone. There's my friend Mrs. Crawford, but she doesn't drive, and her arthritis is worse than mine."

Guidelines for Physical Examination

- Your right arm cannot reach as high as the left with the upper extremity range of motion tests.
- You can pick up a penny without any problem with both hands.
- Students should ask you to perform the "Get-Up-And-Go test," in which you will demonstrate leg weakness and slightly abnormal walking from pain in your knee. (We will train you how to do this.) You will rock three to four times before successfully getting up from the chair, using both hands on the chair arms to lift yourself up.
- In addition, you will have a cane (provided by the simulation center, which you will hold in the hand on the same side as the really bad knee (both hurt) and sometimes in the hand of the stronger knee. Comment during feedback on the student's instruction on proper side to hold the cane (should be on side of strongest leg).

SP General Feedback Guidelines

You should comment on how the encounter made you feel: respected versus angry, safe versus threatened, and engaged and active participant versus feeling left out and ignored.

Did the student express empathy appropriately and acknowledge the challenges your health problem is posing to you?

Was the student respectful of your thoughts and ideas, able to negotiate a plan, willing to compromise (e.g. "Maybe we can address this again during our next appt")?

Your feedback should be specific: give concrete examples versus generalizations (e.g. "I felt reassured when you used the word X" or "when you said xyz," or 'I could tell by the way you looked at me that you understood what it meant to me.")

It is possible that a bit of feedback you planned to share is addressed before you have a chance to speak. You can merely state "I agree with your peers about X,"—or—it is possible you disagree with what was said. Please feel free to say so but be specific as to what you disagree with.

Always offer solutions: "When you said X it made me feel Y. I do not think that was your intention. Can you think now of a better way to say that/state your intention?" or "Perhaps if you had said A instead of B I would have felt more comfortable/in agreement."

Considerations for Working with Older Adult SPs Before the Scenario

- Screen SP candidates for stamina: candidates accustomed to midday rests may not work out.
- Screen SPs for comfort with the subject matter and explain that the encounter provides the students the opportunity to first ask these possibly uncomfortable questions in a protected, safe environment. Likewise, the SP must be willing to deliver the scripted responses correctly and that while she herself does not experience these problems, many others do.
- Assign SPs to this case who have no physical limitations, weakness, or pain associated with the body areas assessed by the physical function examination, so the repeated movements of Get-Up-and-Go and gait assessment do not aggravate existing conditions or challenge the SP's balance.

During the Scenario

- Ensure the SP is comfortable and has their notes with them.
- Check in between students and assist to restroom if needed.
- If SP feedback strays from being brief, concise, supportive, constructive, and focused solely on the student's performance, the preceptor should guide the SP with closed-ended prompts/questions.
- Establish beforehand with the SP exactly how far they are to walk when the student observes their gait and how to turn around with the cane to return to their seat.

After the Scenario

- Solicit feedback from the SP on what, if any, challenges they encountered during the encounters. These can range from physical issues to lack of personal history information to feedback.

Lessons Learned

- Correct cane use is counterintuitive: the cane is to be held in the hand opposite from the bad knee/leg. Many faculty preceptors do not know this, so it is helpful to offer them a guide before the sessions begin that depicts or describes correct use.

References

1. Katz ADL scale. www.ncbi.nlm.nih.gov/books/NBK470404/.
2. Lawton-Brody IADL scale. https://www.alz.org/careplanning/downloads/lawton-iadl.pdf.
3. Get Up and Go Test. pubmed.ncbi.nlm.nih.gov/3487300/.
4. Timed get up and go test. https://www.cdc.gov/steadi/media/pdfs/STEADI-Assessment-TUG-508.pdf.
5. Tips for choosing and using canes. https://www.mayoclinic.org/healthy-lifestyle/healthy-aging/multimedia/canes/sls-20077060?s=4

Resources

Nogoshi M, Williams S, Kasuya R, Sakai D, Masaki K, Blanchette PL. Using standardized patients to assess the geriatrics medicine skills of medical students, internal medicine residents, and geriatrics medicine fellows. Acad Med. 2004;79(7):698–702. https://doi.org/10.1097/00001888-200407000-00018.

Kishimoto M, Nagoishi M, Williams S, Masaki KH, Blanchette PL. Knowledge and attitudes about geriatrics of medical students, internal medicine residents, and geriatric medicine fellows. J Am Geriatric Soc. 2005;53(1):99–102. https://doi.org/10.1111/j.1532-5415.2005.53018.x.

Assessing Falls Risk in Older Adults

16

Target Learner Group: Medical Students Completing Geriatric Training in Internal Medicine Clerkship

Samantha Syms, Sarah Bland, and Maria H. van Zuilen

Background

Falls and mobility assessment are an important competency area for medical trainees [1]. One-third of older adults fall each year. With these falls, they have a higher risk for a severe injury, functional decline, and increased healthcare utilization [2]. The high prevalence of this geriatric syndrome and its potentially serious adverse consequences warrant routine evaluation of mobility and fall risk by healthcare providers. Mobility is one of the four elements of the Age-Friendly Health Systems initiative (in addition to what matters, medication, and mentation), known as the "4Ms," that are critical to providing high-quality care to all older adults [3]. Training on this topic should be included in the medical student curriculum.

As part of the geriatrics curriculum for our medical students, we developed an SP assessment related to falls. Prior to the SP exercise, students participate in a 2-h interactive instructional session for skills practice during which they receive an overview of the SP assessment they will complete 1 week later. As advanced preparation for this session and the subsequent SP exercise, students review (1) an online case-based module on falls from the aquifer geriatrics series, (2) Aquifer Geriatric Series video demonstrating the Timed-Up-and-Go test (TUG) administration, (3) A TUG instruction and scoring sheet with specific elements of gait and balance that can be observed, and (4) a 2-page Falls Evaluation and Management tool developed by the American Geriatrics Society.

S. Syms (✉)
Standardized Patient Program, Gordon Center for Simulation and Innovation in Medical Education, Department of Medical Education, University of Miami Miller School of Medicine, Miami, FL, USA
e-mail: ssyms@med.miami.edu

S. Bland
Phase 2 Clinical Curriculum on the Regional Medical Campus, Department of Medical Education, University of Miami Miller School of Medicine, Miami, FL, USA
e-mail: sbland@med.miami.edu

M. H. van Zuilen
Academy of Medical Education Scholar, Department of Medical Education, University of Miami Miller School of Medicine, Miami, FL, USA
e-mail: rzuilen@med.miami.edu

Our overall learning objectives for the Falls curriculum are the following:

1. Determine if a patient incident meets the criteria for a fall.
2. Take a focused fall risk history from an older adult patient.
3. Perform a Timed-Up-and-Go test to assess mobility and fall risk.
4. Interpret the findings from a fall risk history and Timed-Up-and-Go assessment.
5. Propose a fall risk reduction plan for an older adult patient at high fall risk.

Outline of the SP assessment process and materials

Training of SPs	• Two-hour training session for SPs (repeated each assessment cycle to train new SPs and provide a refresher for existing SPs) • SP role providing a general overview of the scenario as well as specific questions likely to be asked with appropriate responses • Video recording of an encounter demonstrating standard SP responses and overall communication style and SP demeanor
Age range of SP	• SP should appear to be the stated age of the role
Scenario materials	• A curved (straight) cane • Two chairs with armrests (no wheels) • 10 ft. mark on the floor indicating how far the patient should walk • A clipboard with the TUG instruction and scoring sheet (students use the back of this sheet for note taking) • Station instructions (provided in and outside the station) with a brief patient history and pertinent vitals • Medication list (provided by the SP if asked about medications) • Tablet with the form SPs use to evaluate students on their professionalism and communication skills as well as the administration of the TUG

C. M. Smith et al. (eds.), *Comprehensive Healthcare Simulation: Geriatric Simulation*, Comprehensive Healthcare Simulation,
https://doi.org/10.1007/978-3-031-65742-9_16

Postencounter (immediate)	• Postencounter SOAP (subjective, objective, assessment, plan) note template • Student evaluation of the SP, the instructional components, and the timing of the SP session and note station

Key Session Information

Scenario

Students receive the following information on the scenario: Alex Morgan is a 76-year-old patient with hypertension, hyperlipidemia, hypothyroidism, osteoporosis, knee osteoarthritis, and insomnia. The patient has been assigned a gender neutral name so SPs of any gender can portray Alex. For the sake of simplicity, in this chapter, we refer to Mrs. Morgan, however, when preparing for the simulation, use the pronoun salutation that best reflects the SP's gender and pronoun (e.g., Mr. Ms./Mrs./Mx.). Mrs. Morgan is here for a follow-up appointment in the clinic. Mrs. Morgan's daughter could not accompany her to the visit today but left a message for the doctor that she was concerned about her mother's walking. She noticed her mother is shuffling more while walking and at times appears increasingly unsteady. The patient's previous physician has retired. Your attending has just taken over her care.

Vital signs:
Blood pressure: Sitting, 122/72; standing, 90/68
Temperature: 98.5
Respiratory rate: 19
Heart rate: Sitting, 80; standing, 68
BMI: 28

Instructions to Learner

On the day of the SP assessment, students receive a brief overview with instructions for the scenario. Five minutes before the start of the SP encounter, students review the scenario description on the door note which includes the following instructions:

1. Take a targeted history focusing on the daughter's and patient's concerns.
2. Conduct a gait assessment using the Timed-Up-and-Go test (TUG).
3. Interpret the result of the TUG and explain it to the patient.
4. Complete the TUG worksheet noting observed gait/balance abnormalities you observed.
5. Explain to the patient which factors are potentially contributing to the presenting problems and offer a comprehensive and multifactorial plan of care focusing on risk reduction.

You will have 25-min to perform these tasks. You will receive a 10- and 2-min warning. Afterward, you will have 30-min to complete your SOAP (Subjective, Objective, Assessment, Plan) note.

Information for the SPs

General Appearance, Demeanor, and Response Style

The patient is well groomed and casually dressed wearing comfortable walking shoes. The patient's demeanor and response style are pleasant and forthcoming.

History of Current Situation

The patient presents with a progressive history of right knee osteoarthritis with gradually worsening pain and mobility. Over the past year, the patient has fallen twice. In addition to this presenting complaint, the patient expresses concern about frequent nighttime urination with problems falling asleep afterward (this is the issue that "matters most" to the patient). Students are expected to address both issues. Students received prior instruction on the importance of evaluating each of the domains of a comprehensive geriatric assessment—medical, functional, psychological, and socioeconomic. Below is a summary of the key case elements in each of these domains.

Medical Domain

- Mobility history: The patient reports a history of gradually worsening right knee arthritis which is limiting their mobility and agrees with the daughter's noted concerns about gait and balance. The patient borrowed a cane from a neighbor after the last fall and reports feeling "more secure" with this cane.
- Falls history: The patient reports two falls in the past year. Specific elements of the falls are as follows:
  - Events surrounding the falls: During the first fall, the patient tripped over a tree root walking with friends in the park next to their building. The most recent fall occurred 2 weeks ago when the patient had to get up to go to the bathroom in the middle of the night (as happens often). The patient suddenly fell to the ground as they entered the bathroom.
  - Symptoms at the time of the fall (intrinsic risks): The patient acknowledges occasional lightheadedness when standing up too quickly but is unsure if this

happened during the fall. The patient denies any chest pain, sudden weakness, or other preceding symptoms.
  - Environmental factors (extrinsic risks). The patient reports no objects in the way. They did not turn on the light but noted there is a nightlight near the bathroom (see functional domain for additional environmental information).
  - Injuries from the fall: The patient denies loss of consciousness or hitting their head but reports a resolving bruise on their right thigh from hitting the hamper during the fall.
  - Events after the fall (how long were they on the ground, how did they get up?): The patient reports trying to get up on their own unsuccessfully and eventually pushing the call button. A staff member arrived in a few minutes to assist. The patient did not seek additional care.
- Medical history: See description of scenario. All problems are long-standing. Regarding sleep, the patient has no trouble falling asleep initially and denies daytime drowsiness. There is no pertinent family history.
- Medications: Lorazepam for sleep, Ibuprofen for pain, hydrochlorothiazide for hypertension, levothyroxine for hypothyroidism, simvastatin for hyperlipidemia, and alendronate for osteoporosis. When students ask about medications, the patient volunteers that the daughter fills a pill box for the week and that they always take all their medications at night right before bedtime.
- What matters most: The patient expresses concern about having to get up multiple times at night to go to the bathroom with difficulty falling back asleep. The patient only reports urinary frequency at night and reports no other symptoms such as urgency, dysuria, or incontinence.

Socioeconomic Domain

- Living arrangement: The patient currently lives in a small apartment in an assisted living facility (ALF) and moved there 3 years ago after their spouse's death.
- Social support: The patient reports good social support (see functional domain) from the ALF and from the daughter who lives 20 min away, with emotional support from the son who lives out of town.
- Alcohol/tobacco/drug use: The patient drinks one glass of wine nightly after dinner when friends come over but no history of smoking or drug use.
- Economic: The patient has good healthcare insurance and retirement benefits from their elementary school teaching career and no financial concerns.

Functional Domain

- Functional status: The patient is independent in his/her basic activities of daily living (ADLs) but receives assistance with the instrumental activities of daily living (IADLs). The ALF provides all the meals as well as cleaning service, and the daughter assists with finances, shopping and managing the medications. The patient no longer drives.
- Environmental safety: The apartment in the ALF has appropriate safety modifications (e.g., handlebars in the bathroom, a call button), but there are throw rugs in the living room and the apartment is a bit cluttered. The patient lives on the third floor but takes the elevator.
- Footwear: The patient often wears slippers around the apartment but walking shoes when outside.
- Sensory function: The patient reports normal hearing but endorses some blurred vision that gradually developed since their last vision check over 3 years ago.

Psychological Domain

- Memory and mood: The patient denies memory and mood symptoms but expresses concerns about falling again and potentially hurting themselves. The patient has not lost interest in their usual activities.

The Timed-Up-and-Go Test

- The patient completes the TUG in about 25-s (indicating high fall risk) with several attempts to arise, a few seconds to steady themselves before gait initiation, a slow and tentative pace with some shuffling, en bloc turning, and use of the cane on the incorrect side.

The Assessment and Plan

Geriatric syndromes such as falls are usually multifactorial in nature. The following are the main issues that students should recognize and address:

1. Unsafe medications: Both lorazepam (a benzodiazepine) and ibuprofen (a nonsteroidal antiinflammatory agent) are unsafe for older adults. The lorazepam increases fall risk.
2. Timing of the HCTZ (a diuretic): Moving this medication to the AM instead of the PM will help address the nighttime urinary and sleep problems and remove the need for the lorazepam which was prescribed after the patient started the diuretic.
3. Need for physical therapy (PT): The patient would benefit from an exercise regimen focused on strength and balance training and needs an evaluation for a more appropriate assistive device with education on how to use it.
4. Orthostatic hypotension: This is evidenced by the patient's vitals and reported symptoms.

Other issues of concern include excessive alcohol use, vision problems, home safety, unsafe footwear, possible vitamin D deficiency, and potentially other underlying issues.

The Feedback Process

Feedback to learners is essential, especially for a formative assessment [4]. We use a mixed approach. Students review their video encounter and complete a self-assessment using the same communication skills checklist the SP completed and the same rater checklist the faculty uses for the S/O part of the note to evaluate their history-taking. Students reflect on their strengths and develop a SMART goal for an area they want to work on. This self-assessment is the first step in the feedback process. Faculty then provide each student with a detailed feedback report that includes (1) the SP feedback, (2) the faculty feedback on the S/O and A/P parts of the note, and (3) feedback on their self-assessment. Rather than providing a global performance rating, our individually tailored report allows us to give nuanced feedback on different aspects of clinical skills (history taking, reporting, assessment/clinical reasoning, management), identifying areas of weakness as well as areas of strength.

Considerations for Working with Older Adult SPs and Lessons Learned in Running this Scenario

- Given the complexity of the case and the need to train on the appropriate portrayal of the gait during the TUG test, our SP training is significantly longer than for other scenario trainings.
- A significant concern in working with older adult SPs is cognitive overload [5]. Consideration should be given to how many items are on the SP checklist to ensure accurate recall.
- This also pertains to the complexity of the scenario. One strategy to help recall is to provide a quick-reference card reviewing the most important aspects for the SP to review between students.
- There is a clear need for ongoing feedback and retraining. Ideally, feedback would be provided in real time (immediately following the encounter).
- Scenario developers must be aware that learners may bring their preexisting knowledge about common problems in older adult patients into their assessment. For example, learners may assume that an older male patient has benign prostatic hypertrophy (BPH) that contributes to their urinary problems.

References and Resources

1. Leipzig RM, Granville L, Simpson D, Anderson MB, Soriano RP. Keeping granny safe on July 1: A consensus on minimum geriatric competencies for graduating medical students. Acad Med. 2009;84:604–10.
2. Tinetti ME, Gordon C, Sogolow E, Lapin P, Bradley EH. Fall-risk evaluation and management: challenges in adopting geriatric care practices. Gerontologist. 2006;46(6):717–25.
3. Institute for Healthcare Improvement [internet]. What is an Age-Friendly Health System? http://www.ihi.org/Engage/Initiatives/Age-Friendly-Health-Systems/Pages/default.aspx. Accessed 27 Nov 2021.
4. Mitchell O, Cotton N, Leedham-Green K, Elias S, Bartholomew B. Video-assisted reflection: improving OSCE feedback. Clin Teach. 2021;18:409–16.
5. Smith CM, Sokoloff LG, Alsaba N. Collaborative framework for working with older simulated participants (SP). BMJ Simul Technol Enhanc Learn. 2021;7(2):112–5.

Sexual History: The Importance of Social History in Guiding Care of Older Adults

17

Target Learner Group: First Year Medical Students

Catherine Hagele and Lynn Seng

Background

The course in which this case is used, Intro to Clinical Medicine, is intended to prepare students for their clerkship training. This case developed iteratively over a number of years. Students are in the second semester of their first year and have limited experience with simulated participants (SPs).

SPs in this scenario help these students practice before making the transition to their clerkship year by creating a safe, formative, environment for them to practice history taking and by providing feedback to them on their interpersonal skills.

The scenario runs in ten separate rooms over the span of 2 days allowing the entire class of medical students to participate. There is one faculty preceptor, four medical students (this number can vary), and two SPs per room. At the beginning of each session, SPs go to their assigned room and sit together at the back of the room while the preceptor briefs the students. After the faculty overview, students work in pairs, taking turns interviewing the SP and observing an encounter. SPs give interpersonal feedback to the interviewing student after each encounter. The pair of students then rotate to a different social history case with the other SP in the same room and the observing and interviewing students switch roles. SPs perform their case each time they see a pair of students—four times a day.

SPs train to the case within a week of performance and have a half hour of time to brief/refresh the case before interaction with the students. SPs then have another half hour at the end of the sessions to debrief and derole with other SPs and their trainer.

This session provides learners the opportunity to take a social history, including assessing alcohol and substance use, intimate partner violence, and sexual history, in addition to the usual history questions. This is most often the first time a student has asked these kinds of questions of a stranger, the SP. These kinds of conversations can be awkward, embarrassing and challenging for early learners. Learners can practice the skill of this specialized history taking in a neutral, compassionate, nonjudgmental manner in the safe space the SP provides. Feedback from students about this particular session of history-taking practice is typically very positive. Learners often express gratitude for the ability to practice these skills before they see "real patients".

C. Hagele (✉) · L. Seng
Perelman School of Medicine, University of Pennsylvania, Philadelphia, PA, USA
e-mail: hagele@upenn.edu

Key Session Information

Description of the scenario	Anne Jordan, a 65-year-old female, is having unusual vaginal discharge and wants to see the doctor
Setting	Outpatient doctor's office
Learning objectives	Students are introduced to the basic skills of interviewing a patient. Secondary goals include synthesizing this collected data into an oral and written presentation and to begin thinking about the differential diagnosis • Establish rapport with patients • Learn to communicate effectively with patients using known successful techniques • Learn and practice basic and advanced aspects of history taking, including obtaining a chief complaint, taking a full history with a special emphasis on taking a social history
Adjunct materials	• Full history checklist • Communication skills checklist • Social and sexual history checklist
Participants	In one room: • Four first year medical students • Two social history cases—1 SP per case (2 SPs total) • One physician-faculty preceptor Ten rooms, two separate 90-min sessions, over 2 days

C. M. Smith et al. (eds.), *Comprehensive Healthcare Simulation: Geriatric Simulation*, Comprehensive Healthcare Simulation,
https://doi.org/10.1007/978-3-031-65742-9_17

Age of SP	SP should appear to be the stated age of the role
Scenario length	25 min
Session schedule	90 min total: • Preceptor intro—15 min • First student encounter—25 min • SP gives feedback to performing student—5 min • Second student encounter—25 min • SP gives feedback to performing student—5 min • Preceptor wrapup—15 min
	The session is generally a casual environment, with a lot of preceptor variabilities. Some rooms run like clockwork; some rooms run more loosely. Students work in pairs—one student interviews the patient while the other student observes and keeps a checklist of history items the interviewing student asks or misses. After SP feedback, the student pair moves to the other case in the room with students switching who is observer and interviewer. The preceptor moves between the two groups in the room, making their own observations. This ensures each student gets to interview an SP, receive feedback on their interaction from an SP, and observe their peer.
	SPs are in the room for this entire session. SPs also have a 1/2 h before the session for SP briefing and 1/2 h after the session for debriefing/deroling separate from the learners
Room setup	Two "stations" in the classroom • Three chairs—Two facing each other for the interviewer and SP and one off to the side for the observing student
Props	Students may use their checklist and/or paper to write notes
	SPs may carry index cards to unobtrusively jot down feedback notes during any student-to-student discussion or preceptor-to- student discussion. During these times, SPs are in "timeout" mode, where they are neutrally available until needed again in the role or when it is time for feedback. This is a casual enough environment that a few words jotted down on a card is unobtrusive
Wardrobe	Casual clothing
Moulage	None

Instructions to Learners

Prior to the session, learners attend a social/sexual history lecture and review the social/sexual history documents and checklists related to the course. While there is not a particular focus on sexual history taking with older adults, there is mention of the importance of taking a sexual history of all adults, including older adults, no matter how old.

During the session, learners are instructed to take a full history including a full social and sexual history.

Instructions to SPs

Prior to accepting this assignment, the following information is provided for the SPs:

You are portraying a patient presenting to the doctor with vaginal discharge. TRIGGER WARNING: this case deals with intimate partner violence. Please do not accept this case if you feel you cannot perform it. The case does not require a high emotion portrayal, but this character has this subject matter in her social history.

Opening Line

I've noticed some discharge.

History of Current Situation

- It started about a week ago, came on gradually.
- The discharge is from the vagina.
- It is thin and grayish and has a foul odor.
- You are *not* having any pain or urinary symptoms.
- It is noticeable on the tissue every time you go to the bathroom and requires the use of a pad.
- You first noticed it when you went to the bathroom.
- Nothing makes it better or worse.
- There is minimal itching in the vaginal area.

Current and Past Medical History

Certain items, not critical to the learning objectives and therefore not necessary to standardize, are not provided in the SP training case. SPs are instructed to improvise these details as long as they do not conflict or add to the reason for visiting the doctor, for example, do not say you fell down recently because this will complicate the intimate partner violence discussion.

Family Medical History

For this case, family history is intentionally left blank in the SP training case. This section is not critical to the learning objectives and is meant to be something benign and easy for the SPs to remember that is not necessary to standardize. SPs are able to improvise their own family medical history as long as the details do not conflict or add to the reason for visiting the doctor, for example, do not say your mother had any gynecological issues because the interviewer may try to make a familial link to the character's vaginal discharge.

Social/Lifestyle Information

- You live with your husband.
- He is verbally and physically abusive and frequently forces you to have sex with him.
- You do not reveal the abuse unless asked specifically about abuse. "Things are kind of rough at home." Then answer as asked about specifics.
- He physically abuses you by pushing you and sometimes slapping or punching you.
- He has never punched you in the face.
- This has been happening off and on for years.
- Your husband is recently retired or got laid off (SPs choice). Since then, he has been home a lot and the physical and sexual abuse has started up again.
- You do not really have a support system. If asked, you admit to feeling trapped at home with your husband.
- You are not happy.
- You are sexually monogamous with your husband. If asked, you are not sure if your husband is sexually active with others.

Special Instructions for Portraying This Scenario

- You are wearing casual clothing.
- Students are in small groups of four. You will interact with one learner at a time, with another learner observing.
- Give your history sitting in a chair; arrange so it encourages the interviewer to sit next to you, not across the table from you. The proctors will have these chairs set before the session begins. This note is in case the chairs get shifted before SPs arrive.
- Remember, you are not currently in any pain or discomfort.
- Your mood is blunted and expressionless. You are able to answer all the learner's questions.
- You do not appear depressed. You are quiet but willing to talk with the learner.
- Do not ask any unscripted questions. Feel free to improvise any responses that are not indicated directly in the case.
- "Timeouts" are not typical in this setting, but if a learner needs to pause the scene, disengage neutrally and wait for the learner or preceptor to "timein."

Considerations for Working with Older Adult SPs

Some of these points are directly related to working with older adult SPs. While it is important to make sure the needs of this older population are met, we find generally that the robust training time and detailed attention to the full program tend to meet the needs of all SPs, including older adults. We are always open to feedback and incorporate suggestions as the program is able.

Before the Scenario

- Make sure SPs are aware of the subject matter (intimate partner violence) before they are confirmed for this case.
- SPs receive the case, feedback guide, learner checklists,and other session materials approximately a week ahead of inperson training. Provide a video of an encounter if possible. If possible, provide the case with more than the typical week notice, as older adult SPs sometimes want a longer time to study.
- Provide alternative ways of memorizing the case. Flashcards, video version of the case, and online quizzes are some of the strategies that have helped with case fact retention.
- SPs are paid 1 hour for at-home study and preparation.
- Training happens within a week of the session.
- Training is 2.5 hours long with breaks as needed. Allowing time in training for SPs to relate their own personal experience is welcome and necessary. Older adults have a wealth of knowledge to share and greatly enhance the training room, no matter what case is training.
- All SPs demonstrate the ability to portray the case in a standardized fashion with the material provided and have a chance to role-play the scenario and practice giving feedback.
- Make sure all SPs can be heard clearly when other people are also talking in the room. Two cases are running simultaneously; clarity and volume are important, as well as believable portrayal. If any SPs have hearing issues, pairing that SP with a quieter SP (who is running a different case on the other side of the room) seems to help with the overall noise level and is easier for SPs to focus on the sounds of the learner in front of them.
- Provide an opportunity to discuss privately any concerns about the subject matter and how it may affect an SP personally.

- On performance day, provide plenty of time for questions, briefing, and time to use the bathroom and navigate the space to get to the performance room on time.

During the Scenario

- If possible, ensure that chairs are stable and stationary. Rolling chairs can be challenging for SPs that have mobility issues.
- Provide index cards or discreet note-taking opportunity, so SPs can jot down feedback ideas in the event SPs have challenges remembering details.

After the Scenario

- Allow for ample time for debriefing and discussion of the session.
- Provide a brief deroling exercise or other deroling options, for example, deep breathing exercise, reflection on the value of their contribution as a patient, a positive point taken from the session, and inquiry as to how the SP will take care of themselves the rest of that day. A reminder of the impact they have on the student and the learning that is taking place usually is very well received by older adult SPs our experience.
- Remind SPs to communicate any feedback about the program they may think of after the fact and to whom it should be directed.

Lessons Learned

- Because of comments made from SPs themselves before training and comments gleaned from trainers, it is observed that older adult SPs tend to be more aware of their own potential emotional triggers before the encounter occurs. In our experience, they have been more proactive about handling that trigger or removing themselves from the program ahead of time compared to younger SPs.
- Learners tend to believe an older adult SP during the encounter wholeheartedly. It is easier to suspend disbelief it seems. Perhaps the age difference creates an easier ability to see the SP as a patient as opposed to an "actor."
- Learners appreciated SP feedback, especially from older adult SPs. It is unclear if that is because of a generational difference or perhaps a more limited access learners have to hearing how they are perceived by older patients.
- Incorporating deroling is important even for seasoned SPs.
- It is important to check biases before SPs interact with the learners. Remind SPs to wipe the slate clean before interacting with the next learner, so they can mindfully be present for the encounter.

Resources

1. Basile KC, Hertz MF, Back SE. Intimate partner violence and sexual violence victimization assessment instruments for use in healthcare settings: version 1. Atlanta: Centers for Disease Control and Prevention, National Center for Injury Prevention and Control; 2007.
2. Reno R, Park I, Workowski K, Machefsky A, Bachmann L. A guide to taking a sexual history. Atlanta: Division of STD Prevention, National Center for HIV, Viral Hepatitis, STD, and TB Prevention, Centers for Disease Control and Prevention; 2022.
3. Schrier MW, Rougas SC, Schrier EW, Elisseou S, Warrie S. Intimate partner violence screening and counseling: an introductory session for health care professionals. MedEdPORTAL. 2017;13:10622. https://doi.org/10.15766/mep_2374-8265.10622.
4. Moser C. Interviewing a patient about intimate partner violence. Virtual Mentor. 2014;16(11):872–6. https://doi.org/10.1001/virtualmentor.2014.16.11.ecas1-1411.
5. Garbitelli EC, Gerber MR, Williams PN, Heublein M, Watto MF. #218 trauma-informed care with Megan Gerber MD. The Curbsiders Internal Medicine Podcast. https://thecurbsiders.com/curbsiders-podcast/218. Accessed 8 June 2020.

Falls Assessment, Prevention, and Management with Older Adults

18

Target Learner Group: Physiotherapists

Shane A. Pritchard and Felicity C. Blackstock

Background

The learners who engage with this scenario are internationally diverse physiotherapists who obtained physiotherapy qualifications in countries including India, Malaysia, the Philippines, Nepal, Belgium, Italy, Brazil, and Egypt. The scenario is completed as preparation to undertake a practical clinical assessment (performance criteria at entry level to practise thresholds) in a simulation-based environment as the final assessment to be granted full registration to practise in Australia.

In several countries, physiotherapists may work under the direction of physicians. However, in Australia, the clinical reasoning and decision-making practice thresholds for entry-level physiotherapy are set to enable independent practice [1]. Therefore, many physiotherapists are unfamiliar with the expectations of physiotherapy care across the Australian healthcare continuum and must develop new knowledge, skills, and capabilities to be deemed competent to practise in Australia.

Falls are an unfortunately common reason for a person to be admitted to inpatient care in Australian hospitals, and physiotherapists play a major role in the assessment, management, and prevention of falls. A fall is often associated with the culmination of factors related to the person's social situation, medical comorbidity, cognition, physical functioning, pathology, or impairments. Management of a patient following a fall can be a complex clinical decision-making situation requiring a deep understanding of the Australian health and aged care system to promote positive health outcomes. This scenario incorporates many of these factors, resulting in added clinical reasoning complexity to support intervention and discharge planning.

This scenario can also be adapted for other timepoints of someone's care journey to highlight different aspects of falls assessment, prevention, and management relevant to physiotherapy (and allied health) practice. This enables greater individualisation of the learning experience to the varied capabilities and learning needs of the internationally diverse physiotherapists. The progression of timepoints also allows demonstration of how decision-making differs across the continuum of care.

This scenario is designed to encompass the entirety of the expected performance of an entry-level Australian physiotherapist in one session. In short course education programmes, simulation is typically prefaced by knowledge and theory-based activities, including a clinical reasoning framework [2] and review of expected clinical behaviours and management directions. Immediately prior to the simulation activity, learners are briefed on principles and expectations of simulation relating to the session. This is especially important because the course is often the first time that many internationally diverse physiotherapists are learning in simulation-based environments. Principles addressed in the briefing include discussing engagement and realism to support the establishment of "a safe container" [3], the use of timeins and timeouts, roles of observers and therapy assistants, and arrangements for and expectations of feedback and debriefing. Activities for observers within the simulation include completion of a "learning opportunities form" to inform reflection and peer feedback (involving observers documenting examples of high-quality learner behaviour and potential improved behaviours relating to practice threshold competencies) and an adapted version of the SHARP debriefing tool [4] to support debriefing related to concerns, learning points, and action plans for improved future practice. Feedback typically occurs post simulation

S. A. Pritchard (✉)
Monash University, Clayton, VIC, Australia

Physiotherapy Education Australia, Melbourne, VIC, Australia
e-mail: shane.pritchard@monash.edu

F. C. Blackstock
Physiotherapy Education Australia, Melbourne, VIC, Australia

University of Sydney, Sydney, NSW, Australia
e-mail: felicity.blackstock@sydney.edu.au

C. M. Smith et al. (eds.), *Comprehensive Healthcare Simulation: Geriatric Simulation*, Comprehensive Healthcare Simulation,
https://doi.org/10.1007/978-3-031-65742-9_18

and in two phases. Initially feedback is offered from a patient perspective integrated in a facilitator-led debrief, followed by a further facilitator-led debrief incorporating feedback from facilitator and peer perspectives.

Key Session Information

Description of the scenario	Hilda Bernard is an 81-year-old woman who lives alone and sustained a fractured left neck of femur when they fell at home. She underwent surgery on the evening of the fall where the fracture was fixated with a dynamic hip screw. She has just arrived in the rehabilitation ward after a 1-week stay in the acute ward and is waiting for review by the allied health team If a male SP is recruited, the name Harold can be used in place of Hilda
Setting	Patient room of a tertiary rehabilitation hospital
Learning objectives	By the end of this session, learners will be able to: 1. Communicate professionally and effectively with the patient to obtain consent and establish a collaborative, culturally sensitive therapeutic relationship where the patient feels safe and supported 2. Identify and analyse relevant information from medical notes for a patient who has experienced a fall 3. Design and conduct an appropriate physiotherapy assessment, using targeted outcome measures, and interpreting these findings for a patient who has experienced a fall 4. Design, conduct, and monitor an appropriate evidence-based physiotherapy intervention based on all relevant assessment information and aligned with patient goals for a patient who has experienced a fall 5. Apply risk minimisation strategies for safety of self, the patient, and others, including the use of appropriate manual handling
Adjunct materials	Simulated hospital records from various health professions previously involved in the episode of care
Age range of SP	SP should appear to be the stated age of the role
Participants	Learners (three groups of 3–4 comprising): • One physiotherapist learner/physiotherapy student adopting the role of "therapist" • One physiotherapy learner/physiotherapy student adopting the role of "therapy assistant" • 1–2 physiotherapy learners/physiotherapy students observing (with associated observer tasks to complete) Faculty: • Three SPs (one SP interacts with one group of 3–4 learners) • Facilitator
Scenario length	50 min of direct interaction between learners and SPs
Session schedule	1 week prior to the session, training occurs with SPs including provision of instructions 2.5 h total per scenario • 30 min – Faculty conduct rehearsal/dry run with SPs and setup environment • 10 min – Faculty conduct briefing with learners – SPs review preparatory notes and set up environment • 15 min – Learners review medical notes and plan for the interaction – Faculty conduct briefing with SPs • 50 min – Scenario occurs • 10 min – Learners independently complete reflective tasks – Faculty debrief SPs • 15 min – Feedback and debriefing with SPs and learners (regarding the patient perspective) • 20 min – Feedback and debriefing with learners only (regarding clinical performance)
Room setup	• Hospital bed and room set up in a "private room" with three chairs for students and the patient in a wheelchair at the bedside • Rehabilitation space including four chairs for students or SP and space for rehabilitation exercises and equipment • An alternative to the rehabilitation space (if not available) is to have them in a wheelchair sitting in the rehabilitation room with two chairs for observer and therapy assistant and a wheely stool for therapist
Props	• SPs can bring their own phone, magazines, and personal items into the session to replicate what a person might have brought into hospital • Rehabilitation equipment, including gait aids, for the clinical interaction should also be available
Wardrobe	• SP wears casual clothes as would be consistent with a rehabilitation hospital in Australia
Moulage	• Wound dressing applied to the lateral hip region on the affected/operated side • No scar or wound moulage is required due to this being situated underneath the dressing (that will not be removed)

Instructions to Learners

Hilda Bernard is an 81-year-old woman who lives alone and sustained a fractured neck of femur in a fall at home. The scenario focuses on the day of transfer from the acute ward to the rehabilitation hospital 1 week after she has undergone surgery to address the fracture. The surgical procedure was insertion of a dynamic hip screw to stabilise the fracture, conducted under a general anaesthetic.

Hilda Bernard had a routine postoperative period with involvement of nursing and allied health and without unexpected medical complications. She is now awaiting review with the rehabilitation ward physiotherapist, yourself.

Your task today is to conduct a physiotherapy assessment and intervention for Hilda Bernard. Observers will be expected to complete the learning tasks provided.

Instructions to SPs

You will portray the role of Hilda Bernard. You are 81 years old and live alone at home. You had a fall at home 1 week ago and fractured your hip. You underwent surgery on the evening of the fall to put a metal pin in your hip to stabilise the fracture. After 1 week in the acute hospital, you have now been transferred to the rehabilitation ward. You are awaiting your first session with the rehabilitation physiotherapist.

Patient Character Information

Personality traits	• You are a typically anxious person who has noticed these tendencies increase over recent years as your balance has become worse and you have fallen a few times.
	• You also feel an increased need to "rush" (due to urgency to go to the toilet and a fear of incontinence), which means your walking is becoming more difficult.
	• Feeling shortness of breath at times when rushing also increases your anxiety.
Social history	• You live alone in a two-bedroom unit.
	• Your partner died 3 years ago.
	• You do not feel you have a strong social network.
	• Your family live interstate (one daughter and her family) but relationship breakdown has meant there is minimal contact now.
	• You enjoy playing games on your iPad at home (crosswords, sudoku, wordfind, connect-4) and spend many hours of the day completing this or watching TV from their recliner chair.
	• You used to play bowls at the local club but now just go for lunch once per week as bowling became too difficult (the last 2 years).
	• You are increasingly homebound and socially isolated, with few visitors apart from the cleaners who visit once per fortnight.
	• You receive home delivered meals 3 days per week, cleaning for 2 h per fortnight and gardening 2 h per fortnight as part of a funded aged care service package.
Medical history	• High cholesterol (hypercholesterolaemia)
	• COPD (previous smoker of ~5–10 cigarettes per day for 60 years—Stopped 5 years ago after receiving COPD diagnosis—Has had two admissions in the last 5 years when experiencing respiratory infections. They were both pre-2020 when was still getting out of the house. Has not had COVID-19. Takes two puffers once a day.)
	• Diabetes (type 2)
	• Reflux (GORD)
	• Kidney issues (chronic renal failure stage 3)
	• High blood pressure (hypertension)
	• "Heart issues" (atrial fibrillation)
	• "Weak bones" (osteopenia)
	• "Bad knees, hips, and fingers" (osteoarthritis)

The Patient's Health Issue Information

History of the current situation, including a timeline of what has been happening	• This was the third fall that you have had in the past 3 months.
	• You cannot remember how you fell, but you remember using your personal alarm (you wear it around your neck) to call the ambulance immediately.
	• The ambulance arrived shortly after and took you to the emergency department of the local hospital.
	• The leg pain was very intense, and you knew something was very wrong immediately. You could not walk when asked.
	• In the emergency department, you were told that you have a fractured left hip and needed surgery, which occurred later that evening.
	• After waking from surgery, you had considerable pain and could not move around the bed for dressing. The nurses tried to help but your pain was too high.
	• You then saw a physiotherapist who helped you stand, but you became dizzy and the pain increased.
	• Across the week that followed, you managed to take a few steps with the help of the physiotherapist and using a walking frame to be able to reach a chair and sit out of bed for a short time.
	• You were given exercises to strengthen the hip muscles, but these were hard and at times painful, so you did not do them daily.
	• You were then told you needed to go to rehab about a week after surgery.

Current state	• You can stand and turn on the spot (to then sit in a high-backed chair or mobile commode) with one person assisting and a walking frame. • You can walk a few metres with a walking frame and one person assisting for balance. • You spend most of the day resting in bed. Any more than 15 min sitting in the chair once per day (or maybe twice on a good day) is too much. You are reluctant due to pain and fatigue. • Your pain remains quite high, with an ache at rest rated as 2–3/10 that increases to 6–7/10 on movement, and 4–5/10 when putting weight on it (when trying to step with the walking frame). • Due to the pain and noisy hospital environment you have had poor sleep since the fall. This combined with recovering from the surgery has resulted in considerable fatigue.
Person's ideas, goals, concerns, and expectations	• After everything that has happened you very reluctant to walk or move much. • You feel that you need more rest for the pain and fatigue to subside. • You are worried about not being able to go home and terrified of being sent to a nursing home. You cannot bear the thought of being forgotten by the world and not able to play games on your iPad and watch TV on your comfortable chair! • Your primary goal is to be able to return home. You would also like to walk easier, have less pain, and sit for longer.
Physical characteristics	Speaking: • Typically, short sentences with some slow speech because of the fatigue. This is particularly evident after speaking to someone for a lengthy period. Physical tests: • You have full movement in your arms and right leg but have a generalised sense of feeling a bit "weak" due to the fatigue. • You have only slight movement of your left hip (about one-fourth of normal) due to pain, which makes your entire leg feel heavy. Moving around the bed and hospital room: • You can **slide** your heel up the bed about halfway which is quite painful. You need assistance (someone lifting it) to be able to move your leg over the edge of the bed and back again. • You can **roll** to the right side slowly if asked but are unable to roll onto the left side due to pain. • You need assistance (someone supporting the leg and help to push up) to move from **lying to sitting**. • You cannot **stand** without assistance of a person or an aid (if asked). • If an aid (walking frame) is present, then with some assistance, you can **stand up**, but only put about 50% of weight through your left side (with pain going up to about 5/10). • Once standing, you can **walk** a few metres with the frame and someone close by to support balance.
Special instructions for portraying this scenario	• You are compliant with all suggestions and recommendations made by the physiotherapist, but there is considerable anxiety related to anything that "pushes" you a little bit including invoking pain or when doing movement. • With some reassurance, support and assistance you can typically cope. • If prompted for an opening line, consider "hello dear. Oh I'm not doing that well actually."

Session Information

As the patient, you will be resting in bed when the physiotherapist enters. You will then spend time (likely while still in bed) discussing aspects of what has happened to you and how you are doing now.

The physiotherapist is then expected to help you move and complete some exercises in the room or in the rehabilitation area. They will also likely talk with you regarding your understanding of the current problems and discuss some preliminary plans about whether you will be discharged home from hospital or into supported living.

After about 30 min of activity, your pain increases, you become fatigued, and you request to lay down for a rest. The physiotherapist needs to continually connect with you through education, encouragement, and empathy for you to continue with the treatment session beyond the 30 min.

Additional Scenario Information

Learners are provided with simulated hospital records related to the current inpatient stay to review prior to the simulation, as part of the instructions to learners. This occurs following the briefing but prior to commencing the interaction with the patient.

The simulated records can include the following:

- Admission assessment notes from the admitting doctor (e.g. emergency department) with preliminary information on presenting condition, past medical history, medications, and social history
- Postoperative records and surgical recommendations
- Recent nursing staff entries regarding patient progress
- Discharge summary from medical, nursing, and allied health on the acute ward (physiotherapy, social work, and OT)
- A copy of the radiology report and image

The instructions to SPs provided above may be challenging for some SPs to remember due to the length and detail. See below for an alternative presentation of information that might be considered for condensed SP instructions related to "patient character information".

Alternative Condensed Instructions for SPs

Personality traits	You are a typically anxious person who has noticed these tendencies increase over recent years as your balance has become worse, and you have fallen a few times.
Social history	You live alone, as your partner died 3 years ago.
	You do not have a strong social network and typically spent most of the week at home.
	You can make up your own hobbies that you do at home and favourite TV shows.
Medical history	You recall that you are on medication for some health problems but you cannot recall exactly what this are (something about your heart and lungs not being as good these days).

It is difficult to condense the "health issue information" any further due to relevance to the scenario. As such, strategies as described below can be used to assist older adult SPs in learning the content.

For this scenario, SPs who have previously learned and portrayed the role have provided feedback that having predetermined suggestions for hobbies, personality traits, and social behaviours assists them with conceptualising (and remembering) the "person" and their character. As such, we usually provide some example details of these factors to SPs (for which SPs have contributed ideas to the features) but acknowledge in the training that they can be modified by the SP in consultation with the SP educator.

Adapting the Session for Complexity

This scenario can be adapted to be used at various timepoints of the person's care journey to highlight different aspects of falls assessment, prevention, and management relevant to physiotherapy (and allied health) practice. We have previously adapted this scenario across the following timepoints:

- Day 1 postoperatively for initial physiotherapy assessment, primarily focused on cardiorespiratory care post-general anaesthetic and early mobility in the context of acute medical issues.
- Day 5 postoperatively with a focus on discharge planning including decision-making on discharge destination (e.g. suitability for inpatient rehabilitation or not, confirmation of discharge plan and goals).

- Initial physiotherapy assessment upon transfer to the rehabilitation ward (presented in this chapter). This session is timed for Day 7 postoperatively, encompassing initial rehabilitation assessment, fall risk factors, rehabilitation plan, goal setting, and early discharge planning discussions.
- While an inpatient on the rehabilitation ward, with a focus on reassessment of progress, goal setting, reevaluation of discharge plan, and fall prevention strategies to be implemented on discharge.
- Prior to discharge from rehabilitation ward, with a focus on discharge planning (including arranging care and home equipment), reviewing fall prevention strategies to be implemented on discharge, and self-managed progression (exercise, education) postdischarge.
- Family meeting while an inpatient on the rehabilitation ward to address discharge planning, fall risk factors, and navigating the healthcare system.
- Multidisciplinary student opportunity where occupational therapy and physiotherapy students complete a home assessment as a component of rehabilitation and discharge planning. This would require a simulated home environment. The focus of the session is on discharge planning, fall risk assessment, home modifications, and mobility strategies to navigate the home environment.

The scenario characteristics can also be adapted to better align with the learning goals of more advanced or novice learners, the learning objectives of a session, the capabilities/capacity of the SPs, or the setting of practice. Specifically, the medical, social, cognitive, and physical factors can be adjusted on a "spectrum" of complexity creating a multitude of experiences. The scenario is also changed through the emphasis the patient places on their problems and goals.

Table 18.1 presents examples of adjustable factors rated as low, moderate, and high complexity. These factors are incorporated into the instructions to learners and SPs.

Table 18.1 Scenario adaptations for increasing or decreasing complexity for learners

Domain	Lower complexity	Moderate complexity	Higher complexity
Discharge planning—home set up/accessibility	Equipment well set up Easily accessible (e.g. front access, bath/shower) Lives with someone who can provide support for accessibility	Equipment well set up, reasonable accessibility, and no live-in support Live-in support but no equipment set up and poor accessibility	No equipment or modifications at home, poor accessibility (e.g. second story bedroom/bathroom, steps to front access, shower over bath)
Discharge planning—social support	Engaged family close-by who are actively involved in providing support (e.g. meals, household tasks, personal care, community access). Family members are all in good health and close family members working part time only to assist as needed	Some family support for care arrangements, community access and household tasks, but some needs are unable to be addressed without external support. Family members work long hours and live a lengthy distance from the patient	Non-engaged or no involved family members / next of kin to assist with providing support Family disagreement regarding opinion on optimal care arrangements or support required
Discharge planning—social network	Engaged in hobbies with strong social network, friends can come visit	Less social engagement but opportunities exist to enhance this. The person is motivated to connect with people and activities that enhance life	Minimal social engagement and minimal opportunities (many barriers to engagement). Reluctant to talk about and discuss goals as somewhat embarrassed by social isolation
Falls risk factors—previous falls	No previous falls, some near falls. A number of falls prevention strategies already in place (e.g. personal alarm, home modifications). No fear of falling. Enthusiastic to exercise and improve balance and take up all preventative options	Recent falls with some falls prevention strategies implemented (e.g. personal alarm, home modifications). Mild fear of falling	Multiple previous falls without comprehensive falls assessment or prevention plan. Significant fear of falling. Complex home environment that increases falls risk
Falls risk factors—continence	No continence issues that cause "rushing"	Mild/infrequent continence issues that occasionally result in "rushing"	Frequent or severe incontinence requiring frequent rushing to the toilet, including experiencing shortness of breath when rushes to toilet and gets anxious about this
Falls risk factors—vision	Vision not a major falls risk factor, wears eyewear for correction at times	Wears eyewear to correct vision but these can be problematic at times (e.g. multifocals)	Inappropriate eyewear, memory issues impacting use of appropriate eyewear

Table 18.1 (continued)

Domain	Lower complexity	Moderate complexity	Higher complexity
Falls risk factors—cognition	Minimal side effects on memory/ delirium post general anaesthetic (GA)	Some acute memory issues post GA (impacting footwear, corrective eyewear, etc.)	Significant post-GA delirium in the context of previous cognitive decline
Falls risk factors—COPD	Mild COPD which only causes shortness of breath on significant exertion	Stable COPD with shortness of breath associated with occasional rushing in daily tasks	Severe COPD associated frequent SOB and anxiety that significantly increases falls risk as patient rushes when shortness of breath experienced
Falls risk factors—blood pressure	Pre-existing diagnosis of hypertension that has minimal impact on falls risk. Stable blood-pressure post-operatively	Stable blood pressure post-operatively but has intermittent postural hypotension as a side effect of medication	Unstable symptomatic low blood pressure (associated with dizziness) pre-operatively, that is more severe post-operatively influencing mobility and falls risk
Falls risk factors—diabetes	Diagnosis of type 2 diabetes mellitus that is stable and controlled through diet	Pre-existing diagnosis with intermittent unstable blood sugar levels that are rarely intermittent, and mild secondary peripheral neuropathy (25% sensation loss to bilateral feet). Managed with oral hypoglycemics	Unstable and poorly controlled type 2 diabetes mellitus associated with poor peripheral sensation (>75% sensation loss to bilateral feet) and pre-existing skin breakdown requiring dressings. Managed with regular insulin, which patient self-administers
Post-operative recovery (medical)	No significant medical issues prevalent post-operatively	Anaemia post-operatively (Hb below 85 for Day 1 post-op) that is on track to improve (>90 from Day 2) and associated with some light-headedness on mobilizing	Pre-existing anaemia of chronic disease (Hb 90–95) with significant post-operative reduction in Hb requiring blood transfusion, associated with delayed mobilising, exacerbated deconditioning, light-headedness, and increased falls risk
Post-operative recovery (pain)	Well-controlled analgesia with both regular and breakthrough pain relief. Pain scores average 3–4/10, up to 5/10 on movement	Reasonable analgesia effectiveness (3–5/10) but increased pain with movement (up to 6-7/10), causing some hesitation and anxiety with physically demanding tasks	Poorly controlled analgesia (pain fluctuations from 4–5/10 up to 8/10 at rest) resulting in inactivity, maladaptive movements and lack of confidence that increases falls risk

Considerations for Working with Older Adult SPs

The collaborative framework for working with older adult SPs presented by Smith et al. [5] provides helpful strategies relevant to the application of this scenario. We offer the following suggestions regarding how this framework might be implemented for this scenario. These include additional considerations for SPs related to the portrayal of falls risk factors, given that "simulated" physiotherapy intervention may involve genuine exertion of the SP and place them at risk of genuine fall or injury.

Before the Scenario

- Screen the SPs for their own personal falls risk factors that might preclude suitability for the scenario for safety reasons:
  - Previous history of falls
  - Recent falls or near falls (within 3 months)
  - Whether the SP has a fear of falling at present (suggesting higher falls risk)
  - Vision and use of corrective eyewear (including recent checks)
  - Any perceived balance issues
  - Any recent symptoms including dizziness, headspins, light headedness, vertigo, and blood pressure changes
  - Any recent general health concerns for which they have sought medical opinion
- If SPs are portraying fall risk factors that they also have (but to a lesser extent), provide education about how to manage these risk factors (e.g. if balance is an issue for the older SP and the patient role being portrayed, provide strategies to minimise risk of falling when completing balance exercise including but not limited only engaging if there is a support (e.g. chair or bench) nearby, using upper limbs for additional safety if they feel their balance is challenged).
- Practise and check potential exercises (including balance) and functional activities (such as walking, standing, and steps) that might be performed by learners with the SPs in training, to confirm that it is likely to be safe for them to

portray the role and are not going to be placed under unreasonable levels of challenge that might increase risk of a fall within the scenario.

- Simulating a fall is not recommended as part of the scenario. However, with confident SPs who do not possess a large number of falls risk factors, simulated physical characteristics consistent with increased physical risk of falls (e.g. impulsive behaviour when sitting in a chair or attempting to rise from the bed) may be practised and considered by faculty.
- Check the suitability and safety of any props that are to be used (e.g. gait aids/walking frames and therapy equipment) ensuring these do not increase the falls risk of the SP.

During the Scenario

- Ensure room setup is clear of any unnecessary hazards (i.e. that are not a prespecified component of the scenario and learning outcomes) that might increase the fall risk of the SPs. It is worth noting that the scenario may involve the assessment of some hazards, which should be individually addressed before the scenario.
- Observe physical performances of the role closely to monitor for SP fatigue or negative impacts.
- Brief observers or therapy assistants on the imperative to ensure safety in the scenario and provide permission for them to intervene if a safety risk is identified (based on negligence of the "therapist").
- Monitor for appropriate hand and respiratory hygiene related to equipment use, being in close contact (i.e. <1.5 m), and hands-on assistance, with a plan for a session "pause" if a major safety risk is identified.
- Ensure that clothing does not increase the fall risk for the SP. This typically includes well-fitting clothes and shoes that allow freedom of movement without increasing balance demands or creating tripping hazards.
- Provide the actor with a "safe" word that they can use to clearly communicate to you that the scenario is making them feel unsafe and encourage them to use time-outs for their own safety.

After the Scenario

- Debrief with the SP, asking both open- and closed-ended questions regarding SP coping with the role, covering physical symptoms and cognitive impacts at minimum, in addition to any concerns raised in the recruitment process.
- Monitor for fatigue and/or any dizziness that might render the SP at increased risk of falls when they leave the session.
- Have a referral system in place if any issues after the scenario are identified to ensure duty of care with the SP within faculty scope (which could include encouraging SPs to review any new or abnormal concerns with a medical practitioner and informal follow-up with the SP to ensure this has occurred).

The following generic strategies based on the framework presented by Smith et al. [5] are also relevant to this scenario to support older adult SPs in their portrayal:

- Provide information to SPs in a standardised format and structure that SPs have had input on designing.
- Ensure clarity in instructions to SPs on role details to be accurate in remembering and details that can be improvised.
- Complete training sessions in manageable "chunks" to minimise cognitive overload, with clear signposting of what is being covered.
- Provide video demonstration examples of physical characteristics, with associated written instructions for SPs to practise, with the preparatory material.
- Provide SPs with generic responses they can use if they forget aspects of the role.
- Provide SPs with opportunities to meet to discuss aspects of the role and provide feedback to each other regarding physical characteristics (incorporating active and experiential learning principles to task acquisition).
- Ensure SPs are debriefed as a matter of priority on cessation of the simulation.
- Provide SPs with time, resources (e.g. paper, pen) and a framework (e.g. subheadings or sentence prompts) to record feedback and reflections as soon as possible after deroling.

Lessons Learned

When working with a cohort of older adult SPs, it is likely that there will be differences in SPs' strengths and abilities to portray different aspects of the scenario complexity. Recruitment of appropriate SPs and being able to adjust the nature of the complexity of the scenario to suit the SP have been useful strategies for balancing the needs of the learner, the abilities (and falls risk factors) of the SP, and the objectives of the session.

Unlike medicine or nursing where interventions may be more easily substituted for appropriate simulation alternatives (e.g. administration of fake medication or use of a task trainer for suturing), in physiotherapy, many of the interventions are physical and have a direct impact on the person (i.e. the SP) portraying the role. Ideally SPs are not put into a position where their own fall risk factors are significantly challenged in the scenario. As such, safeguards and protections must be implemented to minimise risk of harm to the SP (e.g. musculoskeletal injury from repetitive strains/strains or even genuine falls!).

Risk controls in this scenario have included a safe word if the SP feels they are uncomfortable or not coping, thorough training (including training for poor physiotherapy interventions), and comprehensive reassessment prior to each simulation session to ensure the SP can safely cope with the scenario and potential exercise(s) being completed. If learners do not provide appropriate instructions and the SP is unclear on the activity and/or knows the exercise is going to challenge their balance, they will have insight to speak up as the "patient" and seek further information. Furthermore, if the SP is asked to do something beyond their capabilities, they know to either remain in character and "refuse" or call a time out if they feel unsafe.

In physiotherapy-focused simulation scenarios, the realism of the scenario can rest heavily on the physical performance of the SP; unrealistic portrayal of movement can negatively impact on clinical decision-making as the clinical pattern presented by the SP would not "make sense" to the learner. Preparing to portray physical characteristics can often be optimised by providing training well in advance of the simulation. This enables SPs to comprehensively practise and refine performance of physical abilities, which promotes learning, rather than restricting preparation to short periods that might limit abilities to competently perform new movements or tasks. Additional resources and activities for SPs to complete independently at home or online (e.g. balance training exercises, use of equipment, demonstrations via video) promote learning in an active way. These can be helpful for role preparation through increasing accessibility, promoting engagement and retention, enabling pacing, and allowing independent and supported practice. In addition, if physical characteristic preparation is completed well in advance of the simulation, other SPs can be recruited with sufficient lead in time if a SP is deemed not suitable for the role.

Providing learners with autonomous self-directed reflection or debriefing tasks immediately on cessation of the simulation can provide time and space for faculty to debrief with SPs as a priority after the simulation. Once the SPs have had a "check-in", debriefing with learners can proceed without losing the valuable reflections of the learners in the time-delay.

References and Resources

1. Physiotherapy Board of Australia & Physiotherapy Board of New Zealand. Physiotherapy practice thresholds in Australia and Aotearoa New Zealand. 2015. https://physiocouncil.com.au/wp-content/uploads/2017/10/Physiotherapy-Board-Physiotherapy-practice-thresholds-in-Australia-and-Aotearoa-New-Zealand.pdf.
2. Levett-Jones T, Hoffman K, Dempsey Y, Noble D, Norton C, Roche J, Hickey. The 'five rights' of clinical reasoning: an educational model to enhance nursing students' ability to identify and manage clinically 'at risk' patients. Nurse Educ Today. 2010;30(6):515–20.
3. Rudolph JW, Raemer DB, Simon R. Establishing a safe container for learning in simulation: the role of the presimulation briefing. Simul Healthc. 2014;9(6):339–49.
4. Ahmed M, Arora S, Russ S, Darzi A, Vincent C, Sevdalis N. Operation debrief: a SHARP improvement in performance feedback in the operating room. Ann Surg. 2013;258(6):958–63.
5. Smith CM, Sokoloff LG, Alsaba N. Collaborative framework for working with older simulated participants (SP). BMJ Simul Technol Enhanc Learn. 2021;7(2):112–5.

Supporting Personal Care for Older Adults Living with Dementia

19

Target Learner Group: Healthcare Providers Working with Older Adults

Sandra Parish, Hannah Iannelli, Catherine Wilson, and Chris Attoe

Background

This scenario is suitable for a range of professionals involved in the care of people with dementia exhibiting behaviour that challenges all grades of nurses, occupational therapists, psychologists, psychiatrists, and general practitioners. The scenario allows participants to be involved in a series of simulated situations focusing on the assessment and management of a variety of presentations of behavioural and psychological symptoms of dementia (BPSD). The scenario is informed by the UK National Institute for Health and Care Excellence guidelines for dementia management [1] and incorporates information on assessment and treatment approaches [2]. This scenario aims to get clinicians working together to build skills and confidence in the early recognition and management of these situations. The scenario uses simulation training and debrief models to allow participants to learn positively and constructively from the experience.

To increased fidelity, an older adult professional actor (simulated participant - SP) will undergo training with the mental health simulation faculty. During this course, the actor learns about mental health disorders, clinical pathways, and clinical settings that a patient may experience and engage in. In some circumstances, service users, including patients, family members, or carers, are able to engage in this course to inform actors of their experience of clinical services. The actor will use all of this information to accurately portray patients in simulation scenarios.

For this scenario, learners work in a small group of 12; 2 participants enter the simulation room for approximately 10–15 min and engage with an older adult professional actor while the rest observe from the other room via video link. This scenario is a summative session with no formal assessment providing a safe learning environment for participants, particularly for those entering scenarios.

After 10–15 min, the scenario finishes and the participants rejoin the rest of the group and the debrief immediately begins, led by the course faculty. The Maudsley Debrief Model, which is adapted from the diamond debrief model [3], is our preferred debrief model for this scenario. The debrief follows a structure of Description (5 min), Analysis (20–25 min), and finally Application (5 min). During the application phases, the participants who entered the scenario are instructed to take 5 min to sit and relax before joining the debrief during the application phase. It is integral that during the debrief, personal remarks and critical comments about the participants who entered the scenario are avoided as this will impact the psychological safety of the course.

This scenario can be used as a standalone; it was designed as part of a 1-day simulation course and takes place in the middle of the course day.

This scenario has been running for several years and has been incorporated into different mental health simulation courses that have a focus on dementia. Within all mental health simulation courses, pre- and post evaluation surveys have highlighted a statistically significant improvement in human factor skills such as teamwork and decision-making. Furthermore, this scenario and the course it was integrated within, have received positive feedback from participants emphasising the value to their clinical practice.

S. Parish · H. Iannelli (✉) · C. Wilson · C. Attoe
Maudsley Learning, South London and Maudsley NHS Foundation Trust, London, UK
e-mail: hannah.iannelli@slam.nhs.uk; catherine.wilson@slam.nhs.uk; chris.attoe@slam.nhs.uk

C. M. Smith et al. (eds.), *Comprehensive Healthcare Simulation: Geriatric Simulation*, Comprehensive Healthcare Simulation,
https://doi.org/10.1007/978-3-031-65742-9_19

Key Session Information

Description of the scenario	Personal care for older person with dementia, supporting the older adult to have a face wash, shower, or bath
Setting	Bedroom in care home/acute ward/psych ward/home environment
Learning objectives (please check against SMART learning objective guidelines)	By the end of the session, learners will be able to • Identify a cause of behavioural and psychological symptoms of dementia (BPSD) • Demonstrate management of BPSD • Be able to deliver personal care in a caring and compassionate way • Use effective communication techniques with patients living with dementia
Adjunct materials	N/A
Participants	Learners: Nurse Healthcare assistant Professional working with older adults with dementia Actor/SP: • One female who is an older adult to play Patricia. Faculty: 1–2 facilitators
Age of SP	SP should appear to be the stated age of the role
Scenario length	10–15 min
Session schedule	60 min in total: • 5 min briefing learnings on the scenario • 10–15 min—Running of scenario • 40 min—Debrief of learners
Wardrobe	Actor: • Wearing lots of layers of clothes • A few clothes as options for her to get changed into • Wash bag with items for personal care, for example, comb, pot of cream, and talc

Instructions to Learners

Patricia Scales is a 93-year-old woman with multi infarct vascular dementia who has been on the unit for 3 months. Over the last 2 weeks in particular, staff have been struggling to do personal care in the evening times, and Patricia has been very verbally abusive to staff. You have been allocated to Patricia on this shift and need to try and change her clothes as staff have not managed for the last 2 days due to the level of verbal aggression and her reluctance to allow staff to do so.

Instructions to SPs

You are playing Patricia Scales, a 93-year-old woman with advanced dementia. You are wearing lots of layers of clothes, that is, lots of cardigans and jumpers on top of each other and a nightgown underneath it all. Before your dementia set in, you were always very particular about your appearance and personal care and in the early stages of dementia found the process of being helped with your personal care rather humiliating. This started with people having to help you cut your toenails as you could no longer reach them due to arthritis. Then you did not want people to help you wash although you could not get yourself into the bath without help. Although you are much less cognitively able now, your state of agitation and distress around personal care is an extension of this. Now that you are more confused than previously you often do not understand what people are doing when they come to give you a wash or change your clothes. You particularly find it upsetting when people do not explain to you what they are going to do and just charge in and start to take your clothes off or treat you in a way you perceive as being rough or impolite.

When staff initially approach you in this scenario and say you need to change your clothes, you shout at them. You can be quite rude; even use words that might seem out of character for your personality predementia (e.g. use profanity). If they come near you to try and change your clothes initially really shout at them—either say words or just call out. If they try and touch you initially, even lightly you can shout that they are hurting you.

If you feel reassured by their manner, tone or voice, and what they are saying, then you can respond to what they are saying and be more accommodating, that is, let them come near you. You can be quite changeable in presentation, and if they do anything to upset you, start to shout again and cross your arms or move away so that they cannot get near you.

The facilitator will stop the scenario if the learner does start to manage to actually do personal care, that is, start to remove the cardigans, sweater.

Considerations for Working with Older Adult SPs

When working with an older SP, a number of considerations need to be made.

Before the Scenario

– Approximately 1–2 weeks prior to the course delivery, to support cognition and memory, the SPs are sent a copy of

the course manual which contains information about all the scenarios they would be participating in.
- The SP is given an opportunity to discuss the content and ask any questions to the facilitator delivering the course.
- The facilitator would provide the SP with information about the course, that is, participant numbers, professions, start and finish times, and programme of the day.
- If delivering in person, when the SP arrives, the facilitator will show them the scenario room and introduce them to other staff members teaching or supporting the course, that is, technician, administration, and other course facilitator. This allows SPs to identify any potential risks or physical challenges.
- If delivering online, a technician would be available to visit the SP at their home to support them to set up and explain any necessary technology for the course. They are shown a virtual room.
- When the SP arrives, they have a prebrief with a course facilitator; the facilitator will provide an update on participant information and check that the SP has everything that they need.
- The SP will be given a 15-min warning prior to the scenario starting so they can get into character. The simulation technician will also give a 2–3-min notification before participants enter the scenario.

During the Scenario

- The scenario is observed by course participants, simulation technicians, and course faculty members.
- The facilitator will especially pay attention to stopping the scenario if needed.

After the Scenario

- The SP usually leaves the scenario room after completion of the scenario to minimise fatigue if participating in further scenarios.
- A simulation technician checks in with the SP during this time, to discuss how they felt it went, if they have any questions, and provide feedback.
- If following a scenario, the SP raises any concerns the course facilitator will discuss this with them.

Lessons Learned

- The scenario has improved confidence, knowledge and skills in the assessment, and management of BPSDs of participants.
- Participants better understand the role of nontechnical skills, for example, situational awareness, leadership, teamwork in both psychiatric and medical emergencies and importance of reflecting upon their own capabilities, and role and escalation protocols.
- Participants better recognise when and why safe, high-quality clinical care fails to be delivered when working with persons living with dementia.
- The scenario promotes greater confidence in working as a team or leading a team in the management of challenging situations in dementia care.
- It is crucial that the simulation team recognise the lived experience of the older adults portraying the simulated patients. The simulated patients may require additional debriefs after the scenario if they have a personal experience of being carers or supporting others with their mental health. Acting agencies or other organisations liaising with the simulated patient should also be made aware of this.

References and Resources

1. Nice Dementia Pathways. https://pathways.nice.org.uk/pathways/dementia/dementia-management.
2. James IA. Understanding behaviour that challenges: a guide to assessment and treatment. 2nd ed. London: Jessica Kingsley Publishers; 2011.
3. Jaye P, Thomas L, Reedy G. 'The Diamond': a structure for simulation debrief. Clin Teacher. 2015;12(3):171–5.

Assessing and Supporting Management of an Older Adult's Swallowing Postsurgery

20

Target Learner Group: Speech-Language Pathology Students

Jenni-Lee Rees and Ingrid Scholten

Who Are the Learners?

Students within the Speech-Language Pathology (SLP) program at CQUniversity, Australia, complete this complex scenario in their adult swallowing disorders course.

Why Was This Scenario Developed?

Simulations are used increasingly in SLP to facilitate learning and assess students' competency [1–4]. They allow unlimited portrayal of conditions [5, 6], repeated practice and feedback from multiple sources [5], and preservation of patient well-being and safe management of students' anxiety [5]. This scenario helps establish students' readiness to engage in clinical practicum with older adults in an essential high acuity area [7, 8].

What Is This Scenario About?

Individual students assess and report on an elderly patient's swallowing abilities. This scenario involves Myra Anderson, a 72-year-old with Parkinson's disease who underwent orthopedic surgery for a fractured neck of femur. A swallow assessment was requested following poor response to anesthesia.

J.-L. Rees (✉)
CQUniversity, Rockhampton, QLD, Australia

Rockhampton Hospital, Central Queensland Hospital and Health Service, Queensland, Australia
e-mail: jenni-lee.rees@health.qld.gov.au

I. Scholten
Flinders University of South Australia, Bedford Park, SA, Australia
e-mail: Ingrid.scholten@flinders.edu.au

How Is the Scenario Delivered?

Individual students are randomly assigned one of several potential scenarios in a timed, videorecorded Objective Structured Clinical Exam (OSCE) utilizing paid simulated patients (SPs) aged 65+.

Background

Often SLP students experience limited interaction with the elderly, particularly in situations where they must communicate and negotiate authoritatively and professionally. Independent management of the surrounding clinical environment and equipment during assessment is also crucial. Such combined emotional, communicative, cognitive, and physical loading can be overwhelming.

This simulation concludes a scaffolded experiential education program. Learning occurs over 7 weeks where case-based study, paired role play, verbal scripting practice, group discussion, and theory build clinical confidence and competence in adult dysphagia (swallowing disorders).

The authenticity of this long-established simulation is highly valued by students who report that working with older adult SPs expands their knowledge and prepares them for real-life situations. Comments include "The SP's acting and the whole clinical set-up was so real I kind of forgot I was being examined and could just concentrate on what I had to do"; and "It was really beneficial practicing for the simulation throughout the term so I didn't fall apart, as the SP's condition …felt quite confronting and so real. I really didn't expect that."

C. M. Smith et al. (eds.), *Comprehensive Healthcare Simulation: Geriatric Simulation*, Comprehensive Healthcare Simulation,
https://doi.org/10.1007/978-3-031-65742-9_20

Key Session Information

Description of the scenario	Myra Anderson, a 72-year-old with Parkinson's disease, requires a swallow evaluation post orthopedic surgery.
Setting	Hospital surgical ward
Learning objectives	Students must demonstrate their ability to: 1. Independently analyze swallowing behavior using formal and informal assessment techniques. 2. Negotiate and document ethical, client-centered, evidence-based short- and long-term goals and recommendations for the management and rehabilitation of swallowing disorders. 3. Succinctly provide information and counselling about the swallowing disorder and its implications for safety, nutrition, and hydration, including accurate demonstration of holistic direct and indirect evidence-based treatment options. 4. Explain decisions using clear, logical clinical reasoning that demonstrates self-awareness through identification of gaps in own knowledge and how to improve future learning.
Adjunct materials	• Scenario description • Oromotor checklist • Outcome measure [9] • Documentation checklist
Participants	Learners: • 1 SLP student Faculty/SPs/others: • 1 SP aged ~65 portrays both Myra and nurse Beryl
Scenario length	30 min
Session schedule	60 min: • 10 min—Interview preparation, travel to simulation room • 25 min—Enacting scenario including feedback • 5 min—Student reflection (separate SP debrief occurs during next student preparation period); return to preparation room • 20 min—Clinical documentation.
Room setup	Preparation room: • A desk and chair; blank notepaper and progress notes; SLP stickers for inclusion in notes. Simulation room: • Curtained cubicle containing a hospital bed with rails, chair on one side, bedside cabinet on the other, and overbed tray table. Saline drip. See Supplementary Materials (Fig. 20.1). • Cart containing various test solids and fluids, disposable straws, cutlery and crockery, water jug, measuring cup, and medical equipment (i.e., pulse oximeter, stethoscope, penlight, stopwatch, tongue depressor, personal protective equipment, tissues, hand sanitizer, alcohol wipes). See Supplementary Materials (Fig. 20.2).
Props	Students may bring the following: • Pen • Oromotor checklist • Stethoscope • Penlight • Documentation checklist • Outcome measure [9]
SP wardrobe	Clothing protector, hospital gown/pajama top, nursing vest, and identity lanyard
Others	• Recording equipment • Timer

Instructions to Learners

In the preparation room:

- Read the patient's background notes; will you need further information before conducting a clinical swallow evaluation (CSE)?

In the simulation room (video recorded):

- Enter the "ward" area and approach Beryl, the duty nurse; briefly interview her to address any information gaps.
- Conduct an oromotor assessment (if appropriate) and a CSE.
- Report your findings and recommendations to Beryl.
- Stepping out of the acting role, the SP will ask for a verbal reflection demonstrating your decision-making and the challenges you faced during the simulation. Would you do anything differently; if so, why? What did you do well and why? What might you need to research or include the next time you see Myra? How might this information help your professional development?
- Leave the simulation room.

In the preparation room:

- Document your overall impression with a summary of your findings and outcome measure. List your recommendations and plans.
- Submit your paperwork before leaving.

Instructions to SPs

In this scenario, you play two roles. Firstly, Myra is a 72-year-old woman with Parkinson's disease who broke her hip after falling. She has been slow to recover from the

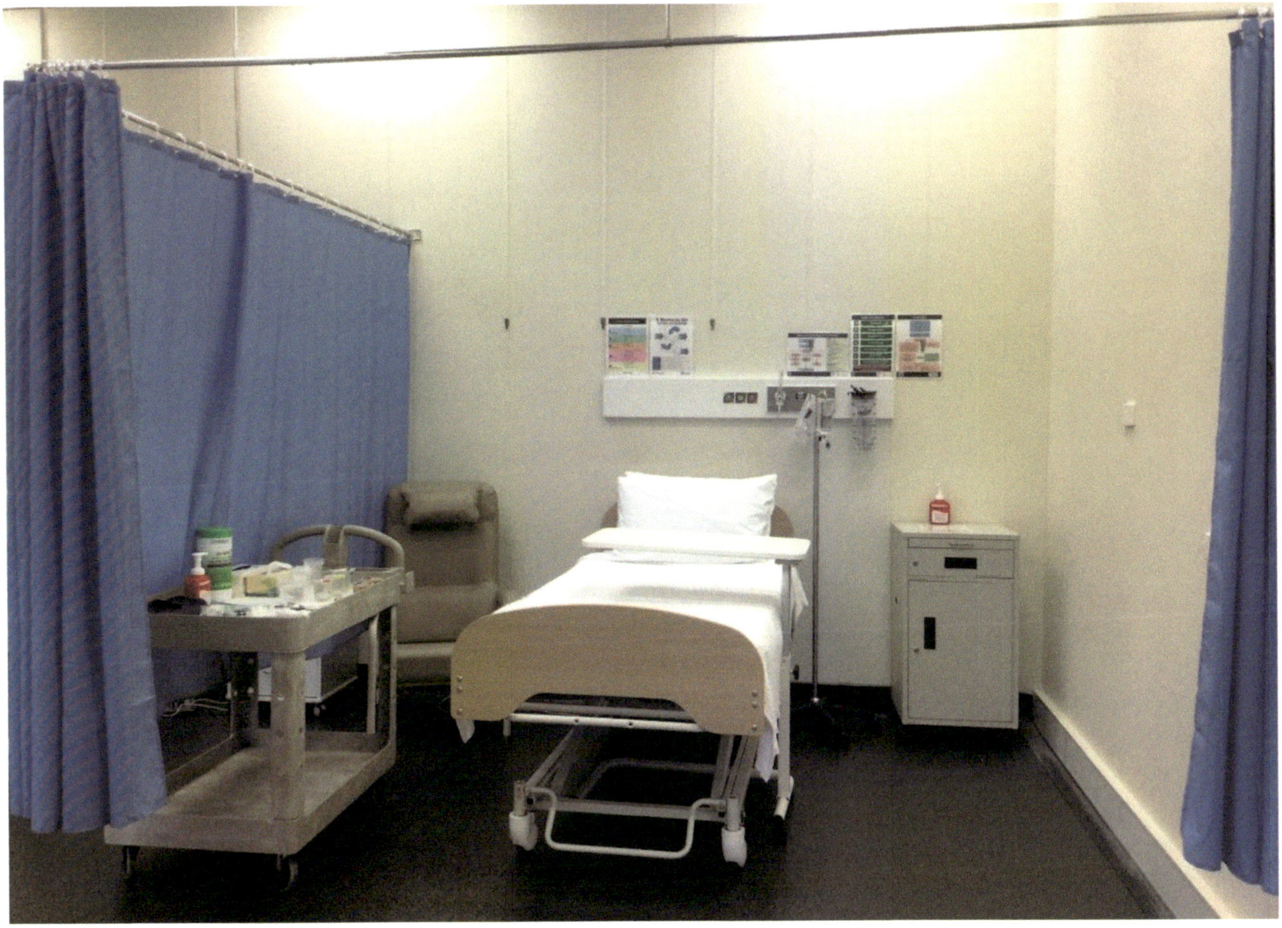

Fig. 20.1 Simulation room. (Photo: J-L Rees)

effects of surgical anesthesia and for 4 days has been "nil by mouth". The doctor needs to know if Myra can swallow her medications safely.

You also portray a registered nurse, Beryl, on the ward. You (Beryl) currently care for Myra and have been liaising with her daughter, Susan. The student will question you regarding Myra's status and care.

The student will then assess you as Myra in her hospital bed, followed by reporting their findings and recommendations to you in your role as nurse Beryl.

This simulation is video recorded for quality assurance purposes. On conclusion of the scenario, you will step out of role and, using a provided script, ask the student to reflect on their performance. Recording will cease once the student has completed this task.

Information for SP as Beryl (nurse) to relay to student:

- Myra was admitted to hospital after falling at home.
- Myra was found 12 h later by her daughter Susan who could not contact her.
- Myra underwent surgery to repair a fractured hip but did not respond well to the anesthesia.
- Since Myra's surgery she has been too drowsy to eat and drink safely, receiving intravenous fluids.
- Myra is asking where she is and how she got there.

Current and past medical history:

- Patient diagnosed with Parkinson's disease 5 years ago.
- Patient unable to take oral medications for high blood pressure (Perindo 8 mg), high cholesterol (Crestor 10 mg), reflux (Nexium 20 mg), and Parkinson's (Madopar 200 mg/50 mg).

Family Medical History: NA
Social/Lifestyle Information
Myra:

- Living independently
- Widow
- Good social support
  - Daughter Susan lives nearby

Person's Ideas, Concerns, and Expectations

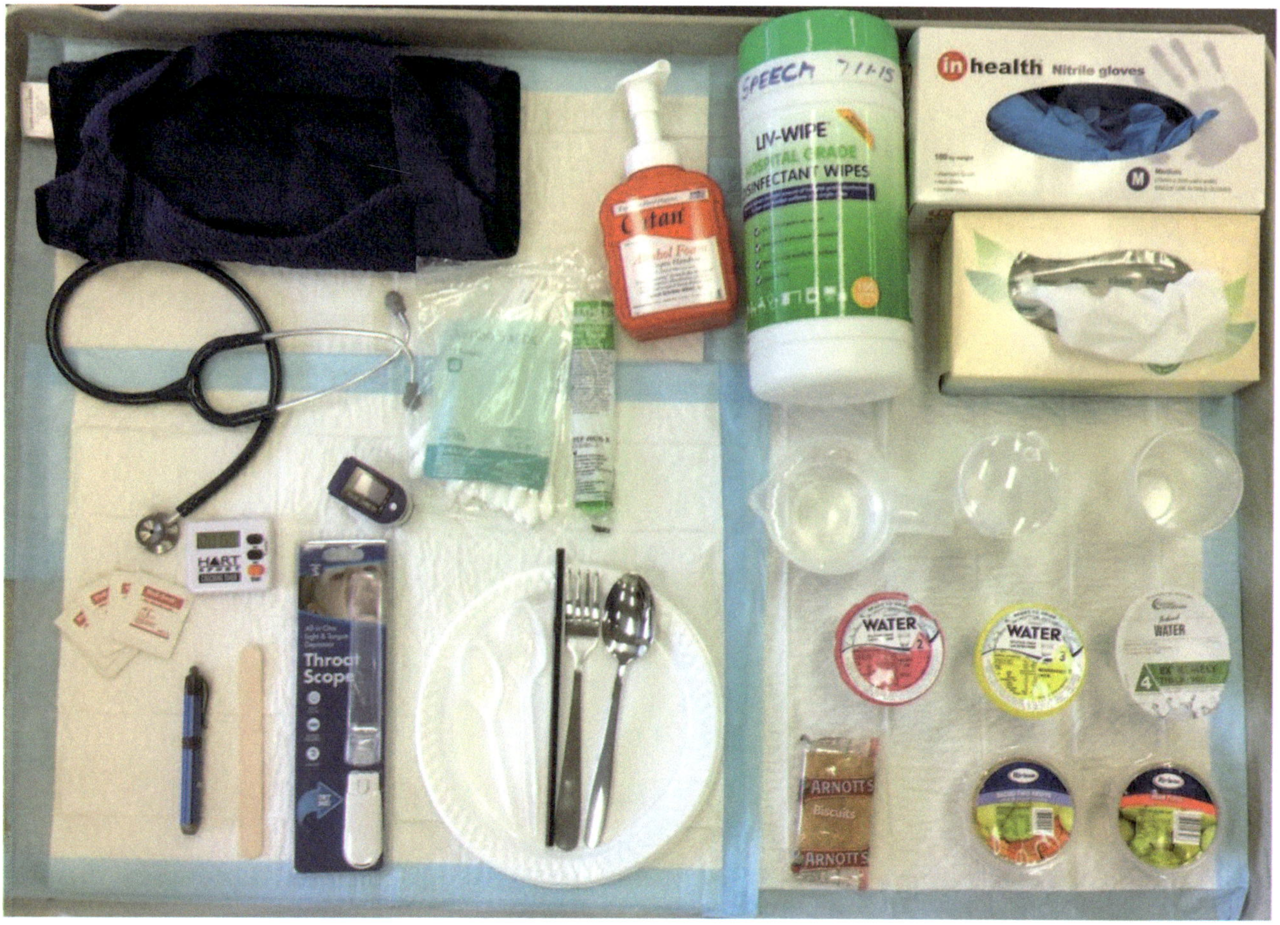

Fig. 20.2 Equipment trolley. (Photo: J-L Rees)

- Myra is confused following surgery and concerned about what has happened.

Opening Line

- (Nurse Beryl) Can I help you?
- (Myra) What do you want? What's happening?

Other Scripted Lines

- (Nurse Beryl after SLP introduction) Yes, we need to see if Myra can take her medications. I have been looking after her for the past 3 days. She seems a bit confused.
- (Myra) Where is Susan?
- (Myra) I'm parched! Can I have a drink of water?
- (Myra) Enough already (in response to bed head elevation).
- (Nurse Beryl) How did you get on with Myra?

Special Instructions for Portraying This Scenario

Action	Myra—patient reaction/symptoms
Presentation	– Lying in bed – Mouth open, snoring quietly – Initially difficult to rouse; gradually open eyes and focus on student – Right hand resting tremor starts once you wake up – You keep looking around, asking for Susan – You grunt with discomfort when the bed head is raised – You need considerable reassurance; you want to go home
Speech/ language/ voice	– A little confused; do not always understand instructions, especially if complex or out of context – Little facial expression – Monotone (flat) weak voice with soft, breathy quality – Mumble, using quick, short sentences; sometimes hard to understand

Action	Myra—patient reaction/symptoms
Respiration	– Short of breath
	– Take a breath every few words
Personality	– Impatient
	– Dislike losing your independence
Oromotor examination	– Fatigue quickly—Examination needs to be brief
	– Can poke out tongue but cannot move it quickly
	– Slow jaw opening
	– Reduced tongue strength, lip movements, and lip seal
	– Diminished smile
	– Weak, breathy cough on command
	– Begin yawning after three tasks
Water trials	**If not placed in an upright position, you do not tolerate any consistency trialed.**
	– You are right-handed and cannot hold utensils due to tremors.
	Teaspoons/dessertspoons of water are not tolerated—You cough weakly immediately after drinking.
	– You struggle to move food/fluids to the back of your mouth to swallow.
	– You cough and splutter drinking from a cup.
	– Even small sips via cup, sipper cup or straw result in coughing.
Thickened fluids	– Mildly thick fluids delivered via spoon, straw, or cup result in throat clearing.
	– You swallow moderately thick fluids from a cup and extremely thick fluids from a dessertspoon quite well but swallow response is slow.
	– Some moderately thick residue remains on your tongue but you swallow successfully with encouragement.
Solids	– Biscuit is chewed slowly and sticks in your throat; you cannot swallow it. If asked to spit it out or you are given thickened fluids to wash it down, you clear your throat.
	– Better on soft diced fruit but if mixed with juice, you cough immediately after swallowing.
	– You tolerate pureed or minced/moist consistency fed via teaspoon or dessertspoon.
	– Ask at the end if you have passed!
	– Ask when you can have a cup of tea and a biscuit.
SP feedback to patient/nurse	– Student is expected to report results and recommendations to you/Myra and you/Beryl. If complex language is used ask the student to explain, for example, "What do you mean?"
	– If told you cannot eat a biscuit and have a cup of tea you (Myra) ask "Why not?" Ask a question such as "Why do I have to have that thickened stuff?" "What if I don't want to?"—The student is required to negotiate to achieve compliance for safe swallowing. "Risk feeding" may be discussed.
	– You/Beryl prompt the student if oral intake recommendations do not include those for swallowing medications
Reflective questions for SLP student	Q1. "Think specifically about the core domains of competence required for speech pathology practice in Australia, namely, professional conduct, reflective practice, and lifelong learning. Reflect on the case, the decisions you have made, and the challenges you were faced with. Discuss your strengths, areas for improvement and learning needs."
	Q2. "How might you use this information in the future to help you become a better clinician? What strategies might you use to help you make these changes and why?"

Considerations for Working with Older Adult SPs

Before the Scenario

- Schedule 1 h of SP training within 1–2 weeks of the simulation; include sufficient practice for SP to memorize main concepts and behaviors.
- Conduct training in simulated environment; highlight all equipment.
- Use multimodal strategies to account for different learning styles and possible age-related cognitive changes and foster consolidation; include detailed notes and audiovisual examples of similar patients.
- Include information about normal aged swallowing and related disorders.
- Consider amount of prior simulation experience and ability to improvise.
- Respect the older SP's mobility and healthcare needs.
- Provide alternative cases should SP struggle to portray key characteristics and/or offer SP a choice of characters; engage the SP in possible alternative suggestions based on their own experiences.
- Check SP food intolerances and personal preferences for texture-modified food/fluid flavors.

During the Scenario

- Consider hospital bed height and possible physical limitations; SP must get in and out of bed during the simulation.
- Ensure easy wardrobe changes, for example, Velcro fastening.
- Permit SP to refer to notes to prevent memory lapses and reduce performance anxiety.

After the Scenario

- Include SP debrief.
- Provide alternative space and seating for SP to rest and prepare for next scenario (if required).
- Hold an SP appreciation event post OSCEs to encourage goodwill and ongoing participation.

Lessons Learned

- Where resources allow, two separate SPs can play the different roles; in that case, the SP playing Myra should appear to be the stated age of the role.
- Engage older adult SPs who can improvise, as students' decision-making is unpredictable.
- Allow older adult SPs to use written prompts to reduce anxiety and ensure accurate case representation.
- A timer is essential; following set timeframes is critical.

References

1. Dudding CC, Brown KK, Estis J, Szymanski C, Zraick RI. Best practices in healthcare simulations in communication sciences and disorders. Indian Hills: Council of Academic Programs in Communication Sciences and Disorders; 2019.
2. Hill AE, Ward E, Heard R, McAllister S, McCabe P, Penman A, et al. Simulation can replace part of speech-language pathology placement time: a randomised controlled trial. Int J Speech Language Pathol. 2021;23(1):92–102.
3. Miles A, Donaldson S, Friary P. Training hospital readiness in speech-language pathology students through simulation. Internet J Allied Health Sci Pract. 2015;13(4):8.
4. Zraick RI. Standardized patients in communication sciences and disorders: past, present and future directions. Teach Learn Commun Sci Disord. 2020;4(3):4.
5. Hewat S, Penman A, Davidson B, Baldac S, Howells S, Walters J, et al. A framework to support the development of quality simulation-based learning programmes in speech–language pathology. Int J Lang Commun Disord. 2020;55(2):287–300.
6. Stead A, Lemoncello R, Fitzgerald C, Fryer M, Frost M, Palmer R. Clinical simulations in academic courses: four case studies across the Medical SLP Graduate Curriculum. Teach Learn Commun Sci Disord. 2020;4(3):6.
7. Bartlett RS, Bruecker S, Eccleston B. High-fidelity simulation improves long-term knowledge of clinical swallow evaluation. Am J Speech Language Pathol. 2021;30(2):673–86.
8. Beaumont-Bowman S. Dysphagia Café [Internet]. Waller J, editor. 2016. https://dysphagiacafe.com/2016/10/21/standardized-patients-bridging-clinical-gap-dysphagia-education/.
9. Ward EC, Conroy AL. Validity, reliability and responsivity of the Royal Brisbane Hospital Outcome Measure for Swallowing. Asia Pacific J Speech Language Hearing. 1999;4(2):109–29.

Collaborating to Promote the Safety of Older Adults in the Community

21

Target Learner Group: Police and Emergency Services

Sandra Parish, Marta Ortega Vega, Megan Fisher, and Marcela Schilderman

Background

Police and ambulance services are often at the frontline of responding to mental health crises; however, professionals from both services have highlighted a lack of training and confidence in mental health knowledge and risk management [1, 2]. Moreover, interprofessional education has been praised for its benefits in improving collaborative care and the quality of mental health outcomes [3]. As such, this scenario was developed as part of a 1-day Police and Ambulance Service Mental Health Awareness simulation course with the aim of supporting emergency service staff to develop mental health awareness and interprofessional working skills.

The scenario was followed by a 35-min debrief using the Maudsley debrief model, which is an adaptation of the Diamond debrief model [4]. This debrief model elicits specific reflections related to human factors developed in the scenario, moving through a process of describing the scenario, analysing the experience and discussing how the learning can be applied to practice.

Participants were asked to complete a pre–/post-course evaluation questionnaire that measured changes using the Human Factors Skills for Healthcare Instrument [5], Mental Illness: Clinicians' Attitudes [6], as well as course-specific scale-based and open-ended questions to understand their experience of the course. An evaluation of the full course has been previously published [7].

The scenario is suitable for a range of professionals working in emergency services that respond to mental health crises, such as police officers, paramedics and other community responders. The scenario and associated handouts should be adapted to align with local policy and emergency protocols.

While the scenario was originally delivered at the end of a course for emergency services, it can also be delivered as a stand-alone scenario or adapted to fit other courses with a focus on safeguarding and risk management.

The scenario has been delivered for several years, with participant feedback noting improvements in interprofessional collaboration, person-centred care, self-efficacy and mental health attitudes.

Key Session Information

Description of the scenario	A neighbour of the patient (Jackie Smith) has just returned from holiday and noticed a male (unknown) has moved into her property, and the neighbour is concerned about this. When they asked Jackie, she was unsure of his name and appeared a little frightened. When the neighbour spoke to Jackie, the man asked for her to return inside The aim of this is for the police and paramedic to assess the situation and attempt to think about safeguarding concerns and determine what actions should be taken to help keep Jackie safe
Setting	Inside of Jackie Smith's, the Simulated Patient's (SP), home
Learning objectives	By the end of this session, learners will have: 1. Improved knowledge and confidence in managing patients with a dementia diagnosis 2. Improved knowledge about dementia and delirium 3. Improved confidence in applying protocols for safeguarding in older adults
Participants	Learners • 1 police officer and 1 paramedic participating (although can be adapted to other emergency service staff) • Remaining participants observe live video Faculty/SPs/others • Facilitator(s) • 1 SP portraying Jackie Smith • 1 SP portraying the unknown male who has moved in
Scenario length	15 min

S. Parish · M. Ortega Vega (✉) · M. Fisher · M. Schilderman
Maudsley Learning, South London and Maudsley NHS Foundation Trust, London, UK
e-mail: Marta.1.ortega_vega@kcl.ac.uk; Meganfisher@nhs.net; marcela.schilderman@slam.nhs.uk

C. M. Smith et al. (eds.), *Comprehensive Healthcare Simulation: Geriatric Simulation*, Comprehensive Healthcare Simulation,
https://doi.org/10.1007/978-3-031-65742-9_21

Session schedule	60 min total: • Scenario set-up and prebrief (10 min) • Scenario (15 min) • Group debrief (35 min)
Room set-up	• Scenario room is to look a little messy with hoarding of old papers • Observers' room is set up with a screen showing the live video and audio feed from the scenario room
Wardrobe	• The SP portraying Jackie Smith should present as an older-looking female dressed in day clothes but looking a little dishevelled • The second SP should present as a male in his 20s, dressed in jeans and a t-shirt

Instructions to Learners

The police received a call from a concerned neighbour regarding Jackie Smith, who is a 77-year-old female with a dementia diagnosis. The neighbour claims to have returned from holiday to see a male now living at the address with Jackie Smith. The neighbour does not know the male, and on asking Jackie about him, she seemed a bit confused as to who he was, and the man then asked Jackie to return inside. The call handlers have sent both a paramedic and a police officer to the scene as they are aware she has a diagnosis of dementia.

- Please go to see Jackie and assess the current situation and address the concerns raised by the neighbour.
- If you need another room, this can be provided.
- This scenario will last approximately 15 min.

Instructions to SP

About the Character

You are a 77-year-old female with memory problems. The emergency services have previously visited you for previous issues related to your memory loss.

Current Medical History

You suffer from moderate dementia (memory difficulties) and were diagnosed a few years ago. You can remember memories from when you are young, but memories from more recent events are more challenging. You are normally generally well although you take some medication for your memory, but you cannot remember what it is called.

Social/Lifestyle Information

- You have one son who lives a number of hours away and you cannot remember where he lives or his phone number.
- Your husband died 10 years ago from cancer and you have lived alone since. You met when you were 18 years old and lived in the same village. You moved to Newbury in your 20s for his work. He retired only a few years before he died.
- You never worked and were a housewife.
- You used to have a cat who died a few years ago and you miss it a lot.

Specific Instructions for Portraying This Scenario

- If the police ask you about the gentleman in front of him, seem a little scared and nervous to speak in front of him, but explain that you do know him but unsure where from.
- If they take you to a separate room, then you can be more open that you do not know who he is and at times he makes you feel scared, but you cannot remember why.
- If asked about him asking for money, you are sure that he has asked for money and you may have given him some.
- He has not been violent towards you but has made you feel as though if you do not do what he says, then he may hurt you.
- You do not remember how he introduced himself, but he is staying here and does not seem to be paying you rent.
- You have not seen your carers for a while either or spoken to your son (suggest to them maybe he has hidden messages from them and your hearing is at times poor and so you may have missed the phone).
- You do not feel safe here with him and would like him to leave but are too worried to tell him.

Instructions to SP 2

About the Character

You are a 25-year-old male, Dante Hughes, who has moved into the house with Jackie Smith. You should dress like a 25-year-old, wearing jeans and a t-shirt.

History of the Situation

You heard from a friend on the street that Jackie lives here and is alone, and you felt this was a good opportunity for you, and so you managed to get her to agree to you living with her; you said you would protect her. You do not pay rent and often try to get her to give you money. You are much stronger than her and could appear threatening although you have not hurt her. You have stopped her seeing her carers to ensure that she does not tell them about your arrangement and have been pretending to be her son.

You do not want to let the police know this and have concocted a story:

- That you are a friend of her son and are staying here for a short time.
- You are helping out and cooking for her and looking after her.

- You are aware that she has memory problems and so are helping out as much as possible.
- You have been attempting to give her rent, but she keeps saying no.
- You are looking for a job as a landscape gardener.
- You have not heard from her son or carers for a while and in fact did not even know she had carers, but you're doing everything they would do anyway, so there's no need to contact them.

Specific Instructions for Portraying This Scenario

You can be overly pleasant towards her and the police.

- Offer tea and apologise for not having cake to offer.
- Act very innocent and keep guiding her to sitting down.
- Seem very surprised when police are there or if they raise any of the concerns, but say 'I can see why, from their point of view, they might be worried, but there is nothing wrong'.
- Try to avoid the police and paramedics taking her off separately.

Considerations for Working with Older Adult SPs

Before the Scenario

- The SP is sent their scenario 1 week prior to the course, and wherever possible, the same SP is scheduled to minimise needing to learn new information.
- The SP is allowed to come in at the break before their scenario to minimise fatigue.
- When the SP arrives, a member of the team pre-briefs them to provide them with information on the participant mix and level of skill and run through the scenario.
- If delivering in person, the facilitator shows the SP the scenario room and introduces them to other staff members teaching or supporting the course to allow them to familiarise themselves with their surroundings. This is also done for online deliveries by showing them the virtual room and faculty.
- If delivering online, a technician is available to visit the SP at their home to support them to set up and explain any necessary technology for the course.
- The SP has water, tea/coffee and food available while they wait.
- A member of the team sits with the SP until their scenario to answer any questions.

During the Scenario

- The scenario room is checked for trip hazards and to ensure that there is some space for the SP to walk/sit comfortably even if the room is set to look messy.
- The room has sufficient lighting to ensure that the SPs can see well.

After the Scenario

- The SP has a debrief with the technicians to de-role, discuss how they felt about the scenario and, if there were any challenges, provide feedback on the scenario.
- The SP is offered the opportunity to watch back their scenario and the post-scenario debrief to see their portrayal of the character for their own development.
- The SP is allowed to leave after their debrief to minimise fatigue.
- If the SP raises any concerns during their debrief, one of the course facilitators schedules a phone call with them after the course to do an additional debrief.

Lessons Learned

- The session is effective at promoting interprofessional collaboration between relevant emergency services to improve the quality of care to patients.
- Longitudinal evaluation was not completed for this scenario, and would be beneficial to understand the long-term impact of training on practice.
- It is crucial that the simulation team recognise the lived experience of the older adults portraying the simulated patients. The simulated patients may require additional debriefs after the scenario if they have a personal experience of being carers or supporting others with their mental health.

References and Resources

1. Emond K, Bish M, Savic M, Lubman DI, McCann T, Smith K, Mnatzaganian G. Characteristics of confidence and preparedness in paramedics in metropolitan, regional, and rural Australia to manage mental-health-related presentations: a cross-sectional study. Int J Environ Res Public Health. 2021;18(4):1882.
2. Scantlebury A, Parker A, Booth A, McDaid C, Mitchell N. Implementing mental health training programmes for non-mental health trained professionals: a qualitative synthesis. PLoS One. 2018;13(6):e0199746.

3. Reeves S. A systematic review of the effects of interprofessional education on staff involved in the care of adults with mental health problems. J Psychiatr Ment Health Nurs. 2001;8(6):533–42.
4. Jaye P, Thomas L, Reedy G. 'The Diamond': a structure for simulation debrief. Clin Teach. 2015;12(3):171–5.
5. Reedy GB, Lavelle M, Simpson T, Anderson JE. Development of the Human Factors Skills for Healthcare Instrument: a valid and reliable tool for assessing interprofessional learning across healthcare practice settings. BMJ Simul Technol Enhanc Learn. 2017;3(4):135–41.
6. Kassam A, Glozier N, Leese M, Henderson C, Thornicroft G. Development and responsiveness of a scale to measure clinicians' attitudes to people with mental illness (medical student version). Acta Psychiatr Scand. 2010;122(2):153–61.
7. Uddin T, Saadi A, Fisher M, Cross S, Attoe C. Simulation training for police and ambulance services to improve mental health practice. J Ment Health Train Educ Pract. 2020;15(5):303–14.

Assessing and Supporting Management of an Older Adult's Aphasia Post-stroke: A Sequential Simulation

22

Target Learner Group: Undergraduate and Postbaccalaureate Speech-Language Pathology Students

Karen L. Lewis and Kari Lim

Background

SLP student clinicians do not have many opportunities for interviewing, interacting with, and/or counselling patients and caregivers prior to graduate school. The scenarios give them the opportunity to practice these skills in a safe environment where they can get feedback from simulated/standardized patients (SPs) and peers [1].

For these formative sessions, students worked in ten groups of three where each student conducted one encounter and watched each of their peers conduct the other two. However, alternative configurations could work as well. Following the encounter, the observing students provided feedback to their peers, while SPs completed a feedback form. SPs then used their written responses as a guide for their verbal feedback. SP feedback is a regular part of the SP Program participation, and SPs had prior training on giving learner feedback.

Immediately following each exercise, all of the students met as a large group to debrief with a faculty member. Students were instructed to enter the histories they had collected on the Speech-Language Pathology Adult Case History Form. (See Fig. 22.2 in Appendix.) This information was then used to inform their language evaluation and report writing in Case 2 (see Fig. 22.5 in Appendix "Evaluations and Results") and their recommendations and therapeutic goals in Case 3 (see Fig. 22.5 in Appendix "Recommendations").

While the students were debriefed by faculty, the SPs were debriefed in a different room by the SP educator who had trained them. They were asked to verbally reflect on their experience with the student, the SP training, the case, the session, and the challenges they had given feedback on. The SP educator recorded this information to improve the scenario for the following year.

The sessions have been delivered for several years, both in person and virtually. Feedback from students has been positive. Comments included the following: the SP experience "prepared me for actual interactions with patients," it "gave me the confidence I needed to embark on my clinical journey the next semester," and the SP feedback was "advice" that I took "with me into graduate school." The SPs in the program predominantly work with medical and physician assistant students and appreciated working with learners from another discipline. The SPs playing the role of Joe enjoyed the challenges of trying to play a character with aphasia [2].

K. L. Lewis (✉)
The University of Texas at Tyler School of Medicine, Tyler, TX, USA
e-mail: Karen.Lewis@uthct.edu

K. Lim
The George Washington University School of Medicine and Health Sciences, Washington, DC, USA

Global Speech Therapy, Washington, DC, USA
e-mail: Kari@GlobalSpeechTherapy.com

C. M. Smith et al. (eds.), *Comprehensive Healthcare Simulation: Geriatric Simulation*, Comprehensive Healthcare Simulation,
https://doi.org/10.1007/978-3-031-65742-9_22

Key Session Information

Description of the scenario	Case 1: Chris Smith, the spouse of Joe Smith, a 75-year-old male, who suffered a mild left hemisphere stroke (cerebrovascular accident, CVA), is attending a meeting with speech-language pathology student clinicians to complete the client's case history Case 2: A 75-year-old male, Joe Smith, who suffered a mild left hemisphere stroke (cerebrovascular accident, CVA), is attending a meeting with speech-language pathology graduate clinicians to complete a full speech and language evaluation Case 3: Chris Smith, the spouse of a 75-year-old male, Joe Smith, who suffered a mild left hemisphere stroke (cerebrovascular accident, CVA), is attending a meeting with speech-language pathology student clinicians to review findings and recommendations from his/her spouse's full speech and language evaluation
Setting	Case 1, 2, 3: Private room in a university speech and hearing clinic
Learning objectives	By the end of the session, learners will be able to: Case 1: Obtain a case history from a client's caregiver Case 2: (a) Complete a full speech and language evaluation (b) Administer and score the Western Aphasia Battery-Revised (WAB-R) (c) Write an evaluation report with findings, recommendations, and therapeutic goals Case 3: Provide caregiver education with findings, recommendations, and therapeutic goals
Adjunct materials See Appendix	Case 1: • Figure 22.1. Speech and Hearing Center Intake/Referral Form- Standard form students receive with any new client in the clinic completed for Joe's referral • Figure 22.2. Adult Case History Form for SLP student clinicians to review with standardized patient (SP); also required for SP training • Figure 22.3. Standardized Patient Case History Write Up for students to complete after the SP encounter • Figure 22.4—Speech Pathology Feedback form for SPs to complete after the encounter Case 2: • Figure 22.5. Speech and Language Evaluation Report. After scoring the full WAB-R, students complete the portions of this report indicated with < > • Figure 22.6. Standardized Patient Diagnostic Write Up for students to complete after the SP encounter • Figure 22.7. WAB-R Summary with example responses entered based on the video of the client that students watch (see below) • A video of the client on which the case is based. (Alternatively, the instructor can model client behaviors.) Students watch the video and complete responses to the Auditory Word Recognition items 1–36 and the Naming and Word Finding: Object Naming sections of the WAB-R. Students complete the rest of the WAB-R during the SP encounter. The SPs watch the video as part of their training to more thoroughly understand and effectively portray the character • Blank WAB-R evaluation protocols [3] for students to complete available at https://www.pearsonassessments.com/store/usassessments/en/Store/Professional-Assessments/Speech-%26-Language/Western-Aphasia-Battery-Revised/p/100000194.html • Expressive aphasia video [4] for SP training available at https://www.youtube.com/watch?v=JWC-cVQmEmY • Speech Pathology Feedback form for SPs to complete after the encounter (same as above) Case 3: • Figure 22.8. Speech and Evaluation Report Example. Completed patient report that students discuss with Chris in the encounter 3 • Figure 22.9. Standardized Patient Education Write Up for students to complete after the SP encounter • Figure 22.4—Speech Pathology Feedback form for SPs to complete after the encounter (same as above)
Participants	Learners: • 1 SLP clinician student who leads the meeting • 2 remaining SLP student clinicians in a small group to observe Faculty/SPs/SP educator: • Faculty facilitator • Case 1 and 3: SPs portray Joe's spouse Chris (male or female, ~70) • Case 2: SPs portray Joe (male 75) • Case 1, 2, 3: SP educator to train and debrief SPs after the encounter
SP age	SPs should appear to be the stated age of the role
Scenario length	The SP encounters are 30-min long, followed by 15-min of SP and peer feedback
Session schedule	• 15-min learner orientation • 30-min SLP student clinician/SP encounter • 15-min peer feedback/SP form completion followed by SP feedback • 15-min learner large group debrief with faculty/15-min SP debrief with SP educator
Room setup	• 2 chairs for SP and learner • Observation space for observing learners • Recording equipment (optional) • Computer for SP feedback form (optional)
Props	Case 2: Pen, comb, book for the WAB-R Sequential Commands section
Wardrobe	SPs wear street clothes

Instructions to Learners

Joe Smith is a 75-year-old male who was admitted to the hospital for a mild left hemisphere CVA. He was hospitalized for 1 week and received occupational therapy, physiotherapy, and speech therapy services. His spouse is concerned about his communication and orientation since being home and has referred him to the University Speech and Hearing Clinic for an evaluation and treatment.

Case 1

You will meet with Joe's spouse, Chris, to complete a case history. There is an Adult Case History Form for you to use as a guide, but it is your responsibility to ask follow-up questions as needed. Following the case history, you will give your recommendations for next steps (i.e., evaluation, suggestions to do at home prior to treatment).

Case 2

You will meet with Joe to complete a full speech and language evaluation. The evaluation tool you will administer is the Western Aphasia Battery-Revised (WAB-R). Following the evaluation, you will score the test and write up your findings in the Speech and Language Evaluation Report. You will also include recommendations and therapeutic goals.

Case 3

You will meet with Joe's spouse, Chris, to review your evaluation report written in Case 2. You must provide your findings, recommendations, and therapeutic goals as well as answer any of their questions.

Instructions to SPs

Case 1

Your spouse, Joe Smith, is a 75-year-old male who was admitted to the hospital for a mild left hemisphere CVA (stroke) 1 month ago. He was hospitalized for 1 week and received occupational therapy, physical therapy, and speech therapy. You have concerns regarding his communication and orientation since being home, so you were referred to the University Speech and Hearing Center. Before speaking with the speech-language pathology (SLP) student clinician today, you completed the Adult Case History Form. The student will review this form with you. You should memorize the information the form contains.

History of Joe's Situation

(Information About Joe's Situation that You May Be Asked)

Joe's stroke left him with receptive and expressive language difficulties (mild difficulty understanding but moderate word finding difficulties). He is mildly hard of hearing and will repeat himself sometimes. He sometimes has difficulty following directions because of his memory and sometimes answers questions incorrectly because of his memory and comprehension. His speech is intact (does not mispronounce or slur words). He has some difficulty with memory, specifically immediate and short-term memory (e.g., dates, errands that need to be done), but you have seen improvement since he came home from the hospital.

Current and Past Medical History

- Joe was relatively healthy his whole life until the stroke.
- He has been mildly hard of hearing the last few years but has not had it checked out.
- The stroke occurred 1 month ago. You found him on the bathroom floor unable to move or speak. You called 911 and he was taken to the hospital.
- Doctors told you it was a left hemisphere stroke.
- Joe received occupational therapy, physical therapy, and speech therapy for 1 week inpatient and then for the last 3 weeks has had home help (therapists came to the house once or twice a week).
- Medications:
  - Keppra—for seizures (since stroke).
  - Coumadin—for preventing blood clots (since stroke).

Social/Lifestyle Information

- Joe is a retired history professor who works as part-time adjunct faculty at a local university. He taught there for 40 years full-time and only recently retired.
- You are a retired high school English teacher.
- Before the stroke, Joe was independent and spent time teaching, reading, staying up on current affairs, and visiting friends/family and was part of a book club.
- Joe still enjoys visiting friends/family, but he cannot go alone. Now, he always goes with you.
- You and Joe have two children, George (45) and Leslie (41), who live close by.
- You are both well-educated, laid-back, and soft-spoken people. You have been happily married for many years (>46).

Chris's Ideas, Concerns, and Expectations

- You are relatively laid-back and optimistic about recovery. You are very accepting of the situation and willing to do whatever is needed for Joe's recovery. You are not worried.

- Both you and Joe have complete trust in the professionals that are working with him and know he will receive good care.
- You have done some research since the stroke.
- Goals: for Joe to be able to better communicate with you, the kids and grandkids, and friends at church.

Opening Line

SLP student clinicians should initiate the encounter by knocking on the door, introducing themselves by name and role, and then asking about the reason for referral. Your response should be as follows: "Joe is having trouble communicating, and I am hoping therapy can help him get better at communicating his thoughts."

Other Scripted Lines

See the Adult Case History Form.

Special Instructions for Portraying This Scenario

- You are wearing casual clothing.
- Students will be in groups of three. One student will conduct the discussion, while the other two students observe.
- The session will last up to 30 min. Students may end it early if they wish.
- Students should follow the questions on the form. If they ask anything not covered in the form, say, "I'm not sure" or "I don't know."
- Once the students have ended the encounter, you may begin the feedback discussion.

SP Feedback Topics

- Patient trust/rapport—How did the learner do at developing a relationship with you and gaining your trust? Would you want to keep working with them? Did you feel they were invested in helping your spouse?
- Communication and listening skills—Did they phrase things clearly, without using jargon? Did they seem to understand what you shared? Did they empathize with you?
- Asking follow-up questions: Did they ask appropriate follow-up questions to the questions on the form?

Case 2

Review Case 1 Instructions for SPs.:

You are Joe Smith, and you are coming to the University Speech and Hearing Center for a speech therapy evaluation and treatment. Your memory has improved since leaving the hospital, but you still have difficulty with receptive and expressive language. The SLP student clinician will complete a full speech and language evaluation using the Western Aphasia Battery-Revised (WAB-R).

Expressive Speech-Language Issues

- During normal conversations, you have trouble thinking of words, particularly complicated words. It feels like they are "on the tip of your tongue."
  - Generally, you can respond with "yes, no, OK," and other short words quickly, but thinking of other words or a sentence can take a little while.
- Sometimes you take long pauses between words (anywhere from a few seconds to occasionally a longer pause of 10–15 s).
- You forget/are not able to remember "filler" words in a sentence.
  - Typically, sentences are not complete, but a string of "key words."
- You use hand motions as you try to come up with words.
- You understand and can answer correctly to most questions, but you may misunderstand and answer incorrectly to longer/complicated questions, or questions spoken with a fast pace.
- You may think of a word that starts with the same sound, but not the actual word (e.g., "spit" for "spoon"), *or* may only think of first the sound or syllable (e.g., "sp" for "spoon").
- You have difficulty expressing some words, but you do not "stutter."

Receptive Speech-Language Issues

- You understand and answer correctly to most questions/directions, but you may misunderstand and answer incorrectly if instructions are too long, include complicated words, or are spoken with a fast pace. (Long sentences or directions can seem like some of the words are in another language, so you miss the full context.)
  - For example, you might hear the word "apprehensive" but process it as "apple."
  - Some of this difficulty might also be because you are moderately hard of hearing.
  - You still enjoy reading, but there are some days it might be hard and a little frustrating for you to understand things.
- You will sometimes forget things, especially short-term memory things like dates, directions, to-do lists, etc. Your memory seems sporadic. (You might remember something one day, and not the next.)
  - For example, Chris might ask you to get a granola bar from the kitchen, but by the time you walk into the kitchen, you can't remember why you're there.
  - For example, you might forget you need to use your walker and try to walk to the bathroom without it.
- You can say "I don't know" frequently as a rote phrase (automatic response).

Details of Social-Personal History

Review Case 1 Instructions for SPs.

Structure of the Encounter

The clinicians should introduce themselves and explain the task. They will be completing an evaluation called the WAB-R (Western Aphasia Battery-Revised). Portions of the tool require interaction with objects that cannot be provided during your encounter. Students see a video of the patient this case is based upon to obtain that information. The portion they will complete with you essentially tests your memory, recall, speech, and language processing. They will be asking questions directly off the packet (which they should not show you) and will not likely ask many additional/follow-up questions. Accordingly, please make the answers you will be giving on the WAB-R as close to the sample as possible.

SP Directions While Completing the WAB-R

- You generally *do not* get visibly frustrated or discouraged when you cannot think of an answer or struggle.
- Pauses to think of an answer should vary between 2 and 5 s on average (somewhat random). Pause slightly longer (4–5 s) for more complex or longer answers.
- Can answer "yes" or "no" questions the quickest, only pausing 2 s.
- Include a few self-corrections.
- When you can't remember things, you feel like they are on the "tip of your tongue" and you may make hand gestures or show that you are trying to remember/express the word.
- Sometimes "sound out" a word you are trying to remember/express. You may think of a word that starts with the same sound, but not the actual word (e.g., "spit" for "spoon"), OR may only think of first sound or syllable (e.g., "sp" for "spoon").
- You understand short instructions the clinician gives you without needing them to repeat or rephrase.
- If the clinician engages in casual conversation, give very short/succinct answers to avoid any difficulties in finding words ("OK, yes, no, mm-hmm, maybe").
- Follow directions written into script (instructions are in parentheses).
- Know which questions you are supposed to get wrong or when to answer "maybe" or "I don't know."
- As the clinician is wrapping up the assessment, ask the clinician some variation of "How long will this take?".
  - Clinicians should be asking you if you have questions, but if they do not, please ask this question at the end of the encounter.

Opening Line

The SLP student clinicians should introduce themselves and explain the task. To avoid difficulties finding words, you will say, "okay."

Other Scripted Lines

See WAB-R protocol.

Special Instructions for Portraying This Scenario

See Expressive and Receptive Speech-Language Issues above.

SP Feedback Topics

- Introduction/explanation—Did the learners professionally and completely introduce themselves and what they would be doing with you today?
- Patient trust/rapport—How did the learner do at developing your trust? Did they show nonjudgmental body language/facial responses? Did they open and close the interview in a friendly, warm way or did they just dive into questions?
- Did they speak to you (tone of voice or pace) like a child? Or did you feel treated with appropriate respect for your age?
- Completing the WAB-R:
  - Did they repeat any of the questions (or answers) to you if you got them wrong or paused? They should *NOT* do this.
  - Did they accidently let you see the form at any point, or the marks they were making on it? They should *NOT* do this.
  - Did they indicate by word, tone, facial expression, etc. when you were getting answers "right" or "wrong"? They should *NOT* do this.

Case 3

Review Case 1 and 2 Instructions for SPs.

Structure of the Encounter

You have returned to the speech and hearing clinic to learn the results of Joe's evaluation. The SLP student clinicians should introduce themselves. They will then be reviewing Joe's patient report with you and reviewing what tests were done and the results with you before sharing their clinical impressions, recommendations, and recommended goals.

SP Directions

- General.
  - You are a supportive spouse and just want to help in Joe's recovery.
  - As the clinician goes through Joe's patient report with you, you will start to show more signs of worry and, at times, frustration with the situation as his main caregiver. You now realize that Joe's condition is his new normal.
  - Clinicians should be checking in with you to see if you have any questions or concerns after they go through each section.

- Clinical Impressions.
  - Generally, nod along with what they are saying as they go through their impressions of Joe's condition (moderate aphasia, has difficulty finding words, etc.). Note: You are familiar with the terms "moderate aphasia" and "CVA" but can question other terms that seem unfamiliar.
  - You agree with the clinician's assessment. When the clinician asks if you have any questions, you will start to show signs of frustration. Example responses are as follows:

    "Joe is really struggling at home. He is really having trouble finding words."

    "I just don't know how to help him and there is so much going on."
- Recommendations.
  - Listen as the clinician goes through their list of recommendations. These will vary by clinician.

    Example: Joe will come to speech therapy three times a week for 50-min sessions.
  - You will start to show growing levels of frustration; it is clear that you are a little overwhelmed with the situation. Example responses are as follows:

    "I'm really worried about the schedule. I'm not sure if I can get him here that many times a week because there is just a lot going on at home."

    "It can be pretty difficult to get him here because getting that walker in the car…it's really heavy!"

    "How long will we have to come to speech therapy? Will it help him in the long run?"
- Goals
  - Clinician will have prepared goals for you in advance (these may vary by clinician) and will check in with you periodically (possibly after sharing each goal).

    Example: Joe will follow two-step directions with cues.
  - Reiterate how these speech therapy goals will affect you and Joe's daily life. Example responses are as follows:

    "What does this look like at home?" or "How do I do this at home?"

Opening Line

Student clinicians should initiate the encounter by knocking on the door, introducing themselves by name and role, and then informing you they will be discussing their plan. You should respond with "I'm looking forward to learning how you can help Joe."

Special Instructions for Portraying This Scenario

Review Case 3 Instructions for SPs.

SP Feedback Topics

- Introduction/explanation—Did the learners professionally and completely introduce themselves and what they would be doing with you today?
- Patient trust/rapport—How did the learner do at developing your trust? Did they open and close the interview in a friendly, warm way or did they just dive into questions? Did you feel they were invested in helping your spouse? Did they periodically check in with you to see if you have any questions? Did they empathize with you?
- Reviewing the information—Did they spend the appropriate amount of time doing the review of your husband's assessment results?
- Communication and listening skills—Did they phrase things clearly, without using jargon?
- Did they "reflect back" after you asked a question or shared an answer to confirm they understood what you mean? Did they ask you if you understand an appropriate number of times?

SP Comments on Portraying Joe Smith

The two most challenging things about portraying the Joe Smith case were (1) the portrayal of aphasia, particularly in terms of getting the hesitations and word-finding difficulty right; and (2) remembering the detail in the part of the interview when the student is filling out the assessment form. There is a lot of very particular detail, and I didn't want to mislead the student with my answers. We saw several videos of aphasia patients in the several times I did the case, and these were tremendously helpful in portraying the aphasia (particularly with the timing of the hesitations and the affect of the patient.) I think we had the tools we needed: the videos were a key element; the trainer's advice on portrayal was also helpful, as well as having a chance to practice part of the material during the training. I guess the one thing I could have wanted more of would be a few more examples of video of aphasia patients, since each of the ones I remember seeing was somewhat different in the presentation of the symptoms--more examples might be better for finding a presentation that isn't just an imitation of one patient.—Glenn

The video was helpful, especially in showing the upbeat and engaged attitude of the patient. Personally, I have had a stroke with temporary effects in speech and have experience with a grandmother and an aunt, who both had word-finding issues. For an SP to know the process of searching the brain rolodex for the right word is helpful. Saying a word that is maybe close, or maybe not, but sounds similar helps with the realism. Doing the test, especially virtually, is challenging. The components of the battery most relevant to the case should be fairly well memorized. Students can be a challenge, especially if they ask compound questions or move a little too fast or get impatient. Most helpful is doing a practice session or two with another SP or instructor.—Tom

Considerations for Working with Older Adult SPs

Before the Scenario

- Aphasia is most commonly seen in older adults. SPs may have life experience with it that could impact their ability to portray the case. Screen SPs for comfort with the subject matter.
- For Case 2, there are scripted responses that SPs deliver with a certain affect which will require significant retention. Screen SPs for memory ability.
- Cognitive load for the case is significant. Form completion should be as easy as possible. If completing an electronic feedback form, screen SPs for ease with the computer.
- Because cognitive load is significant, recruit SPs who are practiced at giving feedback.
- Prior to coming to training, send the SPs the case information, and ask them to read it and imagine how different the Smiths' lives must be since the stroke.
- So the information remains fresh in their minds, train the SPs 1–5 days before the session.
- Plan a 2-h training session for Case 1 and 3. Case 2 may take longer to master the aphasia portrayal. Depending on the SPs' experience, you may need to divide the Case 2 training into two sessions.
- If you record the first time you run the sessions, use the recordings for training future iterations of the session [5]. SLP faculty can highlight portrayals that are especially strong for other SPs to emulate.

During the Scenario

- Consider the mobility of the SPs, and ensure the room is free of hazards and SPs know where to sit (if videoing scenario).
- Consider the hearing capacity of the SPs, and ensure they can hear overhead announcements (if facilities have this equipment).
- If using a computer, consider SPs' familiarity with technology and ensure they know how to access the feedback form.

After the Scenario

- For their psychological safety, provide the SPs an opportunity to de-role and discuss their emotional response to the case portrayal.
- Include the opportunity for SPs to provide case and training feedback during the debriefing session so that it can be incorporated into future iterations of the case.

Lessons Learned

- Including the SLP faculty in the SP training enabled the SPs to fully understand what to expect from the SLP patient visit.
- Educating SPs about aphasia and its characteristics helped them to fully understand the impact of Joe's stroke on their characters' lives.
- Incorporating videos of patients with aphasia answering questions enabled the SPs to perform more realistically.
- SPs playing Joe need time for practice and feedback to successfully perform the role. They need guidance in understanding the difference between word finding and stuttering. A study by Baylor et al. [6] suggests that training may need to focus on auditory comprehension as well.

Appendix

Speech and Hearing Center

SPEECH AND HEARING CENTER INTAKE/REFERRAL FORM

CONTACT INFORMATION

Name: Joe Smith ____ Age: 75 ____ Date Of Birth: January 14, 1948 ____

Gender: Male ____ Pronouns: he, him, his ____ Name Of Contact Person: Chris Smith ____

Relationship To Person Seeking Services: ☐ Self ☐ Parent/Guardian ☑ Spouse ☐ Other ____

Address: 123 17th St NW Alexandria, VA 22304 ____

Phone: 202-123-4567 ____ Alternate Number: NA ____

Email Address: Joe&ChrisSmith@gmail.com ____

Do you prefer in-person or virtual appointments? ☐ In-Person ☑ Virtual ☐ No Preference ☐ Both

HISTORY

What is the primary language used? English ____

Is there a medical diagnosis? ☑ Yes ☐ No If yes, what? Stroke ____ Date of onset? 1 mo ago

Has person had evaluation before? ☑ Yes ☐ No If yes, when? 1 month ago ____ Where? Hospital ____

Has person ever had such therapy in the past? ☑ Yes ☐ No If yes, what for? ____

Has person had a hearing exam? ☐ Yes ☑ No If yes, when? ____ Results? ____

Does person use hearing aids? ☐ Yes ☑ No

PROBLEMS/ SYMPTOMS

Please describe why person is interested in services:

☐ Stuttering ☐ Articulation ☐ Hearing Aids

☐ Social Skills ☐ Reading - Decoding ☐ Lip-reading

☐ Apraxia/Dysarthria ☐ Reading - Comprehension ☐ Voice

☑ CVA ☐ Receptive Language ☐ Gender Affirming Voice Training

☐ TBI ☐ Expressive Language ☐ Accent Modification

☑ Aphasia ☐ Auditory Processing ☐ Laryngectomee

☐ Dysphagia ☐ Hearing ☐ Other ____

TYPES OF SERVICES INTERESTED IN:

☐ Evaluation Only ☐ Treatment Only ☑ Evaluation & Treatment ☐ Individual ☐ Group

REFERRED BY: Check all that apply.

☐ Children's Hospital ☐ Doctor ____

☐ Newspaper ____ ☐ Personal Acquaintance ____

Which one? ____ How did they hear about the Speech and Hearing Center? ____

☑ Internet ☐ Other ____

FOR OFFICE USE ONLY

Date ____ Admin/GTA initials ____ Track ____ Clinician ____

Wait List Time ____ Provided Other Facilities for Services ☐ Yes ☐ No

Fig. 22.1 Speech and Hearing Center Intake/Referral Form

ADULT CASE HISTORY FORM

SPEECH-LANGUAGE PATHOLOGY

Client Name: Joe Smith **Date of birth:** January 14

Person Interviewed: Chris Smith **Relationship:** Spouse

Student instructions: Ask the following questions. It is your responsibility to ask follow up questions as necessary.

What do you hope to get out of speech therapy for client?

- To get better at communicating thoughts and needs

What is client's primary language? Other languages spoken?

- English only

MEDICAL HISTORY

Please check all that apply. Please provide dates where applicable.

☑ Stroke (1 month ago)
☐ Head injury
☑ Hearing loss (ongoing)
☑ Voice issues or changes (1 month ago)
☑ Swallowing issues or changes (1 month ago)
☐ Any neurological or degenerative diseases

How would you describe client's current state of health?

☐ Excellent
☑ Average-fair
☐ Poor

Has client been hospitalized within the last 5 years? If so, why? Where?

- 1 month ago, Joe had a mild stroke. Was in hospital for one week

Please list any medications taken at this time and reason:

- Keppra for seizures
- Coumadin for preventing blood clots

Fig. 22.2 Adult Case History Form

Does client use any of the following assistance devices?

- ☐ Wheelchair
- ☑ Walker (forgets to use it sometimes)
- ☐ Cane
- ☐ Other
- ☐ None

Is client able to climb stairs: __X___ Yes _____ No (with help)

SPEECH-LANGUAGE HISTORY

Does the client have difficulty with:	Never	Sometimes	Frequently
Swallowing		X	
Drooling	X		
Expressing thoughts			X
Being understood by others		X	
Understanding what others are saying to you		X	
Orientation/memory		X	
Problem solving		X	
Focusing/attention	X		
Reading/writing		X	
Finding words			X
Maintaining topic of conversation		X	
Fluent speech (stuttering)	X		
Following directions		X	
Voice difficulties		X	

Are there any other difficulties besides what is listed above?

- No

Did the problem begin suddenly or develop over time?

- 1 month ago, after stroke (but he has been hard of hearing for a while)

Has client been seen by any other rehabilitation professionals?

☑ Speech therapy: where: Hospital when: 1 month ago

☑ Physical Therapy: where: Hospital when: 1 month ago

Fig. 22.2 (continued)

☑ Occupational Therapy: where: Hospital when: 1 month ago

☐ Other:

Does this speech-language difficulty impact the client's ability to function in daily life?

- Yes, we can't always understand him
- He has difficulty thinking of words and sometimes the day
- Sometimes he repeats himself after 5-10 minutes
- Doesn't always answer questions correctly but he is hard of hearing
- He has difficulty following directions, but I think he forgets what I told him

How or where does the speech-language difficulty impact the client the most?

- With other family members or people less familiar with him, especially in loud and crowded places

Describe the client's daily communication needs:

- Talking with spouse throughout the day as well as children, grandchildren, friends, and visitors

SOCIAL AND EDUCATIONAL HISTORY

Client's marital Status:

☐ Single ☐ Divorced
☑ Married ☐ Widowed

Spouse or partner's name:

- Chris Smith

Children:

- George Smith; age 45
- Leslie (Smith) Carroll; age 41
- They both live nearby

Fig. 22.2 (continued)

Occupation:

- Retired history professor

Employer:

- Retired from the George Washington University

Highest level of education (grade or degree) completed.

- Master's

Any additional information gathered:

Fig. 22.2 (continued)

Fig. 22.3 Standardized Patient Case History Write Up

Standardized Patient-Case History Write Up

Name: ______________________________

(Your responses below will be graded based on the length, content, and your reflective insight)

1. In 1-2 paragraphs, summarize your experience.(_________/10points)
   Include the following
   -what went well/what did not
   -were you able to answer the spouse's questions
   -did you notice any inconsistencies with responses from the caregiver
   -what additional information did you feel was missing from the background information provided, case history form, or caregiver report
   -how would you ask for the additional information you need
   -how did the experience differ from your expectations as a clinician
   -how will you use this experience professionally

2. In 1-2 paragraphs, summarize your professional recommendations for the patient. (_________/5points)
   Include the following:
   -does the patient need a full evaluation and what areas will you want to evaluate (be specific)
   -do you expect the patient to present with mild, moderate, or severe deficits and why
   -what recommendations do you have now for the caregiver

Speech Pathology Feedback

-

(Master Evaluation)

Greeting and Opening

1. **The clinician introduced him/herself by name and title:**

◯ Yes	P.V.: 1.0
◯ No	P.V.: 0.0
◯ Inconsistent	P.V.: 0.5

Category: Communication

Question Point Value: 1.0

2. **The clinician seated him/herself at eye level with the patient:**

◯ Yes	P.V.: 1.0
◯ No	P.V.: 0.0
◯ Inconsistent	P.V.: 0.5

Category: Communication

Question Point Value: 1.0

3. **The clinician briefly explained what he/she would be doing before the beginning of the session:**

◯ Yes	P.V.: 1.0
◯ No	P.V.: 0.0
◯ Inconsistent	P.V.: 0.5

Category: Communication

Question Point Value: 1.0

Professionalism

4. **The clinician maintained appropriate eye contact with the patient throughout the session:**

◯ Yes	P.V.: 1.0
◯ No	P.V.: 0.0
◯ Inconsistent	P.V.: 0.5

Category: Communication

Question Point Value: 1.0

5. **The clinician maintained facial expressions that were appropriate to the context:**

◯ Yes	P.V.: 1.0
◯ No	P.V.: 0.0
◯ Inconsistent	P.V.: 0.5

Category: Communication

Question Point Value: 1.0

6. **The clinician maintained an attentive and relaxed posture throughout the session:**

◯ Yes	P.V.: 1.0
◯ No	P.V.: 0.0
◯ Inconsistent	P.V.: 0.5

Category: Communication

Question Point Value: 1.0

7. **The clinician spoke at an appropriate rate and volume throughout the session:**

◯ Yes	P.V.: 1.0
◯ No	P.V.: 0.0
◯ Inconsistent	P.V.: 0.5

Category: Communication

Question Point Value: 1.0

Fig. 22.4 Speech Pathology Feedback form

Speech Pathology Feedback

-

(Master Evaluation)

8. The clinician used professional language throught the session (avoided "um, yea"):

- ◯ Yes P.V.: 1.0
- ◯ No P.V.: 0.0
- ◯ Inconsistent P.V.: 0.5

Category: Communication

Question Point Value: 1.0

9. The clinician acknowledged the patient/spouse's feelings:

- ◯ Yes P.V.: 1.0
- ◯ No P.V.: 0.0
- ◯ Inconsistent P.V.: 0.5

Category: Communication

Question Point Value: 1.0

Content

10. The clinician rephrased patient responses to ensure understanding of patient responses:

- ◯ Yes P.V.: 1.0
- ◯ No P.V.: 0.0
- ◯ Inconsistent P.V.: 0.5

Category: Communication

Question Point Value: 1.0

11. The clinician made attempts to build rapport and connect with the patient/spouse:

- ◯ Yes P.V.: 1.0
- ◯ No P.V.: 0.0
- ◯ Inconsistent P.V.: 0.5

Category: Communication

Question Point Value: 1.0

12. The clinician addressed the concerns of the spouse/patient:

- ◯ Yes P.V.: 1.0
- ◯ No P.V.: 0.0
- ◯ Inconsistent P.V.: 0.5

Category: Communication

Question Point Value: 1.0

13. The clinician explained his/her recommendations:

- ◯ Yes P.V.: 1.0
- ◯ No P.V.: 0.0
- ◯ Inconsistent P.V.: 0.5

Category: Communication

Question Point Value: 1.0

14. The clinician obtained patient/spouse consent (verbally or nonverbally) following given recommendations:

- ◯ Yes P.V.: 1.0
- ◯ No P.V.: 0.0
- ◯ Inconsistent P.V.: 0.5

Category: Communication

Question Point Value: 1.0

Wrap-Up and Farewell

Fig. 22.4 (continued)

Speech Pathology Feedback

-

(Master Evaluation)

15. The clinician informed the patient or family member of the next step:

◯ Yes	P.V.: 1.0
◯ No	P.V.: 0.0
◯ Inconsistent	P.V.: 0.5

Category: Communication

Question Point Value: 1.0

16. The clinician asked for and answered any questions from the patient or family member:

◯ Yes	P.V.: 1.0
◯ No	P.V.: 0.0
◯ Inconsistent	P.V.: 0.5

Category: Communication

Question Point Value: 1.0

17. The clinician stated that they are available for any future questions or concerns:

◯ Yes	P.V.: 1.0
◯ No	P.V.: 0.0
◯ Inconsistent	P.V.: 0.5

Category: Communication

Question Point Value: 1.0

Additional Comments

18. Comments

Category: Comments

Question Point Value: 0.0

Fig. 22.4 (continued)

Speech and Language Evaluation Report

Student instructions: Complete the areas noted with < > below.

CLIENT INFORMATION

Client Name: Joe Smith
Date of Birth: January 14, 1948

Date of Evaluation: January 15, 2023
Chronological Age: 75 years, 0 months

Evaluating Therapist:
Evaluation Location: Speech and Hearing Clinic

REASON FOR REFERRAL:
Joe, a 75-year-old male, was referred to the GWU Speech & Hearing Center by his spouse due to concerns regarding communication and orientation.

BACKGROUND INFORMATION

History
An interview and case history were completed by Chris Smith, Joe's spouse. The following information was provided:

Speech and Language History
Chris reported that since Joe's stroke, other family members sometimes have difficulty understanding Joe, especially in loud and crowded places. He often has difficulty thinking of words. He will sometimes repeat himself after 5-10 minutes in a conversation. Chris also reported that Joe sometimes has difficulty following directions and remembering the day of the week.

Medical History
Joe suffered a left hemisphere CVA one month ago. He received OT, PT, and ST during his one week stay at the hospital. He is currently taking Keppra to control seizures and Coumadin to prevent blood clots. He has a walker but according to his spouse, he forgets to use it. He is hard of hearing but does not wear a hearing aid.

Family, Social, and Educational History
Joe lives in Virginia with his spouse, Chris. He is a retired history professor. He has two grown children, George and Leslie, who live nearby.

EVALUATIONS AND RESULTS

The following assessment tools were administered in English:
1. Hearing Screening

Fig. 22.5 Speech and Language Evaluation Report

2. Oral Mechanism Examination
3. *Western Aphasia Battery- Revised (WAB-R)*
4. Informal Observations

The assessment description and results are as follows:

1. Hearing Screening

A hearing screening was not completed during the evaluation. Joe's spouse reports that he is hard of hearing but does not have hearing aids.

2. Oral Mechanism Examination

An oral mechanism examination was administered to evaluate the structural and functional integrity of Joe's oral mechanism for speech production.

Results are as follows:

Face: Overall appearance, symmetry, and tone appear to be within normal limits.
Jaw: Range of motion and strength appear to be within normal limits.
Lips: Range of motion, coordination, and strength appear to be within normal limits.
Teeth: Occlusion and structure appear to be within normal limits.
Tongue: Range of motion, coordination, and strength appear to be within normal limits.
Hard Palate: Structure and symmetry structure appear to be within normal limits.
Soft Palate: Structure, symmetry, and mobility appear to be within normal limits.
Diadochokinesis (DDK): Joe's ability to coordinate production of syllables in rapid succession ("papapapa") and rapidly alternate speech movements ("pataka") is within normal limits.

3. Language

The *Western Aphasia Battery-Revised (WAB-R)* is a standardized measure used to evaluate a person's language function following an acquired neurological disorder. The WAB includes the following series of subtests:

- Spontaneous Speech: the person must respond verbally to 6 personal questions and describe a black and white picture.
- Yes/No Questions: the person must answer personal, environmental, and general yes/no questions
- Auditory Word Recognition: the person must point to items from an array of objects and pictures in the same category
- Sequential Commands: the person must follow verbal commands of increasing length and complexity
- Repetition: the person must repeat words, phrases, & sentences of increasing length and complexity
- Object Naming: the person must name common objects from a variety of categories
- Word Fluency: the person must name as many animals as able in one minute
- Sentence Completion: the person must complete five orally presented sentences
- Responsive Speech: the person must respond verbally to five simple questions

Fig. 22.5 (continued)

The WAB was administered to assess Joe's language function following his CVA. Joe's scores are as follows:

Subtest	Scores
Spontaneous Speech	<#>
Yes/No Questions	<#>
Auditory Word Recognition	<#>
Sequential Commands	<#>
Repetition	<#>
Object Naming	<#>
Word Fluency	<#>
Sentence Completion	<#>
Responsive Speech	<#>

The subtest scores are combined and transferred to section scores, to determine the type of aphasia. The section scores are as follows:

- <u>Spontaneous Speech</u>: Measures ability to produce functional communication in conversation and picture description.
- <u>Auditory Verbal Comprehension</u>: Measures ability to comprehend yes/no questions and sequential commands with increasingly complex grammatical constructions.
- <u>Repetition</u>: Measures ability to repeat words, phrases, and sentences of increasing length and complexity.
- <u>Naming and Word Finding</u>: Measures ability to name items in a category, complete a sentence, and name an item described.

Area	Score
Spontaneous Speech	<#>
Auditory Verbal Comprehension	<#>
Repetition	<#>
Naming and Word Finding	<#>

Based on Joe's above scores, he has <type> aphasia. Section scores are also converted to the Aphasia Quotient (AQ) to determine the severity of aphasia. Joe's AQ is <#> which indicates he has <mild, moderate, severe, profound> aphasia.

CLINICAL OBSERVATIONS:

1. Voice and Fluency

Fig. 22.5 (continued)

Vocal parameters and fluency were informally assessed during conversation. Joe's pitch, vocal quality, loudness, and fluency were judged to be within normal limits for his age and gender.

2. Language Sample

An informal language sample was obtained to assess various aspects of Joe's language use and understanding including morphology and syntax (word and sentence structure), semantics (vocabulary and meaning), and pragmatics (social use of language) in conversation.

Verbal language refers to one's ability to express (expressive language) and understand (receptive language) thoughts and ideas through verbal communication.

Joe frequently spoke in 1–3-word phrases that primarily consisted of nouns. He did not consistently use verbs, linking words to connect phrases, or descriptive concepts (temporal, qualitative, quantitative). Joe shows relative strength with receptive language, such as following simple verbal commands or answering simple questions. He did show difficulty as the commands and questions grew in complexity and length.

Pragmatics is the use of language in socially communicative interactions with others and includes certain communicative behaviors that are expected (e.g., eye contact, personal space, etc.).

Joe used appropriate eye contact and was friendly with the examiner. He maintained appropriate personal space and showed good verbal turn taking in conversation and during testing. Joe appears motivated and ready for speech therapy. He completed all tasks given within a 2-hour time span without showing fatigue. Despite having difficulty with word finding, Joe remained in good spirits, even laughing at himself at times when he realized he had used the wrong word.

SUMMARY

Joe Smith is a 75-year-old male who presents with <mild, moderate, severe> aphasia characterized by difficulty with <describe difficulties> This negatively impacts his ability to communicate his wants and needs with his family members and medical team.

RECOMMENDATIONS

The following is recommended for Joe Smith

1. Speech therapy is recommended
2. See below for recommended speech and language goals

Fig. 22.5 (continued)

Recommended Goals
Below is a list of short-term and long-term goals for Joe based on the evaluation results above:

Long Term Goal 1: Joe will improve expressive language skills to a more functional level

Short Term Goal:
1.1 <State short term goal >
1.2 <State short term goal >
1.3 <State short term goal >

Long Term Goal 2: Joe will improve receptive language skills to a more functional level

Short Term Goal:
2.1 <State short term goal >
2.2 <State short term goal >
2.3 <State short term goal >

____
< Name >
< Title >

Fig. 22.5 (continued)

Fig. 22.6 Standardized Patient Diagnostic Write Up

Standardized Patient-Diagnostic Write Up

Name: ____

(Your responses below will be graded based on the length, content, and your reflective insight)

1. In 1-2 paragraphs, summarize your experience.(________/10 points)
   Include the following
   -what went well/ what did not
   -did you notice any inconsistencies with patient responses
   -what additional information did you feel was missing from this measure
   -did you follow protocol or did you cue the patient in any way
   -how did the experience differ from your expectations as a clinician
   -how will you use this experience professionally

2. Complete: *clinical impressions, recommendations, and recommended goals* sections on the *Patient Report*. (15 points)

2a. List goals and evidence-based practice rationale below for **each** short term goal:

Section	Description	SP Instructions
Spontaneous Speech	A. Conversational Questions: Client must respond to 6 personal questions. B. Picture Description: Client must describe a black and white picture.	A. Joe answers most of these questions correctly but uses single words or short, telegraphic phrases. B. Joe uses single words or short, telegraphic phrases. He has difficulty thinking of some words and may gesture to indicate the word. He may say a word that sounds like the target word or starts with the same sound.
Auditory Verbal Comprehension	A. Yes/No Questions: Client must answer personal, environmental, and general yes/no questions B. Auditory Word Recognition: Client must point to items from an array of objects and pictures in the same category. There are 6 items in each category: real objects, drawn objects, forms, letters, numbers, colors, furniture, body parts, fingers, and right-left body parts. C. Sequential Commands: Client must follow verbal commands of increasing length and complexity.	A. Joe answers approximately 50% of the questions correctly (all types). He may use fillers and pause to think ("um," "uh"). He may also look around the room or use gestures to help think of answers. B. Joe identifies all of the real objects, pictured objects, forms, letters, numbers, and colors accurately (with a few self-corrections). He misses a few of the other categories (12 per category). C. Joe is able to follow the first half of verbal directions given. He struggles with the second half. He may be able to complete part of a complex direction.
Repetition	Client must repeat words, phrases, & sentences of increasing length and complexity.	Joe is able to repeat the first half of the words given. Once the stimuli moves to phrases and sentences, he has difficulty, often leaving out words or whole phrases.
Naming and Word Finding	A. Object Naming: Client must name common objects from a variety of categories B. Word Fluency: Client must name as many animals as able in one minute. C. Sentence Completion: Client must complete five sentences D. Responsive Speech: Client must respond to five simple questions.	A. Joe has the most difficulty with object naming. He is able to think of names for about 5 common objects (e.g., ball, book, key) but struggles with all of the other objects. With phonemic cues: (the first sound—"s" for stairs, or the first sounds—"st" for stairs) and semantic cues (e.g., for "knife": "it's used to cut food"), he is able to name about 5 items but is unable to name the rest. B. Joe is able to think of about 10 animals in 60 seconds, but he uses lots of pauses and fillers (e.g., "um," "uh"). He may use gestures or produce sounds to help think of names. C. Joe completes the first one accurately, uses phonemic paraphasias for two questions (e.g., "swhite" for "white" and misses the remaining two. D. Joe does not answer any accurately. He is able to answer two questions with alternative response or phonemic paraphasia (e.g., "paint" for "white") and misses the other three.

Fig. 22.7 WAB-R Summary with example responses

Speech and Language Evaluation Report Example

CLIENT INFORMATION

Client Name: Joe Smith
Date of Birth: January 14, 1948
Date of Evaluation: January 15, 2023
Chronological Age: 75 years, 0 months

Evaluating Therapist:
Evaluation Location: Speech and Hearing Clinic

REASON FOR REFERRAL:
Joe, a 75-year-old male, was referred to the GWU Speech & Hearing Center by his spouse due to concerns regarding communication and orientation.

BACKGROUND INFORMATION

History
An interview and case history were completed by Chris Smith, Joe's spouse. The following information was provided:

Speech and LanguageHistory
Chris reported that since Joe's stroke, other family members sometimes have difficulty understanding Joe, especially in loud and crowded places. He often has difficulty thinking of words. He will sometimes repeat himself after 5-10 minutes in a conversation. Chris also reported that Joe sometimes has difficulty following directions and remembering the day of the week.

Medical History
Joe suffered a left hemisphere CVA one month ago. He received OT, PT, and ST during his one week stay at the hospital. He is currently taking Keppra to control seizures and Coumadin to prevent blood clots. He has a walker but according to his spouse, he forgets to use it. He is hard of hearing but does not wear a hearing aid.

Family, Social, and Educational History
Joe lives in Virginia with his spouse, Chris. He is a retired history professor. He has two grown children, George and Leslie, who live nearby.

EVALUATIONS AND RESULTS

The following assessment tools were administered in English:
1. Hearing Screening
2. Oral Mechanism Examination
3. *Western Aphasia Battery-Revised (WAB-R)*

Fig. 22.8 Speech and Evaluation Report Example

4. Informal Observations
The assessment description and results are as follows:

1. Hearing Screening
A hearing screening was not completed during the evaluation. Joe's spouse reports that he is hard of hearing but does not have hearing aids.

2. Oral Mechanism Examination
An oral mechanism examination was administered to evaluate the structural and functional integrity of Joe's oral mechanism for speech production.

Resultsare as follows:

Face: Overall appearance, symmetry, and tone appear to be within normal limits.
Jaw: Range of motion and strength appear to be within normal limits.
Lips: Range of motion, coordination, and strength appear to be within normal limits.
Teeth: Occlusion and structure appear to be within normal limits.
Tongue: Range of motion, coordination, and strength appear to be within normal limits.
Hard Palate: Structure and symmetry structure appear to be within normal limits.
Soft Palate: Structure, symmetry, and mobility appear to be within normal limits.
Diadochokinesis (DDK): Joe's ability to coordinate production of syllables in rapid succession ("papapapa") and rapidly alternate speech movements ("pataka") is within normal limits.

3. Language
The *Western Aphasia Battery-Revised (WAB-R)* is a standardized measure used to evaluate a person's language function following an acquired neurological disorder. The WAB-R includes the following series of subtests:

Spontaneous Speech: the person must respond verbally to 6 personal questions and describe a black and white picture.
Yes/No Questions: the person must answer personal, environmental, and general yes/no questions
Auditory Word Recognition: the person must point to items from an array of objects and pictures in the same category
Sequential Commands: the person must follow verbal commands of increasing length and complexity
Repetition: the person must repeat words, phrases, & sentences of increasing length and complexity
Object Naming: the person must name common objects from a variety of categories
Word Fluency: the person must name as many animals as able in one minute
Sentence Completion: the person must complete five orally presented sentences
Responsive Speech: the person must respond verbally to five simple questions

The WAB-R was administered to assess Joe's language function following his CVA. Joe's scores are as follows:

Fig. 22.8 (continued)

Subtest	Scores
Spontaneous Speech	12
Yes/No Questions	36
Auditory Word Recognition	53
Sequential Commands	32
Repetition	48
Object Naming	22
Word Fluency	9
Sentence Completion	4
Responsive Speech	2

The subtests cores are combined and transferred to section scores, to determine the type of aphasia. The section scores are as follows:

<u>Spontaneous Speech</u>: Measures ability to produce functional communication in conversation and picture description.
<u>Auditory Verbal Comprehension</u>: Measures ability to comprehend yes/no questions and sequential commands with increasingly complex grammatical constructions.
<u>Repetition</u>: Measures ability to repeat words, phrases, and sentences of increasing length and complexity.
<u>Naming and Word Finding</u>: Measures ability to name items in a category, complete a sentence, and name an item described.

Area	Score
Spontaneous Speech	12
Auditory Verbal Comprehension	6.05
Repetition	4.8
Naming and Word Finding	3.7

Based on Joe's above scores, he has Broca's aphasia. Section scores are also converted to the Aphasia Quotient (AQ) to determine the severity of aphasia. Joe's AQ is 53.1 which indicates he has moderate aphasia.

CLINICAL OBSERVATIONS:

1. Voice and Fluency

Vocal parameters and fluency were informally assessed during conversation. Joe's pitch, vocal quality, loudness, and fluency were judged to be within normal limits for hisage and gender.

Fig. 22.8 (continued)

2. Language Sample

An informal language sample was obtained to assessvarious aspects of Joe's language use and understanding including morphology and syntax (word and sentence structure), semantics (vocabulary and meaning), and pragmatics (social use of language) in conversation.

Verbal language refers to one's ability to express (expressive language) and understand (receptive language) thoughts and ideas through verbal communication.

Joe frequently spoke in 1–3-word phrases that primarily consisted of nouns. He did not consistently use verbs, linking words to connect phrases, or descriptive concepts (temporal, qualitative, quantitative). Joe shows relative strength with receptive language, such as following simple verbal commands or answering simple questions. He did show difficulty as the commands and questions grew in complexity and length.

Pragmatics is the use of language in socially communicative interactions with others and includes certain communicative behaviors that are expected (e.g., eye contact, personal space, etc.).

Joe used appropriate eye contact and was friendly with the examiner. He maintained appropriate personal space and showed good verbal turn taking in conversation and during testing. Joe appears motivated and ready for speech therapy. He completed all tasks given within a 2-hour time span without showing fatigue. Despite having difficulty with word finding, Joe remained in good spirits, even laughing at himself at times when he realized he had used the wrong word.

SUMMARY

Joe Smith is a 75-year-old male who presents with moderate aphasia characterized by difficulty with word finding, speaking in sentences in fluently, and relative strengths in auditory verbal comprehension. This negatively impacts his ability to communicate his wants and needs with his family members and medical team.

RECOMMENDATIONS

The following is recommended for Joe Smith

1. Speech therapy is recommended
2. See below for recommended speech and language goals

Fig. 22.8 (continued)

Recommended Goals

Below is a list of short-term and long-term goals for Joe based on the evaluation results above:

Long Term Goal 1: Joe will improve expressive language skills to a more functional level

Short Term Goals:
1.1 Joe will independently label household items or pictures in 8/10 trials.
1.2 Joe will imitate 5–7-word sentences with only one model in 8/10 trials.
1.3 Joe will independently produce qualifier + noun when shown an item or object in 8/10 trials.

Long Term Goal 2: Joe will improve receptive language skills to a more functional level

Short Term Goals:
2.1 Joe will independently follow 2-3 step simple verbal directions in 8/10 trials.
2.2 Joe will independently point to house hold items or pictures when named in 8/10 trials.
2.3 Joe will independently answer general yes/no questions in 8/10 trials.

Kari Lim, M.S., CCC-SLP

Kari Lim, M.S., CCGSLP
Speech Language Pathologist & Evaluator

Fig. 22.8 (continued)

Standardized Patient-Education Write Up

Names: ____
Length of encounter with SP: ___________________________
Amount of time group spent on write up: ____________________

*One write-up to be turned in PER GROUP but everyone is expected to contribute to the assignment.

(Your responses below will be graded based on the length, content, and your reflective insight)

1. In 1-2 paragraphs, summarize your personal experiences.(________/5 points)
   Include the following
   -how do you think the session went
   -did you cover all of the areas in the report
   -how would you judge your rate of speech
   -what was the hardest information to cover from the report
   -what emotions did thepatient experience after you shared your recommendations and why do you think she felt those emotions
   -how did you feel when the patient was explaining her feelings

2. In 1-2 paragraphs, summarize your professional experiences. (________/5 points)
   Include the following:
   -what were you thinking/feeling before the session
   -how would you go about building more rapport with the patient in such a short amount of time
   -how did the experience differ from your expectations as a clinician
   -how will you use this experience professionally
   -do you feel like you were an empathetic listener
   -did you answer all of the patient's questions
   -how would this session differ if the patient was present with the spouse
   -what would you say or do differently next time

Fig. 22.9 Standardized Patient Education Write Up

References and Resources

1. Zraick RI. Standardized patients in communication science and disorders: past, present, future directions. Commun Sci and Disord. 2020;4(3):1–20. https://doi.org/10.30707/TLCSD4.3/KHSI3441.
2. American Speech-Language-Hearing Association. Aphasia. Cited 01/03/23. Available from: https://www.asha.org/public/speech/disorders/aphasia/
3. Pearson Assessments. Aphasia Battery—Revised (WAB-R) Cited 01/03/23. Available from: https://www.pearsonassessments.com/store/usassessments/en/Store/Professional-Assessments/Speech-%26-Language/Western-Aphasia-Battery-Revised/p/100000194.html
4. Tactus Therapy. Broca's Aphasia (Non-Fluent Aphasia). Cited 01/03/23. Available from: https://www.youtube.com/watch?v=JWC-cVQmEmY
5. Schlegel C, Bonvin R, Rethans JJ, van der Vleuten C. The use of video in standardized patient training to improve portrayal accuracy: a randomized post-test control group study. Med Teach. 2015;37(8):730–7. https://doi.org/10.3109/0142159X.2014.970989.
6. Baylor C, Burns MI, Struijk J, Herron L, Mach H, Yorkston K. Assessing the believability of standardized patients trained to portray communication disorders. Am J Speech Lang Pathol. 2017;26:791–805.

Part V

Applications: Older Adult Care in an Acute setting

Trauma in an Older Adult: Small Accidents, Big Injuries

23

Target Learner Group: Emergency Department Team

Nemat Alsaba and Jane Schweitzer

Background

Care of trauma patients is a cornerstone of emergency medicine. Trauma assessment and management in older person is more complex than in younger people due to age-related anatomical and physiological changes and polypharmacy, including anticoagulation, affecting all aspects of trauma assessment and management [1]. Based on this concept, it is not surprising that injured older adults have higher mortality, longer intensive care stays, and more prolonged hospital admissions than younger people [2]. Furthermore, this also unfortunately highlights that even a minor trauma for an older adult can be associated with significant injuries that lead to functional decline and loss of independence [1]. Hence it is essential to practice as a team on how best to approach geriatric trauma. In addition, there are crucial practice points to consider, including understanding typical injuries in this age group and common geriatric trauma resuscitation pearls and pitfalls [3].

Although the most common geriatric trauma is a fall from a standing height [4], we have chosen another low-speed injury, such as a golf cart (buggy) injury, for our geriatric trauma case scenario, as falls are covered in other chapters in this book. Falls from a golf cart remain an essential source of injury for people of all ages, including older adults. The rate of golf cart injuries to older adults significantly increased from 2007 to 2017 by 67.6%, as noted by a US study [5]. Traumatic brain injury (TBI) in injured older adults is a common cause of hospital admission [6]. Recognizing a significant TBI in older adults might be tricky to detect initially, especially when older adults present with a normal level of consciousness, i.e. normal Glasgow Coma Scale (GCS) [1].

The high use of antiplatelet/anticoagulation medications in this age group can add another layer of complexity to managing the injured older adult, which this scenario also highlights.

Key Session Information

Description of the scenario	The scenario has 2 phases Phase 1: 70-year-old Kiran Sharma was involved in a golf cart rollover. They were brought in by ambulance with an obvious forehead wound. Initial assessment indicates a normal Glasgow Coma Scale (GCS) of 15, but the patient becomes slightly confused and agitated during the simulation Phase 2: The patient becomes progressively confused with a reduced level of consciousness and signs of increased intracranial pressure (bradycardia and high blood pressure), requiring intubation. Head/brain imaging shows an intracranial bleed requiring intubation and urgent referral to neurosurgical team. The emergency department (ED) team is also expected to discuss and manage the reversal of the patient anticoagulation medication (applicable to the choice of anticoagulation drug chosen for the scenario). The patient's partner, Alex Lee, arrives in the ED, and the team is expected to give a clinical update while communicating effectively and compassionately with the partner.
Setting	Resuscitation bay

Supplementary Information The online version contains supplementary material available at https://doi.org/10.1007/978-3-031-65742-9_23.

N. Alsaba (✉)
Department of Emergency Medicine, Gold Coast Hospital and Health Service, Gold Coast, QLD, Australia

Faculty of Health Sciences and Medicine, Bond University, Gold Coast, QLD, Australia
e-mail: nalsaba@bond.edu.au

J. Schweitzer
Gold Coast Health Simulation Service and Nursing Midwifery Education and Research Unit (NMERU), Gold Coast, QLD, Australia
e-mail: jane.schweitzer@health.qld.gov.au

C. M. Smith et al. (eds.), *Comprehensive Healthcare Simulation: Geriatric Simulation*, Comprehensive Healthcare Simulation,
https://doi.org/10.1007/978-3-031-65742-9_23

Learning objectives	By the end of the session, learners will be able to: 1. Collaborate with fellow learners to apply a team-based approach for the assessment and management of geriatric trauma 2. Recognize different approaches and management of the reversal of various anticoagulation medications in the trauma setting 3. Prepare and perform safe intubation for the injured older adult with severe traumatic brain injury 4. Demonstrate effective and compassionate communication with the partner, including breaking bad news
Adjunct materials	**Pre-reading resources for participants** • https://gedcollaborative.com/podcast/trauma-in-older-adults/ • Geriatric Trauma and Medical illness: Pearls and Pitfalls • https://litfl.com/anticoagulated-patients-in-the-ed/ • Older Person Trauma-Primary Survey I Trauma Victoria (reach.vic.gov.au) • https://emergencymedicinecases.com/geriatric-trauma-under-triaging-resuscitation-airway-head-c-spine-imaging-clearing-c-spine/
Participants	**Learners:** 3 medical staff 3 nursing staff Allied health relevant to your workflows and depending on your ED size and setting (optional). Examples of allied health that we have involved in when running this simulation in the past are: • Radiographers (to assess how to perform fast and safe imaging in a geriatric trauma setting). • Social workers (how best to integrate and support extra family support in the ED workflow). • ED pharmacist (how to order and administer anticoagulation reversal agents in the resuscitation bay safely and promptly). **Educators:** 2 debriefers (1 medical and 1 nursing) 2 older adult SPs (the injured patient and their partner) 1 registered nurse (RN) as an embedded participant 1 sim technician

Age of SP	SP should appear to be the stated age of the role
Scenario length	70 min
Session schedule	Pre-brief 10 min Scenario 20 min Debrief 40 min
Room setup	Simulated resuscitation bay
Props	**Clinical equipment:** • Patient monitoring (BP cuff/pulse oximeter/ECG leads/monitor)—we use simulated cardiac monitors such as Laerdal SimPad PLUS or iSimulate. See Fig. 23.1. • IV line • IV cannula x 2—one for each arm. See Fig. 23.2 on how to attach a simulated IV cannula onto the SP that allows the participant to administer fluid or "simulated" medication • Airway part-task trainer • Intubation trolley and equipment • Cervical spine collar (soft) **Medications** (such as analgesia, sedation, paralytic, etc.) appropriate to your site/region **Investigations:** • X-rays (chest and pelvic); both have no signs of fractures • Focused Assessment with Sonography for Trauma (FAST) scan—normal • CT head (shows intracranial bleeding requiring decompression) • Blood results (venous blood gas (VBG) including site-specific lab investigation) Images and results can be sourced from your own clinical cases or from FOAMed (Free Open Access Medical Education)
Wardrobe	Golf clothes—simulated blood on the patient's shirt Everyday clothing for the partner
Moulage	Forehead bruising Multiple bruises and abrasions over the forearms (see Resource 26.03 in Chap. 26 on how to create bruises) Blood on the shirt (see Resource 1 on how to moulage blood)

Instructions to Learners

During the pre-brief time, we recommend asking learners to share a thought or top tip on navigating the trauma care of the older person, what "trauma" looks like in this population, and factors impacting assessment and management, e.g. pathophysiological changes of aging, polypharmacy, and communication challenges.

The following handover is presented by the embedded participant to the team at the start of the simulation activity:

> The ambulance brought a 70-year-old person after their golf cart rolled over. They are in c-spine collar and had an Initial GCS 15 but now they appear confused.
>
> Vital signs seem normal (HR 75, BP115/75).
>
> There were no obvious injuries apart from a forehead abrasion and a couple of abrasions on the left side of the chest and arm.

Your task is to assess and manage the patient as a team.

Instructions to the Embedded RN Participant

During the faculty pre-brief, it is helpful to plan with the older adult SP and embedded RN participant how the transition to a part-task trainer for intubation will work.

Your tasks as an embedded participant are:

- To give clinical handover of the case to the team at the start of the scenario
- To facilitate the smooth running of the scenario and transitions between scenario stages/phases
- To ensure safety of the older adult SP

You will also need to be observant and know the team plan for administering medications, procedures, and any patient transfers, e.g. from trolley to CT scan or if the team plans to proceed with intubation due to clinical deterioration. This situational awareness will help you anticipate what support the older adult SP might need or what resources and information the participants might require. In phase 2, the patient is more confused, GCS is dropping, and the vital signs are changing (HR 50, BP 180/100), indicating catastrophic intracranial bleed; make it explicit to the older adult SP that the team will now proceed with intubation so the SP would start portraying the "deeply sedated" patient.

Instructions to SPs

The simulation delivery method will affect the instructions for the older adult SP in this case. As this scenario is set in a potentially high-stress environment (i.e. the resuscitation room), there is limited benefit of having a sophisticated backstory for the older adult SP to remember, with much of the action during the scenario about focused patient assessment and treatment. Details of the case are sent to older adult SPs 1–2 weeks prior to the day of the simulation. The script will usually include a brief description of the role and a timeline for the scenario.

Patient Role

Current and Past Medical History

Current: You are an active person who visits your general practice doctor quarterly for routine medication review and general health checks. You are allergic to aspirin. You take prescribed blood thinners for a heart condition *(sim educators can choose anticoagulation class drug appropriate to your regional guidelines)* and pain relief medications for osteoarthritic joints.

Past: Coronary angioplasty 8 years ago and right total knee replacement 4 years ago.

Social/Lifestyle Information

Your name is Kiran Sharma and you live with your partner. You play golf 3 days a week. You have a full driver's license with no restrictions.

Person's Ideas, Concerns, and Expectations

Backstory: You are an active 70-year-old person. Today you were having your usual golf day. You were involved in a golf cart accident. While driving the golf cart and attempting to turn left, you saw a rock on the road that you tried to avoid, but the cart hit the rock and rolled over to the side. You were not speeding. You hit your head and felt blood oozing down your forehead. You also had pain in your chest after the fall. Paramedics arrived quickly, assessed you while bandaging your head, and explained that you'd need to go to the hospital.

Scenario start: You are positioned on a trolley, with your head bandaged, and appear uncomfortable and slightly agitated (you are becoming more fidgety, not following conversations, and wanting to get up and walk away, but you are not aggressive). You will also have a soft neck collar applied. You have slight chest discomfort with bruising across your left chest and abdomen.

Opening Line

> Can I get up and take this thing off my neck?

Expectations

Phase 1: You are cooperative when the team starts examining you and compliant when the team puts on monitoring equipment (BP/ECG/pulse oximeter).

You are initially quite talkative, but you are unable to answer some of the questions correctly, e.g. you give the wrong name of the hospital, or you can't remember the date.

The team is trying to decide the extent of your head injury. When the team examines you, you are sore across the abdomen and chest and your head is very painful.

Once the first set of observations is done and with appropriate reassurance, you become less agitated. Once you have answered a few questions, you become drowsier and less talkative. The embedded nurse will let you know when to change your behavior from phase 1 to phase 2. There will be no pause to transition to phase 2 as it will be a natural progression of the scenario.

Phase 2: You appear drowsy with a decreased level of consciousness; you feel nauseous and may even dry retch or try to vomit. Your blood pressure is elevated, and you feel very unwell. You should expect the team to continue assessing you and planning to take you to have a scan of your head. If the team decides to intervene and place a breathing tube, that will happen on a piece of equipment the embedded nurse will provide to the team. You will stay in bed with your eyes closed and not engage in any conversation (as if you are deeply sedated). The embedded nurse will explicitly tell you when the simulation activity is over.

Partner Role

Person's Ideas, Concerns, and Expectations

Your name is Alex Lee. You were at home when your partner left for golf this morning and were quite surprised to get the call from the emergency services. You are very concerned about what has happened and their current condition. Your partner has some medical problems but is generally well and is only on a couple of medications.

Despite being 70 years old, you live an active life and you both manage well at home. You are unaware of your partner's injuries and what procedures or interventions will be provided to him by the ED team.

The learner should inform you that your partner likely has a brain injury and a bleed on their brain and has been intubated (they have a tube in the windpipe to help them breathe). The current situation is that they are awaiting reviews by the neurosurgical and intensive care unit (ICU) teams to decide the next critical step in their management. They should inform you that the prognosis in this case may be poor but that your partner's condition is currently being actively managed.

If they ask you what your partner's wishes are about resuscitation, inform them that you have never discussed this.

Ask for further clarification when the ED team uses medical jargon rather than simple terms to explain his management or prognosis.

You should be upset but calm during the discussion.

Opening Line

Yes, I'm the partner of Kiran Sharma.

Considerations for Working with Older Adult SPs

Before the Scenario

- Check in with the older adult SPs to see if they or their friends or families have any previous experiences with road trauma and if they feel comfortable portraying the injured older adult or the partner of the severely injured patient.
- Email the scenario and SP script 2 weeks before the simulation activity. You might consider using a larger font for the scenario. You might also consider chunking phase 1 and 2 information to help with older adult SP's memory retention.
- Discuss with the older adult SP any physical challenges that might require consideration. This includes back, neck, or joint pain that may affect the older adult SP positioning on trolleys, equipment used, such as cervical collars, and moulage application.
- Communicate with the older adult SPs again 1 week before the simulation activity and clarify any further concerns or questions about the case.
- Ensure SPs arrive 1 h before the start of the simulation to rehearse and apply the moulage.
- Ensure SPs are part of the simulation pre-brief mental rehearsal.
- Have a plan for how the older adult SP will communicate with the embedded RN, including key points to transition each scenario stage. This may differ each time depending on who is taking each role; examples include a touch on the foot or arm with a short sentence such as "Are they drowsier than before?".

During the Scenario

- Use a soft neck collar with an appropriate size to prevent neck pain or discomfort.
- Avoid using a rigid stretcher for the injured older adult SP, which can cause back pain, and substitute that with your regular ED bed/trolley.
- The embedded RN observes both SPs (patient and partner) for any signs of unexpected distress (physical or psychological).
- Empower the older adult SPs and the simulation team to stop the scenario if SP safety is at stake.

After the Scenario

- Ask the older adult SPs if they have any immediate concerns from the scenario.
- Ensure you allow time for older adult SPs to de-role and come out of the role before they leave the session; this could be done by providing a quiet space for them to sit and offering them a cup of water before they join the debriefing room.
- Ensure the moulage is removed safely before older adult SP leaves the simulation service.
- Plan to follow up with the older adult SPs to check their well-being and capture further feedback on improving this simulation activity.

Lessons Learned

- We ran this scenario with multiple options of scenario progression depending on various factors (the focus of the skill acquisition of the participants, the availability of resources to run the scenario, whether it is time, availability of equipment, or human resources). Figure 23.3 gives the readers multiple scenario progression options depending on resources and the focus of the simulation activity.
- One of the unintended consequences and benefits for the older adult SPs while running this simulation is the impact on their health literacy and self-awareness of safety measures during driving and other activities to prevent injuries. This effect has been explored and documented in the literature in similar simulation activities [7].
- While the scenario template gives a normal progression and expectation of the scenario plan and outcome, it is essential to be flexible and embrace any unexpected outcome during the scenario, e.g. faculty can't control the conversations between the team and the patient during the scenario, so be ready to tackle awkward interactions in the debrief if necessary.
- An SP voice and reflection during the debrief provide valuable insight into our patients' experience of a resuscitation situation.
- Equity, diversity, and inclusion considerations—each hospital has unique populations; we have found that choosing a diverse SP group supports diverse communities, e.g. same-sex partnerships, partnerships with significant age gaps, or biracial couples, enabling exploration of cultural factors during simulation debrief. We have found from running this scenario multiple times how changing the partner's age and sex affected the learner's behaviour and interactions and has enriched our debriefing sessions and learning conversations. The patient and their partner have been assigned gender-neutral names so SPs of any gender can portray the roles.

Appendix

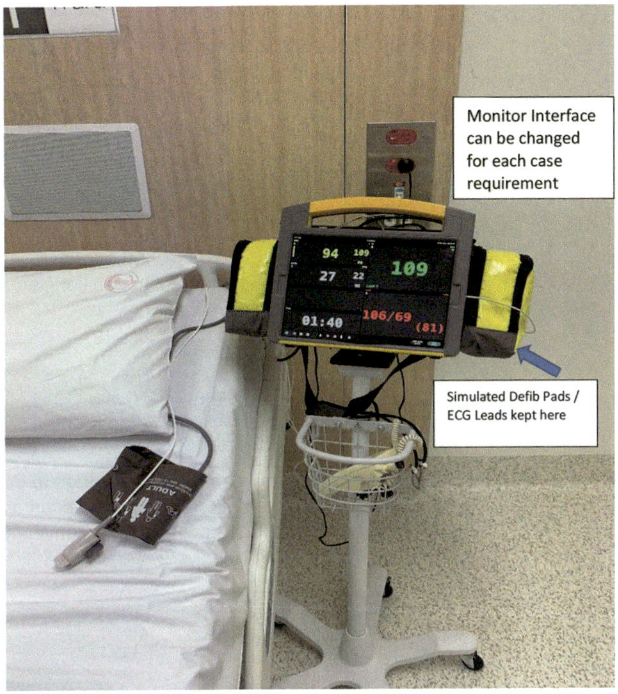

Fig. 23.1 Example of simulated patient monitor

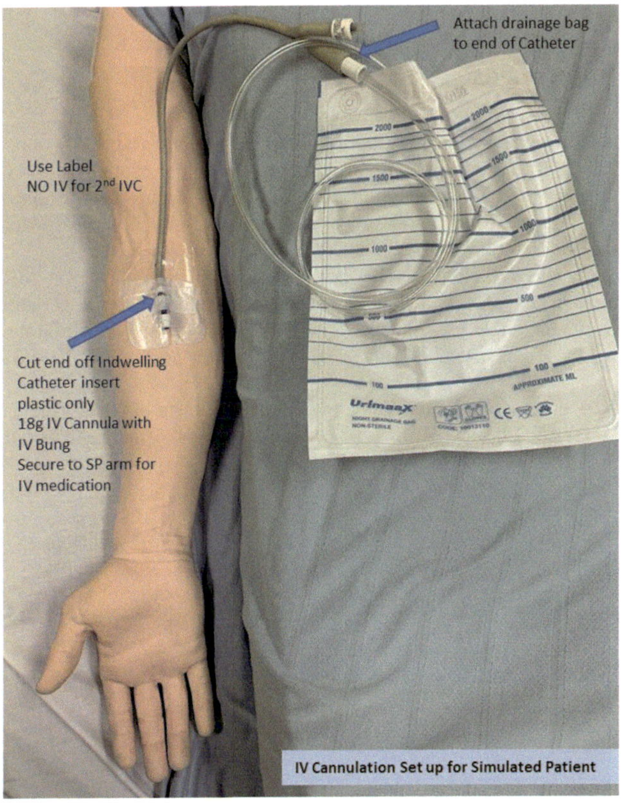

Fig. 23.2 Example of intravenous (IV) cannulation setup

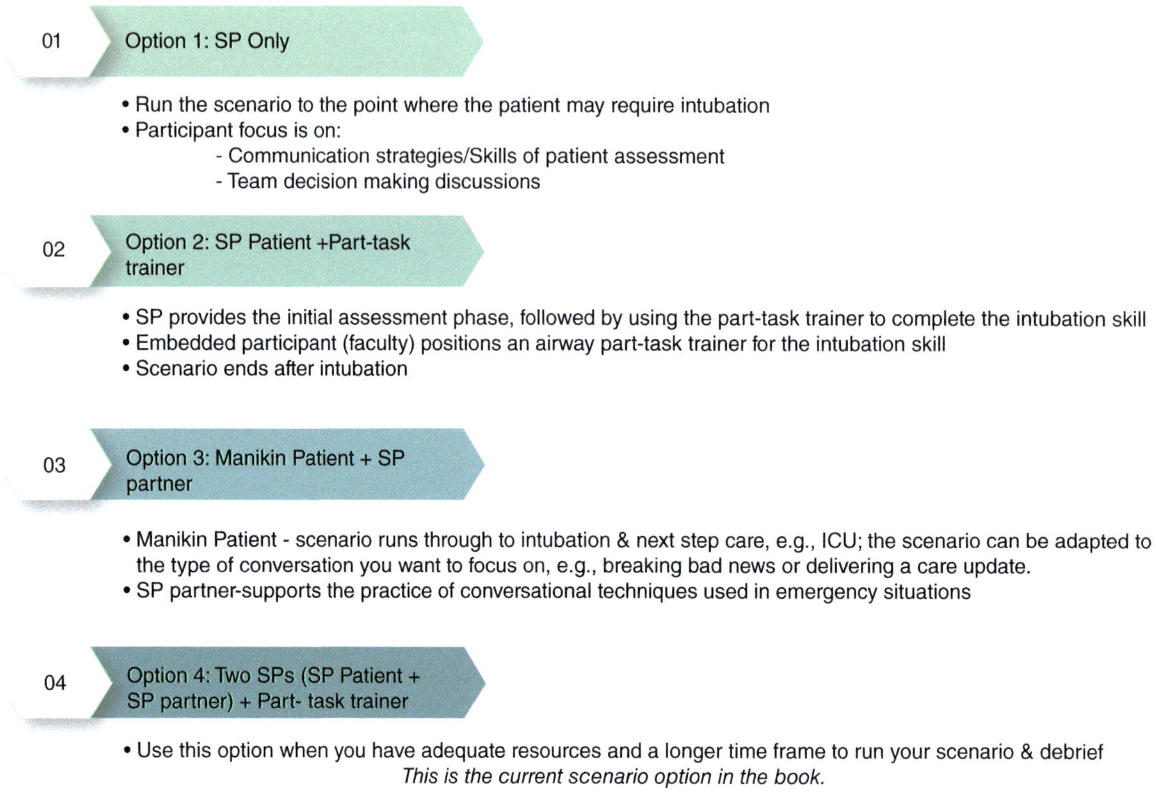

Fig. 23.3 Scenario progression options

References

1. Carpenter CR, Arendts G, Hullick C, Nagaraj G, Cooper Z, Burkett E. Major trauma in the older patient: evolving trauma care beyond management of bumps and bruises. Emerg Med Australas. 2017;29(4):450–5. https://doi.org/10.1111/1742-6723.12785.
2. Jacobs DG, Plaisier BR, Barie PS, Hammond JS, Holevar MR, Sinclair KE, et al. Practice management guidelines for geriatric trauma: The East Practice Management Guidelines Work Group. J Trauma. 2003;54(2):391–416. https://doi.org/10.1097/01.ta.0000042015.54022.be.
3. Pan London Major Trauma System Management of Older Trauma. Third Edition, April 2021. https://www.c4ts.qmul.ac.uk/downloads/london-major-trauma-system-older-traumaguidance_ third-editionApril2021.pdf
4. Atinga A, Shekkeris A, Fertleman M, Batrick N, Kashef E, Dick E. Trauma in the elderly patient. Br J Radiol. 2018:20170739. https://doi.org/10.1259/bjr.20170739.
5. Horvath KZ, McAdams RJ, Roberts KJ, Zhu M, McKenzie LB. Fun Ride or risky transport: Golf cart-related injuries treated in U.S. emergency departments from 2007 through 2017. J Saf Res. 2020;75:1–7. https://doi.org/10.1016/j.jsr.2020.10.002.
6. Hawley C, Sakr M, Scapinello S, Salvo J, Wrenn P. Traumatic brain injuries in older adults—6 years of data for one UK trauma centre: retrospective analysis of prospectively collected data. Emerg Med J. 2017;34(8):509–16. https://doi.org/10.1136/emermed-2016-2065.
7. Lee DA, Maxwell CA, Miller S. "This Is Me!" Perceptions of older adult simulated participants in an aging and injury simulation experience. J Trauma Nurs. 2021;28(1):10–20.

Older Adult Falls in the Emergency Department: Keeping Everyone Safe

24

Target Learner Group: Emergency Department and Other Hospital Teams

Hemal Patel and Carolyn Hullick

Background

Falls are one of the most common reasons for older persons to present to the emergency department (ED) [1]. Falls are the leading cause of trauma-related mortality and morbidity in both the United States and Australia [2–4]. Unfortunately, despite high-quality health systems, falls in hospitals are one of the leading causes of hospital-acquired complications, particularly for older Australians [5].

As we have moved through the COVID-19 pandemic, hospitals, particularly EDs, have experienced overcrowding worldwide [6–8]. As increasing numbers of patients remain in EDs, the risk of hospital falls will remain significant [9].

Preventing falls within hospitals is a top patient safety priority. Clinicians must also have the confidence, expertise and skills to manage a patient after falling [10]. The acute management of falls can be confronting and physically challenging. There is a risk of staff-related injuries. Therefore, it is essential to have a team-based, coordinated approach to manage potential subsequent injuries and contemporaneous reporting of adverse events.

There is evidence that older persons are less likely to receive pain relief in the ED than younger persons. Although inadequate pain relief is associated with increased risk of delirium, opioid medications are also associated with delirium. Older persons are more likely to have multiple chronic conditions and cognitive impairment which can be exacerbated within an ED environment that is increasingly overcrowded. All of these factors contribute to older persons not receiving optimal pain management [11].

In this scenario, the learners, two doctors and two nurses, find a patient on the floor next to the patient's bed. The patient is complaining of severe hip pain due to a hip fracture. The majority of hip fractures occur in people aged 65 years and over because of increased risk of osteoporosis and increased risk of falls [12].

The learners work together to address the situation. Observers are asked to take notes and comment on the learner's technical, cognitive and behavioural skills within this acute situation.

This scenario is delivered as a planned in situ simulation session for clinicians to deal with the unique challenges in the ED. More importantly, this scenario is undertaken by the interprofessional team that often responds to acute medical problems. Although this scenario is designed to train clinicians on how to assess and manage an older person after a fall, the in situ nature of this simulation provides the clinicians with the opportunity to undertake training in finding and using the equipment available in the work environment with their colleagues. It also offers an opportunity for the team involved in the scenario to contribute to process change and quality improvement within the environment in which they operate.

Supplementary Information The online version contains supplementary material available at https://doi.org/10.1007/978-3-031-65742-9_24.

H. Patel (✉)
Wyong Hospital, Central Coast Local Health District, Wyong, NSW, Australia

New South Wales Ambulance, Clinical Capability, Quality and Safety, State Headquarters, Homebush, Sydney, NSW, Australia

School of Medicine and Public Health, University of Newcastle, Newcastle, NSW, Australia
e-mail: Hemal.patel@health.nsw.gov.au

C. Hullick
School of Medicine and Public Health, University of Newcastle, Newcastle, NSW, Australia

Belmont Hospital, Hunter New England Local Health District, Belmont, NSW, Australia

Australian Commission on Safety and Quality in Health Care, Sydney, NSW, Australia
e-mail: Carolyn.hullick@health.nsw.gov.au

C. M. Smith et al. (eds.), *Comprehensive Healthcare Simulation: Geriatric Simulation*, Comprehensive Healthcare Simulation,
https://doi.org/10.1007/978-3-031-65742-9_24

Key Session Information

Description of the scenario	An 80-year-old male presents to the ED with abdominal pain. While waiting to be seen, he tries to get out of bed to go to the toilet. He is found on the floor complaining of severe right hip pain
Setting	ED cubicle [it could also be in an inpatient ward]
Learning objectives	By the end of the session, learners will be able to: 1. Manage a patient immediately after they have fallen, including: • Delivering basic life support • Providing reassurance • Completing primary and secondary trauma survey • Moving the patient safely back to bed • Monitoring the patient 2. Assess older person's pain and provide appropriate pain management for a patient with a fractured neck of femur in the ED 3. Document and report clinical incidents that occur in a healthcare setting 4. Recognise the importance of teamwork and interprofessional communication in healthcare
Adjunct materials	See Supplementary Material
Participants	Learners: • Two medical staff and two nursing staff Faculty: • One simulated participant (SP) • Facilitator • Simulation educator • Hospital orderly or patient care assistant who helps move patients around the hospitals
Age of SP	SP should appear to be the stated age of the role
Scenario length	70 min
Session schedule	• 15-min briefing • 20-min scenario • 35-min debriefing
Room setup	• Clinical bed space • Video link can be set up in a separate room for observers or they can stand back and observe • If there is no direct video link available, a live video feed to the observers' room can be established using a smart device set up on a tripod and a videoconferencing (VC) platform as you would set up for a meeting **Setting up videoconferencing for the simulation:** This can be set up using personal devices and a computer screen (with or without a projector). Like any virtual meeting, the setup will depend on your organisation's videoconferencing (VC) subscription and equipment. From previous experience having a mobile phone setup in the clinical space on a tripod will get a very good vantage point on the communication and workflow of the learners. This is then video-conferenced to a separate room/space with a computer and projector screen where observers can watch the simulation activity. There will be challenges to looking at what is happening with the cardiac monitor. A second device can be used for this. Additionally, having a separate microphone plugged into the personal device will help improve the sound quality for observers
Props	• Patient medication list written on a small piece of paper which the older adult SP can hand over to the learners • Observation chart for documenting observations—this can also include the patient's medical, social and drug history **Clinical equipment:** • Intravenous lines and intravenous fluids • Analgesia • Syringes • Blood pressure cuff, pulse oximeter and cardiac monitor. Most simulation services have a cardiac monitor for simulation like iSimulate© to display the abnormal vital signs of the SP during the simulation scenario. If not available, vital signs can be written on a piece of paper or whiteboard **Other equipment:** • Patient transfer equipment including a board and sheet for managing the patient who has a fall in the hospital • Lifting equipment that is available and used in the organisation • Soft mat for the older adult SP to lie on the floor during the scenario **Patient investigation results:** • X-ray of right impacted neck of femur fracture • Electrocardiograph—normal sinus rhythm *Note*: FOAMed (Free Open Access Medical Education) sites are excellent as a resource for investigation props for all our simulation cases. Some examples of FOAMed include *Radiopaedia* for imaging, *Emergency Medicine Cases and Life in the Fast Lane*
Wardrobe	Patient gown
Moulage	• Bruise moulage over the right hip—refer to Resource 26.03, *Elder abuse moulage* "what and how", in Chap. 26 • Simulated IV cannula in the hand—refer to Resource 1

Instructions to Learners

Mr. David Jones, an 80-year-old man, has presented to the ED with abdominal pain. He has not opened his bowels for 4 days but has been otherwise well. He lives with his partner in their own home. They are both independent. Mr. Jones continues to drive and has a healthy lifestyle. He has hypertension and hypercholesterolaemia treated with medication (ramipril and rosuvastatin). He is not on any other prescription or over the counter medications. Mr. Jones has no previous surgical history. Mr. Jones has been waiting for 4 h to be reviewed by the medical team as the ED is overcrowded. You hear a thud and find your patient groaning in pain on the floor next to his cubicle bed in the ED.

Your task as a team is to:

- Ensure the safety of Mr. Jones and the staff
- Provide basic life support

- Safely transfer Mr. Jones into his bed and subsequently manage his injuries from the fall
- Undertake accurate and timely documentation and reporting of critical patient incidents at the hospital

Instructions to SP

You are portraying an 80-year-old patient, Mr. David Jones, who attends the ED with abdominal (stomach) pain and then falls while in the hospital waiting to be seen. The scenario will start with you on the floor on a soft mat beside the bed. You do not need to portray the fall from the bed. The learners will arrive to assess and manage you after the fall.

The following explains what happened at home and then in the ED before the fall:

You have not opened your bowels in the last couple of days. You have not had any vomiting. You are prone to developing constipation. You took some laxatives this morning but have not passed a bowel motion. You are concerned that your pain is worsening and that you have something major wrong, so you decide to go to the hospital.

When you arrived at the hospital, a nurse took you to a bed in the ED. You have changed into a gown and your blood pressure, pulse and oxygen levels have been recorded (all are normal). An intravenous cannula was placed in your left hand, and blood was taken. You do not know the results of these blood tests.

You were waiting in a bed to be seen by a doctor when you urgently needed to go to the toilet to open your bowels. After pressing the buzzer, no one came to assist you. You were worried you might soil yourself if you did not get to the toilet quickly. You decided to take yourself to the bathroom. Unfortunately, you have fallen onto the floor beside your bed, injuring your right hip. Your hip pain is severe. You cannot walk and cannot stand up. However, you have no pain from the fall other than your right hip.

After your fall in the ED, the treating doctors and nurses are expected to:

- Offer you pain relief.
- Move you safely from the floor to the bed. This will be done by either supported mobilisation or a patient transfer device if available.
- Request X-rays to help diagnose your injuries.
- Ensure you understand what has happened and the likely subsequent medical treatment.

Current and Past Medical History

- You are diagnosed with high blood pressure and high cholesterol, which are well controlled with medication.
- You have not had any previous surgery.
- You have not had any other medical problems.
- You do not have any drug or food allergies.

Family Medical History

- You do not recall any major family health problems.

Social/Lifestyle Information

- You live at home with your partner. You are both independent.
- You have no children.
- You drive and do your own shopping.
- You play golf three times a week to keep yourself healthy and fit.
- You do not smoke, and you do not drink any alcohol.

SP Ideas, Concerns and Expectations

- You enjoy your independence.
- Your expectations are that the injury may just be a severe bruise to the right hip area and with some tablets it will feel better and you will be able to go home.
- You are concerned that if you cannot go home, your partner will be alone.

Opening Line

I have fallen over; I was trying to rush to the toilet and tripped. I have bad pain in my hip.

Special Instructions for Portraying This Scenario

- You will wear a patient gown with shorts underneath to maintain dignity.
- You will start the scenario by lying on the floor on a soft mat.
- A minimum of two doctors and two nurses (the learners) will help you get back into bed, while the other participants (four to six, including one facilitator) will be observing.
- The scenario will last no more than 20 min. The learners should have you back into the bed within 5 min. If this does not occur within the time frame, the facilitator and simulation educator will prompt the learners to safely get you back into bed.
- Stress the importance of the pain in your right hip—you cannot stand or move your legs at all. If the learners try to move you without giving you pain relief, you should make this known by raising your voice and wincing with pain.
- If pain relief is given (ideally through an intravenous cannula), you should feel slightly more comfortable.

- The learners will be guided to perform an X-ray as you cannot move your right leg without a significant amount of pain. If this does not occur within a few minutes of being placed back into your bed, you may provide a prompt, e.g. “Do I need an X-ray?”.
- If the learners tell you that your right hip is broken, you may ask relevant questions or portray feelings that come to mind. Feel free to use your own words. Here are some examples of questions that you may want to ask:

Related to the Diagnosis

- What does the X-ray show?
- I was just trying to go to the toilet, why didn’t someone answer my buzzer?
- Ask for clarification if a learner expresses something in a way that you do not understand, such as:
  - What does that word mean?
  - Could you explain this more clearly?
  - Can someone let my partner know?

Related to the Treatment Plan

- Does this mean I need an operation?
- When will the operation happen?
- When can I go back to playing golf?
- Will I have to go into a nursing home?

Considerations for Working with Older Adult SPs

Before the Scenario

- Hip fractures more commonly occur in older persons who are more likely to have weakened bones and more likely to fall. When recruiting older adult SPs for this scenario, check whether they have had a previous lower limb bony injury or hip dislocation, including pelvic fractures, as this might carry physical, psychological and emotional risks. We recommend offering this scenario to an older adult SP without a history of the above conditions.
- Ideally for this scenario, the older adult SP will have reasonable fitness and not be considered frail. They should be able to lie on the floor for 5 min while waiting to be moved back into bed. We also recommend that a soft mat is placed beside the bed for the older adult SP to lie on to ensure their comfort while they are on the floor during the scenario.
- Send the scenario and the scripted lines to the older adult SP a week before. This allows them to prepare for the role and may assist if they have memory or cognitive changes. The older adult SP needs to know explicitly that they will be required to lie on the floor and be physically manoeuvred by the ED nurses and doctors.
- A phone call to the older adult SP 24–48 h before the scenario is useful in mitigating any issues. This will allow the opportunity for a verbal run through the scenario, clarify expectations and address concerns regarding the simulation activity as well as assist if they have memory changes.
- Undertake a simulation pre-brief immediately prior to the simulation activity to do a final test run and address any concerns raised by the older adult SP.
- It is essential to ensure a safe environment for older adult SPs and learners. Facilitator needs to be confident that the appropriate equipment is available to transfer a patient from the floor to the bed using relevant work health and safety techniques.
- If you plan to repeat the scenario on the same day, we recommend recruiting two older adult SPs. This takes into consideration that the scenario may be physically challenging for older adult SPs to play the role twice. In addition, two older adult SPs allow multiple learners to experience the simulation in 1 day. It also allows the learners to repeat the scenario after reviewing their performance.

During the Scenario

- For this scenario, the patient is initially not attached to cardiac monitors and alarms. When the simulation starts, the learners may ask that monitoring is attached to the older adult SP. This may add to the ambient noise and make it harder for the SP to understand the flow of the scenario, particularly if they have hearing challenges. If monitoring is attached, facilitator should ensure the monitors are set to low volume.
- Ensure that the room is free of hazards and comfortable and accessible for the older adult SP. Also, consider the room’s temperature, given that the SP may be on the mat on the floor for a while.

After the Scenario

- Older adult SP is encouraged to give feedback and reflections immediately after this scenario ends to promote retention and avoid relying on their memory to provide commentary.
- It is valuable to have older adult SP involved in the debrief to share the insights of the scenario from a patient’s perspective. It also allows refining this simulated activity for next time.

Lessons Learned

- This activity is enhanced when run as an in situ as it helps engage learners in identifying where equipment for patient transfer would be best kept, thereby improving processes within the clinical space. Staff may not know where the equipment is when they urgently need it for patient care and safety.
- While running this scenario, we recognised the importance of training all staff in manual handling. It is difficult for staff to safely lift patients from the floor if they have not planned how to undertake the task. Lack of training puts staff at risk of injuring themselves and others.
- Pain management in older persons is complex. The scenario allowed learners to consider the importance of ensuring patients have timely access to pain relief.
- Working with older adult SPs in this scenario offered invaluable benefits. It provided real-time feedback from the older adult SP around the behavioural and communication skills of the treating team, in addition to contributing to the authenticity of the simulation. This encouraged further learner engagement in the simulation activity.

Acknowledgements We would like to acknowledge the wonderful people who have helped design this simulation activity and helped contribute to improving patient care. The Belmont Hospital Education Team nursing leaders, Catherine MacDonald and Nathan Sharrock, and the Belmont Hospital Emergency Department have continued to support a culture of education and interprofessional learning.

References

1. Nagaraj G, Hullick C, Arendts G, Burkett E, Hill KD, Carpenter CR. Avoiding anchoring bias by moving beyond 'mechanical falls' in geriatric emergency medicine. Emerg Med Australas. 2018;30(6):843–50.
2. Australian Institute for Health and Welfare (AIHW). Falls Canberra 2022 [updated 25/11/2022; cited 2022. Available from: https://www.aihw.gov.au/reports/injury/falls.
3. Cubitt M, Braitberg G, Curtis K, Maier AB. Models of acute care for injured older patients-Australia and New Zealand practice. Injury. 2023;54(1):223–31.
4. Hammouda N, Carpenter CR, Hung WW, Lesser A, Nyamu S, Liu S, et al. Moving the needle on fall prevention: a Geriatric Emergency Care Applied Research (GEAR) Network scoping review and consensus statement. Acad Emerg Med. 2021;28(11):1214–27.
5. Fernando-Canavan L, Gust A, Hsueh A, Tran-Duy A, Kirk M, Brooks P, et al. Measuring the economic impact of hospital-acquired complications on an acute health service. Aust Health Rev. 2021;45(2):135–42.
6. Lindner G, Woitok BK. Emergency department overcrowding: analysis and strategies to manage an international phenomenon. Wien Klin Wochenschr. 2021;133(5–6):229–33.
7. Dinh MM, Berendsen RS. Overcrowding kills: How COVID-19 could reshape emergency department patient flow in the new normal. Emerg Med Australas. 2021;33(1):175–7.
8. Javidan AP, Hansen K, Higginson I, Jones P, Lang E, International Federation Emergency Department C, et al. The International Federation for Emergency Medicine report on emergency department crowding and access block: a brief summary. Emerg Med J. 2021;38(3):245–6.
9. McErlean DR, Hughes JA. Who falls in an adult emergency department and why-A retrospective review. Australas Emerg Nurs J. 2017;20(1):12–6.
10. Morris ME, Webster K, Jones C, Hill A-M, Haines T, McPhail S, et al. Interventions to reduce falls in hospitals: a systematic review and meta-analysis. Age Ageing. 2022;51(5):afac077.
11. Tyler KR, Hullick C, Newton BA, Adams CB, Arendts G. Emergency department pain management in older patients. Emerg Med Australas. 2020;32(5):840–6.
12. Australian Commission on Safety and Quality in Health Care. Hip Fracture Clinical Care Standard Sydney: ACSQHC; 2016 [Available from: https://www.safetyandquality.gov.au/sites/default/files/migrated/Hip-Fracture-Care-Clinical-Care-Standard_tagged.pdf.

25 Recognizing and Responding to Sepsis and Delirium in an Older Adult Living in a Care Facility

Target Learner Group: Emergency Medicine Trainees

Alice Gray

Background

For the most part, emergency medicine (EM) trainees have limited formal teaching on geriatric medicine topics. However, older adult patients are encountered daily on shift and older adult patients are at a high risk of developing delirium. The ability to detect delirium in the emergency department (ED) is paramount as evidence shows that if emergency providers miss delirium, admitting services may also miss the diagnosis [1]. The diagnosis of delirium is especially challenging when there is a baseline of dementia or other cognitive impairments, as cognitive changes are often cited for the patient's presentation. However, missing delirium has a very high mortality rate, and patients who have dementia are at a much higher risk of developing delirium.

When there is suspicion of delirium, gaining collateral information is of paramount importance. An integral aspect of this scenario is calling the long-term care (LTC) facility for collateral information, as the older adult with delirium cannot give relevant information. If learners call the LTC facility, they will be able to gather a detailed history from a caregiver about the patient's functional baseline. One of the debriefers will be asked to portray the caregiver in the LTC facility on the phone. As part of their workup to uncover the cause of the delirium, learners are expected to examine the patient thoroughly. An older adult simulated participant (SP) portrays the patient. If learners examine the patient, a picture of an infected sacral pressure ulcer is given to the participants. This is the underlying cause of the patient sepsis and delirium. Older adult patients with sepsis may have a very subtle presentation without fever and hypotension [2].

The debriefing focuses on the diagnosis and identification of delirium, atypical presentations in older adult patients (infection and sepsis), and how to collect appropriate collateral information on patients with cognitive impairment or delirium.

Key Session Information

Description of the scenario	87-year-old Jamie Gordon presents to the emergency department with a concern about a decreased level of consciousness They are from an LTC facility. Their initial vital signs: HR 92, BP 115/74, RR 20, T 35.1 °C SpO_2 95% room air, GCS 13–14
Setting	Simulated emergency room setting
Learning objectives	By the end of this session, learners will be able to: 1. Recognize and diagnose delirium and sepsis in an older adult 2. Manage delirium using non-pharmacologic strategies 3. Recognize the importance of calling for collateral information about a patient's condition in a timely manner
Adjunct materials	• Cardiac and respiratory monitoring equipment • IV access with fluids • Medications for treating the infection and managing delirium • Telephone • LTC transfer sheet with contact number
Participants	Learners: • 4–5 learners, one to be "team leader" Faculty/SPs/others: • Facilitator(s)—one to answer the phone as a caregiver • 1 SP to portray patient
Age of SP	SP should appear to be the stated age of the role
Scenario length	40 min
Session schedule	5 min pre-brief, 15 min scenario, 20 min debrief
Room setup	• Stretcher in the middle of the room • Debriefers behind the glass (or off to the side of the room) • Separate room for debriefing with chairs in a circle
Props	Learners may carry notes/pens and their phones

A. Gray (✉)
University Health Network, Toronto, ON, Canada
e-mail: alice.gray@uhn.ca

C. M. Smith et al. (eds.), *Comprehensive Healthcare Simulation: Geriatric Simulation*, Comprehensive Healthcare Simulation,
https://doi.org/10.1007/978-3-031-65742-9_25

Instructions to Learners

You are working in a community hospital. You are about to see an 87-year-old, Jamie Gordon, sent from an LTC facility for altered mental status. The patient has been in the department for a few hours.
Please manage the patient as you normally would in the emergency department.

Instructions to SP

You are portraying a patient with moderate dementia who is also more confused and agitated due to delirium.

Special Instructions for Portraying This Scenario

- You are in a hospital gown on a stretcher in a room. However, you will be wearing appropriate clothing underneath the gown. You will be lethargic and very drowsy during the assessment. Your eyes will close intermittently but you will wake to voice. You cannot pay attention for very long periods of time. You are unable to give any information. You can state your first name but not your birthday or where you live. You are not oriented to time or place. You are distracted during the interview. You get off-topic frequently. Otherwise, you have a slightly high respiratory rate (20–24) but do not appear in much distress unless they try to turn you in bed or move you in bed. If asked, you will say that you have some pain around your "bottom".
- There is a picture of a sacral pressure ulcer underneath you that the faculty will give to the learners if they attempt to examine you.

Instructions to the Caregiver at LTC (on the Phone)

Patient's Medical History

- The patient moved into the LTC home 1 year ago. They have mild to moderate dementia.
- They normally can dress themselves. They use a walker. They require some help with bathing. They normally have some confusion around dates and times but can hold a basic conversation.
- In the last few days, they have been less mobile and refusing to come down for dinner, so they have had meals in their room. They tend to scream and moan when caregivers are attempting self-care. They have been agitated recently and normally this is not the case.
- No medication changes.
- No falls or other trauma.
- No outbreaks at the long-term care facility.

Social/Lifestyle Information

- They have one grown child who lives in the area.

Past Medical History

- Dementia, hypertension, dyslipidaemia, diabetes, hysterectomy, breast cancer treated remotely with mastectomy and radiation, heart failure with preserved ejection fraction, osteoarthritis, anxiety.

Your Ideas, Concerns, and Expectations

- It upsets you to see the patient this way.
- You are sure something has changed, as they are more confused than normal.
- If learners do not suspect any infection, you mention that they seem to be in pain when staff attempt to change their clothing or bathe them.

Special Instructions for Portraying the Caregiver from the LTC (on the Phone)

- If the learners ask about something you are unsure of, say "I don't know" or "I can get that information for you".
- Ask questions that flow from the learner's behaviours. Do not drive the interview forward with questions if the learners get stuck. Quietly wait until they get on track again.
- You may ask any relevant questions that come to mind. Feel free to use your own words.

Considerations for Working with Older Adult SPs

Before the Scenario

- Screen older adult SPs for comfort with subject matter and memory ability.
- Train less than 1 week prior to the session. Training should be no more than 2 h long with a break half-way through the session.
- Send a video of a patient with delirium (on YouTube) if possible, to give the older adult SP an idea on how best to portray the confused older person with delirium.
- Review (frequently) the etiquette to be followed before, during, and after the session (e.g. stay in role until out of the room; how to handle requests for feedback).
- Simplify the older adult SP role details.

During the Scenario

- Ensure that the room is free of fall hazards and that chairs are comfortable and accessible for older adult SPs
- Ensure there is a comfortable bed for older adult SPs to use during the session
- Ensure facilitators face older adult SP when calling a time in or time out so older adult SP with hearing challenges is clear when the simulation starts and stops

After the Scenario

- Provide an opportunity for older adult SP to de-role
- Provide an opportunity for older adult SP to give feedback about the session for future iterations of the session if appropriate

Lessons Learned

- Many learners do not attempt to call the LTC home despite having easy access to the phone number on the transfer sheet. If this happens, we prompt them by having the patient's "daughter" call in to check on her mother. When learners attempt to elicit information from the daughter, she will encourage them to call the LTC home.
- Learners infrequently exposed the patient to examine the skin integrity despite no other clear source of infection. To prompt this, the caregiver can mention that there was something of concern on their lower back. We also ensured that the SP was clothed underneath the hospital gown, that they were comfortable being examined by the learners, and that a printed picture of the sacral pressure ulcer was provided when they attempted to examine the older adult SP back.
- Much of the debrief focused on barriers to calling for collateral information. While many learners understand the importance, it's important to tease out ways to facilitate communication.
- This can be a difficult role to play for an older adult SP, as portraying a confused patient with delirium is challenging. Having an experienced older adult SP helps facilitate this portrayal. Also using videos to demonstrate delirium can be extremely helpful to prepare the older adult SP for role portrayal.

References

1. Han JH, Wilson A, Ely WE. Delirium in the older emergency department patient – a quiet epidemic. Emerg Med Clin North Am. 2010;28(3):611–31.
2. Rowe TA, McKoy JM. Sepsis in older adults. Infect Dis Clin N Am. 2017;31(4):731–42.

26 Recognizing and Managing Abuse and Mistreatment of Older Adults

Target Learner Group: Emergency Department Team

Clare Scott and Nemat Alsaba

Background

Elder abuse and mistreatment are defined as a single or repeated act or lack of action (negligence) within a perceived trusty relationship that results in distress, harm, or risk of harm to the older person. Elder abuse and mistreatment can take multiple shapes and forms, ranging from physical, psychological, and sexual abuse, including neglect and financial exploitation (1–3).

Unfortunately, although elder abuse and mistreatment are common in emergency department (ED) presentation, they go under-recognized and underreported due to multiple challenges, including failure to identify elder abuse by clinicians (1, 2). Furthermore, delays in recognizing and responding to elder abuse and mistreatment are linked to high abuse-related morbidity and mortality. These issues highlight the need to understand the subtle signs and symptoms along with risk factors for elder abuse and mistreatment (4).

The scenario allows ED staff with different experience levels to practice the challenges of recognizing and responding to elder abuse cases together. It also helps with skill application and knowledge translation, such as having difficult conversations and applying strategies to obtain personal information while establishing an agreed understanding and plan of care with the older person.

Supplementary Information The online version contains supplementary material available at https://doi.org/10.1007/978-3-031-65742-9_26.

C. Scott
Gold Coast Health Simulation Service, Gold Coast Hospital and Health Service, Gold Coast, QLD, Australia
e-mail: clare.scott@health.qld.gov.au

N. Alsaba (✉)
Department of Emergency Medicine, Gold Coast Hospital and Health Service, QLD, Australia

Faculty of Health Sciences and Medicine, Bond University, Gold Coast, QLD, Australia
e-mail: nalsaba@bond.edu.au

Key Session Information

Description of the scenario	Daphne Davies, a 79-year-old woman, presented to ED with abdominal pain. Initial assessment revealed that she had a fall 2 days ago and sustained multiple bruises. She has been experiencing intermittent dizziness prior to and after the fall Participants are expected to: • Recognize the cause of the fall is due to elder abuse • Identify risk factors for elder abuse in this case • Manage and treat the complexity of this presentation (medical issues, elder abuse with its physical and psychological injuries) with professionalism, compassion, and empathy
Setting	Simulated ED room
Learning objectives	By the end of this session, learners will be able to: 1. Demonstrate effective team-based communication and assessment of an older person presenting with a fall 2. Recognize unique and subtle signs and symptoms of elder abuse presentation and appropriate management 3. Illustrate a sensitive discussion and approach to a patient with a complex and challenging situation, such as an elder abuse case
Adjunct materials	Pre-reading resources are sent to the participants a week before the simulation activity. Here are some resources we found helpful and included in our pre-reading: • https://gedcollaborative.com/podcast/how-to-identify-and-intervene-in-cases-of-elder-abuse/ • https://litfl.com/elder-abuse/ • https://www.ncbi.nlm.nih.gov/pmc/articles/PMC5391043/ • Participant information (Resource 1).

C. M. Smith et al. (eds.), *Comprehensive Healthcare Simulation: Geriatric Simulation*, Comprehensive Healthcare Simulation,
https://doi.org/10.1007/978-3-031-65742-9_26

Participants	Learners:
	• 2 doctors and 3 nurses
	Faculty/SPs/others:
	• 2 facilitators/debrief leads (1 medical and 1 nursing)
	• 1 older adult SP
	• Sim technician
	• Embedded participants
	  • Family member accessible via phone
	  • Registered nurse (RN).
	  • ICU/trauma team (if applicable to your hospital setting) is available via phone for participants requesting ICU/trauma review and input

Age of SP	SP should appear to be the stated age of the role
Scenario length	60 min
Session schedule	10 min of pre-briefing 15 min for simulation 35 min of debriefing
Room setup	Emergency patient bed space

Props	**Clinical equipment and consumables:**
	• IV line and IV fluid
	• Syringes
	• REALITi 360 or any other simulation cardiac monitor
	Investigation:
	Utilize either:
	• Your own clinical database for investigation results/images
	Or
	• Free Open Access Medical Education (FOAMed) resources
	  • Chest X-ray → within normal limits
	  • Pelvic X-rays → normal with no fractures
	  • CT head → normal CT head
	  • Focused Assessment with Sonography for Trauma (FAST) scan → free fluid in the hepatorenal angle signifying an internal injury and bleeding
	  • ECG → fast atrial fibrillation (AF)
	  • Venous blood gas (VBG) →see Fig. 26.1)
	Others:
	Patient medication list, handwritten by SP and in their handbag
	Simulated room video streamed to debrief room. If your simulation room has no video streaming device, please refer to Key Session Information in Chap. 24 on how to set up videoconferencing in your simulation cubicle

Wardrobe	An old nightgown with coffee and food stains for the SP
Moulage	A mixture of old and new bruising Bruising includes: • Handprint bruises to upper arms indicating patient being grabbed • Handprint bruises to the anterior chest wall indicating the perpetrator pinned the patient down • Bruising to the right upper quadrant of the abdomen and thigh due to direct, blunt injury (kick) and/or fall • Bruising over the forehead Resource 3 has comprehensive moulage information including what, why, and how

Instructions to Learners

In our simulation service, we have adopted sending an email to the participants 1 week before the simulation activity with information detailing the following:

- Time and format of events
- Aim of the simulation activity
- FAQs, i.e., "How to administer the simulated medications?", "Who can we call?", and "What information is available—pathology, X-rays, etc.?"
- Hyperlinks to resources and pre-reading, including guidelines, podcasts, and articles
- Participant information (Resource 1)

This aligns with our philosophy of setting learners up for success while reducing cognitive load and providing a psychologically safe learning environment to maximize their simulation learning experience.

The following information will be given to the participants as a handover by the embedded participant RN:

> Thanks for taking over; I have just triaged Daphne, a 79-year-old who had a fall 2 days ago and is now complaining of vague abdominal pain. She is slightly tachycardic. Can you review her, please?

Instructions to Embedded Participant RN

Your simulation responsibilities are to:

- Maintain the safety of participants
- Maintain the safety of older adult SP by implementing a planned pre-simulation safety code with them
- Initiate the simulation with the handover scripted above
- Bridge any simulation knowledge gaps, i.e., equipment access and sourcing blood products
- Guide participants with prompts if required, i.e., phone calls to family
- Provide investigation results as requested, i.e., pathology or radiology

Instructions to SPs

You are portraying Daphne Davies, a 79-year-old woman, dropped off at the emergency department by your adult child because you have abdominal pain. The abdominal pain started after you fell at home 2 days ago. The pain is on the right side of the abdomen. There is no history of vomiting. Initially, state you fell a few stairs in the garden, but later, if asked to explain more about the fall, reveal your child was drunk and accidentally pushed you down the stairs. You don't think they meant to push you.

Be cagey about what happened and withdrawn throughout the encounter with the ED team. Withdraw physically when touched; this is one of the subtle signs of elder abuse as the patient's unconscious reaction to simple physical touch is withdrawal. During assessment and conversation, avoid eye-to-eye contact. This is also another subtle sign of elder abuse and mistreatment.

Be reluctant to answer questions but inform them you have gradually worsening pain in your abdomen since the fall. You also hit your head when you fell 2 days ago.

The team will assess and examine you, and the inspection of the bruising patterns on your body suggesting physical abuse should trigger more questions about whether you feel safe at home living with your adult child.

Current and Past Medical History

You've been experiencing palpitations for 3 days before the fall. You have a history of atrial fibrillation (racing or irregular heartbeats), hypertension, COPD (breathing problem), and type 2 diabetes.

You take multiple medications: blood thinner, diabetic and BP medications, and puffers/inhalers. Your medication list is in your bag (rivaroxaban, atenolol, Seretide, candesartan, and metformin). You don't need to remember the names of the medications.

Social/Lifestyle Information

You live with your 50-year-old child.

They have a few whiskeys most nights. They get angry when drunk, sometimes grabbing your arm and telling you to go to your room and leave them alone.

They accidentally pushed you over while drunk 6 months ago; you were fine and didn't want to cause a fuss. You don't want to get them in trouble as they mean well and let you stay home with them. They have been struggling since their partner left them 3 years ago. They often blame you, saying you're a burden.

Some of your medications ran out a week ago. They have been too busy to collect it from the pharmacy. You've been having on-and-off racing heartbeats and dizziness since.

If asked about your home situation, you often don't have lunch when they are at work, as you have difficulty making your food.

You rarely go out. You spend most of your time at home alone.

> **Tip**
> When writing a script for the SP role, invite older adult SPs to be part of the design and write-up to reflect true collaboration. Ensure the scenario narrative is simple but informative. Some older adult SPs might not have a clinical background, so avoid using medical or technical terminology. For example, words like tachycardia, tachypnea, and rebound tenderness could be replaced with simple descriptions.

History of Current Situation

What brings this person to a healthcare provider at the starting point of the scenario?

- Concerns about the current symptoms (the abdominal pain and dizziness) are getting worse.

Person's Ideas, Concerns, and Expectations

You are concerned about the pain in the right side of your abdomen. You are also worried you may fall again because you feel dizzy and your heart is racing.

You don't want to end up in a nursing home and want to go back home with your child. You are happy managing as you are.

Opening Line

I feel dizzy, and my belly pain is not going away.

Embedded Participant Family Member Script

At the 10-min mark of the simulation, the embedded RN will prompt the participants to call their son/daughter if they have not done so already.

You dropped your mother off at the ED but had to leave to go to work. You plan to come and pick her up when you finish. When the participants call you for further information, you will offer a different story (she fell in the supermarket on slippery wet tiles, has been forgetful lately and can make up some stories).

You become rattled and annoyed by some of the questions but then apologize.

Examples are as follows:

I just told you that she fell in the supermarket; why do you keep asking the same question?
I don't know….sorry, I had a very hectic day at work.
I can't remember.

Considerations for Working with Older Adult SPs

Before the Scenario

- Screen older adult SPs for comfort when involved in a confronting scenario or difficult conversation.
- Send older adult SP the scenario 1 week before the training.
- Give older adult SP permission to contact you and freely discuss the case and how to portray the role.
- Be patient and mindful of SP's learning process. Some may interpret information faster than others. Ensuring adequate time to process and develop one's storyline is important.
- Provide older adult SPs with a contact person and their phone number to call when arriving at the department in case they have difficulties finding the simulation room.
- As the role has a considerable amount of moulage (multiple bruising patterns and different ages), ensure the older adult SP has no current skin condition that might be affected by using makeup and applying moulage. Extra care should be taken during the application and removal of the moulage for older adult SPs with thin and dry skin.
- On the day prior to the simulation activity, ensure the following with the older adult SP:
  - Meet and greet them at the entrance of your department.
  - Ensure they have their own visual or hearing aids.
  - Ensure they have eaten, are well hydrated, and feel well.
  - Orient them to the department amenities and remind them to use the toilet just before the activity, as they will be immersed in it for approximately 60 min from the start to the end.
  - Establish an agreed safety code/word/action to be utilized if an apparent risk presents.

During the Scenario

The embedded RN encouraged to:

- Remain vigilant of the safety and comfort of the older adult SP, intervening if apparent risks appear
- Give previously agreed-upon verbal or physical cues to trigger the older adult SP's reaction, i.e., prompting with keywords to escalate a patient response or a physical touch to subdue their responses

After the Scenario

- Encourage older adult SP to de-role and support them during this process.
- Assist older adult SP with removing all monitoring and IV therapy attachments with care due to their frail and thin skin to prevent skin breaks. Utilize this task to hear the older adult SP's initial thoughts and reactions to the interaction between them and the participants. This will help them verbalize their feelings and thoughts before debriefing.
- Assist older adult SP with removing the moulage (bruising patterns) to protect their skin.
- Encourage older adult SP to provide additional feedback about the simulation activity in a follow-up phone call or email.

Lessons Learned

- Identifying one simulation team member on the day whom the older adult SP can refer to for information and queries will reduce multiple versions of instructions and answers and prevent older adult SPs from becoming potentially overwhelmed.
- Including older adult SPs in simulation-related creative development activities is paramount in building relationships and improving the delivery of the simulations. For instance, most SPs found moulage workshops enjoyable and informative, giving them a sense of pride and autonomy to create their "look" to fit the scenario narrative. (See Resource 2) However, this is optional; we continue to offer moulage applications to those who prefer not to apply their moulage.
- Choosing the right older adult SP for this confronting and challenging role is crucial. An experienced older adult SP who can critically analyze the participant's body language, facial expressions, and verbal cues, react immediately and appropriately, and give feedback eloquently will help achieve the intended learning outcome.
- Running this simulation activity in our emergency department has normalized the sensitive conversations about elder abuse amongst the staff. We have noticed an increase in identified elder abuse cases in our ED.

Disclaimer The authors declare they have no financial affiliation with any moulage products cited in these resources.

Appendix

Fig. 26.1 VBG

Venous blood gas (VBG)

RADIOMETRY ABL800 FLEX

Identifications	
Patient ID	123456
Patient Last Name	
Patient First Name	
Sample Type	**Venous**
T	37.2
FiO2 (0.21)	Room Air
Operator	Simulation Service

Blood Gases			
pH	7.33		7.350 - 7.450
pCO2	45	mmHg	35.0 - 45.0
pO2	60	mmHg	75.0 - 100
cHCO3-(P)c	19	mmol/L	21.0 - 27.0
cBase(B)c		mmol/L	-3.0 - 3.0
P50c		mmHg	
Baro		mmHg	
Oximetry Values			
aO2		%	
clHb	79	g/L	105 - 135
Hcl		%	
FO2Hb		%	94.0 - 98.0
FCOHb		%	0.0 - 1.5
FMelHb		%	
FHHb		%	
Electrolyte Values			
cNa+	129	mmol/L	135 - 145
cK+	4.9	mmol/L	3.2 - 4.5
cCl-	99	mmol/L	100 - 110
cCa2+	1.20	mmol/L	1.15 - 1.36
AnionGap K+c		mmol/L	
Metabolite Values			
cGlu	4.9	mmol/L	3.0 - 7.8
cLac	2.9	mmol/L	0.7 - 2.5
cCrea	178	µmol/L	36 - 82

References

1. Rosen T, Hargarten S, Flomenbaum NE, Platts-Mills TF. Identifying elder abuse in the emergency department: toward a multidisciplinary team-based approach. Ann Emerg Med. 2016;68(3):378–82.
2. Hullick C, Carpenter CR, Critchlow R, Burkett E, Arendts G, Nagaraj G, et al. Abuse of the older person: is this the case you missed last shift? Emerg Med Australas. 2017;29(2):223–8.
3. Abuse of older people [Internet]. World Health Organization. World Health Organization; 2022 [cited 2023Jan6]. Available from: https://www.who.int/news-room/fact-sheets/detail/abuse-of-older-people
4. Kaspiew R, Carson R, Rhoades H. Elder abuse: understanding issues, frameworks and responses. Australian Institute of Family Studies: Melbourne; 2016.

Toxicology Emergencies in Older Adults: Slow Is Smooth, Smooth Is Fast

27

Target Learner Group: Pre-hospital Physicians, Paramedics, Emergency Department and Other Hospital Teams

Hemal Patel and Carolyn Hullick

Background

As modern scientific and medical advances continue to contribute to healthier and longer lives for humanity, a problem that health professionals encounter regularly is the complications of polypharmacy in an older person [1–3]. This is largely due to the fact that seemingly benign symptoms that older persons have can reflect the profound effect of drug pharmacokinetics and lead to life-threatening complications [4, 5].

Unfortunately, geriatric toxicology is challenging to recognise early in the Emergency Department (ED) as most overdoses are unintentional, and presentations to the ED can be non-specific, mimicking other clinical presentations. Mimics of geriatric toxicology can include sepsis, heart failure and gastrointestinal and neurological presentations, such as stroke, leading to delays in diagnosis and treatment and thus contributing to morbidity and mortality in this population [6, 7].

Supplementary Information The online version contains supplementary material available at https://doi.org/10.1007/978-3-031-65742-9_27.

H. Patel (✉)
Wyong Hospital, Central Coast Local Health District, Wyong, NSW, Australia

New South Wales Ambulance, Clinical Capability, Safety and Quality, State Headquarters, Homebush, Sydney, NSW, Australia

School of Medicine and Public Health, University of Newcastle, Newcastle, NSW, Australia
e-mail: Hemal.patel@health.nsw.gov.au

C. Hullick
School of Medicine and Public Health, University of Newcastle, Newcastle, NSW, Australia

Belmont Hospital, Hunter New England Local Health District, Belmont, NSW, Australia

Australian Commission on Safety and Quality in Health Care, Sydney, NSW, Australia
e-mail: Carolyn.hullick@health.nsw.gov.au

A significant proportion of older persons take cardiac medications [8], and the toxicological effects of these medications, including beta-blockers, can manifest as cardiac ischaemia, profound cardiogenic shock and life-threatening bradyarrhythmia (e.g. complete heart block) [9].

For the purposes of this chapter, the focus is on bradyarrhythmia caused by beta-blocker overdose and toxicity. The management of bradyarrhythmia in the ED involves chemical and electrical pacing [10]. Traditionally, pre-hospital teams have managed bradyarrhythmia, including complete heart block with medications including atropine and adrenaline in an attempt to stabilise the patient enough for transfer to the hospital [11]. More recently, pre-hospital teams in Australia have instituted pre-hospital transcutaneous cardiac pacing for bradyarrhythmia in addition to the standard drug therapy used. This practice falls within the scope of intensive care paramedics who can institute transcutaneous pacing for patients.

The transfer of care of critically unwell patients from the pre-hospital setting into the hospital is always high-risk, involving complex communication and equipment and multiple personnel [12]. The addition of transcutaneous cardiac pacing adds a layer of complexity and risk to the transfer of care which needs to be practiced so that the patient who has been stabilised in the pre-hospital environment does not deteriorate in a time-critical window during the transfer of care [13].

Traditionally, medical, nursing and paramedic teams tend to undertake education in isolation, with content and simulation specific to the group's scope of practice. Learning in clinical silos is a missed opportunity to fully appreciate the perspectives and skill sets of other members of the clinical workforce [14]. Interdisciplinary in situ simulation allows learners to appreciate different frames of reference from all members of the multidisciplinary and interprofessional teams who contribute to the patient's care in an environment where they usually practice as clinicians.

C. M. Smith et al. (eds.), *Comprehensive Healthcare Simulation: Geriatric Simulation*, Comprehensive Healthcare Simulation,
https://doi.org/10.1007/978-3-031-65742-9_27

In this scenario, the pre-hospital paramedic team brings the patient into the ED. The aim is to provide clinical handover and transfer the patient onto the hospital bed while maintaining cardiac output. This scenario was run as a planned session within the ED with a videoconferencing link for the hospital team to observe and appreciate bradyarrhythmia management in the pre-hospital setting, including attachment to transcutaneous pacing.

The hospital and pre-hospital team work together to transfer the patient attached to transcutaneous pacing to receive definitive management. Other team members are observers who comment on technical, cognitive and behavioural skills in this acute time-critical situation. This was a particularly important scenario to ensure purposeful practice was undertaken, as receiving patients already initiated on transcutaneous pacing into the ED is not a common occurrence. Interdisciplinary training was critical to ensure patient safety while maintaining confidence within the whole treating team in an uncommon but emergent scenario.

Key Session Information

Description of the scenario	75-year-old Riley Bird presents to the ED with the ambulance service with complete heart block. The patient is attached to transcutaneous pacing. They are bradycardic (rate 40) and hypotensive (BP 80/40)
Setting	ED resuscitation cubicle
Learning objectives	By the end of the session, learners will be able to: 1. Provide safe transition from pre-hospital care to hospital care, including: • Giving a structured clinical handover • Transferring from the pre-hospital transcutaneous pacing device to the hospital transcutaneous pacing device effectively • Anticipating and managing complications of transfer from one external pacing device to another 2. Recognise and address analgesic requirements of the externally paced, critically unwell patient 3. Demonstrate a systemic approach to the assessment and management of the bradycardic older person 4. Demonstrate an understanding of beta-blocker toxicity management (initial supportive care, appropriate management of severe toxicity) 5. Develop an appreciation and understanding of the pre-hospital setting for ED clinicians and the critical importance of structured handovers
Adjunct materials	See Resources below
Participants	Learners: • 2 paramedics • 2–3 medical staff • 2 nursing staff Educators: • 1 simulation equipment technician (helps with parameters on the monitoring) • 1–2 facilitators • 1 simulated patient (SP)
Age of SP	SP should appear to be the stated age of the role
Scenario length	90-min
Session schedule	• 20-min briefing • 30-min scenario (including pre-hospital assessment and initiation of management) • 40-min debriefing
Room set-up	Clinical bed space, ideally resuscitation bed space Videoconferencing linked to a separate room for observers (see Resource 2)
Props	**Ambulance trolley** • Blood pressure cuff, pulse oximeter, cardiac monitor **Clinical equipment:** *Pre-hospital:* • Nasal prongs • IV line • Cardiac pacing pads, leads and defibrillator/pacer • Intravenous fluids *Emergency department:* • Nasal prongs • IV line • Cardiac pacing pads, leads and defibrillator/pacer • Intravenous fluids • Drugs/infusions—atropine, adrenaline, isoprenaline, noradrenaline, antiemetics, insulin/dextrose • Two pacing devices are preferable as clinicians will need to transfer the simulated patient from the first device to the second • Management/guideline of beta-blocker toxicity • Complete heart block ECG • Paced ECG, rate 60–70 bpm • Normal chest X-ray
Wardrobe	Casual clothing
Moulage	• Create sweat to support the "sick" look by combining three parts glycerin (available at drug stores) with one part water in a spray bottle. Then spray onto the forehead

Instructions to Learners

You receive a pre-hospital notification phone call from the ambulance coordinator. A 75-year-old Riley Bird is being transferred to your ED with the paramedics. They had diarrhoea for 5 days and have not been drinking very much. This morning, Riley felt lightheaded and had a brief loss of consciousness. They take daily metoprolol and apixaban for paroxysmal atrial fibrillation. Riley is not on other medications and has no other medical or surgical problems. The paramedic team found an abnormal ECG showing a complete heart block and instituted cardiac pacing in the pre-hospital setting.

Riley lives at home with their partner who is also independent. Riley has no allergies.

Your task is to:

- Transfer the patient from the ambulance stretcher to the hospital bed safely.
- Maintain the cardiac output of the patient.
- Ensure safe clinical handover of the patient.
- Continue clinical assessment and management of the patient.

Instructions to Simulated Participant (SP)

You are portraying a 75-year-old person, Riley Bird. You have come to the emergency department (ED) via ambulance because you have had diarrhoea and have not been consuming much food and fluid over the last 5 days. You have not had any vomiting. This morning you were feeling lightheaded and had an episode where you had a brief loss of consciousness while sitting with your partner in the living room. You had no pain. Despite feeling unwell in the last few days, you have continued to take your medications for your irregular heartbeat.

You have never had episodes of loss of consciousness or feeling lightheaded before this morning. Your partner reported that you went very pale and sweaty prior to losing consciousness. Your partner says you passed out for a few seconds and then woke up. You had no abnormal shakes or movements and no seizure-like activity.

You have not been taking any medications for your diarrhoea as you thought it would pass. You have been feeling thirsty. You have not been urinating as much. You have had no fever, no blood in your diarrhoea and no abdominal pain. You have had no shortness of breath, cough or runny nose. You had no speech disturbance or other weakness in your arms, legs or face.

The scenario will start while you are at home. The paramedics will assess and manage you so they can transfer you safely to the hospital.

The scenario will end after the ED team receives the handover and safely transfers you to their cardiac machine.

When the paramedics arrive, you feel lightheaded but know exactly where you are. They will inform you that your blood pressure is low and your heart rate is slow.

The paramedics will place a simulated intravenous cannula in your right arm. They will also give you medication to speed up your heart and give you fluid through the cannula to increase your blood pressure. They will place two large cardiac pads on your chest.

You will be transferred to the ED for definite treatment of your abnormal heart rate.

On arrival, you continue to feel lightheaded, sweaty and vague in the ED. The paramedic team will hand over the care to the hospital team while transferring the connection of the two large cardiac pads to the hospital machine. If you are attached to the machine controlling your heart rate, you complain of discomfort around the placement of the pads. You should ask for pain relief.

Current and Past Medical History

- You have paroxysmal atrial fibrillation which is well controlled with medication (metoprolol to slow your heart and apixaban as a blood thinner).
- You have not had any previous surgery or other medical problems.
- You do not have any drug or food allergies.

Family Medical History

- You do not recall any major family health problems.

Social/Lifestyle Information

- You live at home with your partner. You are both independent.
- You play tennis three times a week to keep yourself healthy and fit.
- You do not smoke and you do not drink any alcohol.

Person's Ideas, Concerns and Expectations

- You enjoy your independence.
- You are concerned that the diarrhoea is making your blood pressure low.
- Your expectation is that you will improve and go home soon after the hospital team gives you fluid through the drip.

Opening Line

I am feeling very lightheaded and weak.

Special Instructions for Portraying This Scenario

- You will be wearing casual clothes.
- In this scenario, two to three ambulance officers, two doctors and two nurses will participate, and other learners will observe.
- You will start the scenario on a chair in a room outside of the ED.
- When the ambulance officers arrive, they will assess you and you will tell them that you are feeling lightheaded and weak.
- You will be moved onto an ambulance stretcher, and further treatment will be started, including medication and fluids to improve your low blood pressure and slow heart rate.
- Two large "cardiac pads" connected to a machine may be placed on your chest to help speed up your heart. In real life, these pads tend to cause pain, so if they are placed on you, you should complain of pain and ask for pain relief.
- You will be transferred on the ambulance trolley to the ED, where the hospital team will take over your care following the handover of information about what happened before you arrived at the ED.
- In the ED, you will continue your treatment with the cardiac pads on your chest, and extra medication will need to be initiated to help your condition improve.
- The hospital team may perform further tracing of your heart and take blood tests from the simulated intravenous drip placed in your arm. The hospital team will be provided with these results. You may provide a prompt, e.g. "Do I need any blood tests?" or "Do I need another tracing of my heart?".
- You may ask any relevant questions that come to mind. Feel free to use your own words. Here are some examples of questions that you might ask:

Related to the Diagnosis

- What does the ECG/heart tracing show?
- Why are my heart rate and blood pressure low?
- What are the pads on my chest for?
- Have I had a stroke?
- Ask for clarification if the learners express something in a way that you do not understand, such as:
  - What does that word mean?
  - Could you explain this more?
  - Can someone let my partner know? Where are they?

Related to the Treatment Plan

- Does this mean I need an operation?
- When will I get better?
- Will I be able to play tennis on Thursday?
- Will I have to take more medication?

Considerations for Working with Older Adult SPs

Before the Scenario

- Recruit the right older adult SPs for this scenario, and check whether they have a history of severe osteoarthritis, back pain or joint replacement, as these conditions may restrict the transfer of the older adult SP from the ambulance stretcher to the hospital bed.
- Identify if the older adult SP has had severe heart problems with conduction abnormalities requiring a pacemaker. This may require caution when recruiting an older adult SP for this scenario due to the potential provocation of previously experienced negative emotions.
- Ensure the older adult SP is not allergic to the adhesive in the pad and ECG dots. When removing them, take care to avoid causing any skin damage.
- Screen older adult SPs for hearing challenges. In this scenario, noise from both the monitors and multiple participants may make it harder for the older adult SP to understand what is going on.
- Send the scenario to the older adult SP 1 week before the training date so that they can familiarise themselves with the script and flow of the scenario. Include pictures of some of the equipment you will use, such as the transcutaneous pacing and the cardiac "electrical" pads.
- Arrange a session with the SP 48 h before the simulation activity, either in person or via videoconference, to offer them the opportunity for a verbal run-through of the scenario, clarify expectations and address any concerns.
- Perform a test run with the older adult SP and faculty facilitating the scenario on the day of the simulation activity before the participants' arrival.
- Give the older adult SP a small piece of paper with a list of their medications to hand to the learners instead of memorising the medication list. This can reduce the cognitive burden on the older adult SP.

During the Scenario

- Ensure that the simulation space is a safe environment and that fall risks and further harm are prevented, including having adequate personnel to help move the older adult SP from the ambulance trolley to the hospital bed.
- If the older adult SP suffers from hearing challenges, it is important to ensure that all communication with them is paired with a gentle touch on the shoulder and eye-to-eye contact is used to gain the SP's attention and to communicate effectively.
- Consider the room's temperature, given that the older adult SP may be on the hospital bed for some time and provide them with warm blankets.

After the Scenario

- Allow the older adult SP to provide feedback and reflections immediately after the scenario has ended to promote retention and avoid relying on their memory to provide commentary.
- Engage and support the older adult SP to join the learning conversation so learners understand the insights of the scenario from the patient's perspective. It also gives an opportunity to refine the simulated activity for next time.

Lessons Learned

- The inclusion of the pre-hospital phase as a prequel to the hospital-based simulation has facilitated holistic learning. It offers valuable insight into the factors affecting patient care before hospital arrival and in the ED. Bringing the team together has allowed us to share collective knowledge through simulation.
- Familiarising the older adult SP with the equipment used during the simulation and how it will be applied is important to ensure a shared understanding of the activity and familiarity to guarantee the SP's physical and psychological safety and the activity's success.
- The scenario was purposefully practiced in real time with skills delivered as would be performed in the field. The learning outcomes for this training day focused on a safe, structured process for the transfer of care of the patient from the paramedical team to the hospital resuscitation team.
- During the simulation activity, stronger and more respectful working relationships were formed, which directly transferred to improved patient care.

IPE Reflection

Learning together and practicing together builds strong working relationships and a deeper appreciation of the skills that other teams possess. It is very much a knowledge-sharing activity on many levels.—Intensive care paramedic

I truly believe it has a massive impact on both my clinical and critical thinking skills, made me more approachable and built rapport with the medical team.—Nurse, simulation coordinator

Resources

Many of the resources for this scenario can be sourced from free open access medical resources through Internet search engines. This includes the chest X-ray, ECGs and the management of beta-blocker toxicity. These can be downloaded and printed depending on the needs of the team participating in the scenario.

Below are some resources developed from practicing the simulation activity with the interprofessional team that might be useful for the readers to consider.

1. **ISBAR tool:** The transfer of care of critically unwell patients from the pre-hospital setting into the hospital is a high-risk setting. It involves complex communication, equipment and multiple personnel. It is important to have a structured clinical handover tool like ISBAR (Introduction, Situation, Background, Assessment, Recommendations) [15]. ISBAR provides a framework to ensure that relevant information is effectively communicated. A timely, relevant and structured process that results in transfer of responsibility and accountability of care is required (Microsoft Word—Hunter New England Health ISBAR toolkit text Final.doc (safetyandquality.gov.au) last accessed 31/7/2023).
2. **Setting up videoconferencing in the resuscitation bay:** This can be done using personal devices and a computer screen (with or without a projector). Like any virtual meeting, the set-up will depend on your organisation's videoconferencing (VC) subscription and equipment. From previous experience, having a mobile phone set up in the clinical space on a tripod will give a very good vantage point for the communication and workflow of the learners. This is then video-conferenced to a separate room/space with a computer and projector screen where observers can watch the simulation activity. There will be challenges to looking at what is happening with the cardiac monitor. A second device can be used for this. Additionally, having a separate microphone plugged into the personal device will help improve the sound quality for observers.

Acknowledgements We would like to acknowledge the wonderful people who have helped design this simulation activity and helped contribute to improving patient care—the Belmont Hospital Education Team leads, Catherine MacDonald and Nathan Sharrock, along with Bradley Taylor (Clinical Training Officer), Jeanine Bond and Graham Andrews (Intensive Care Paramedics) with NSW Ambulance who continue to contribute to multidisciplinary simulation.

References

1. Davies LE, Spiers G, Kingston A, Todd A, Adamson J, Hanratty B. Adverse outcomes of polypharmacy in older people: systematic review of reviews. J Am Med Dir Assoc. 2020;21(2):181–7.
2. Khezrian M, McNeil CJ, Murray AD, Myint PK. An overview of prevalence, determinants and health outcomes of polypharmacy. Ther Adv Drug Saf. 2020;11:204209862093374.

3. Page AT, Falster MO, Litchfield M, Pearson SA, Etherton-Beer C. Polypharmacy among older Australians, 2006–2017: a population-based study. Med J Aust. 2019;211(2):71–5.
4. Luttikhuis HM, Blomaard LC, Van Der Kaaij MAE, Gombert-Handoko KB, De Groot B, Mooijaart SP. Geriatric characteristics and the risk of drug-related hospital admissions in older Emergency Department patients. Eur Geriatr Med. 2022;13(2):329–37.
5. Maher D, Ailabouni N, Mangoni AA, Wiese MD, Reeve E. Alterations in drug disposition in older adults: a focus on geriatric syndromes. Expert Opin Drug Metab Toxicol. 2021;17(1):41–52.
6. Coleman JJ, Pontefract SK. Adverse drug reactions. Clin Med. 2016;16(5):481–5.
7. Just KS, Dormann H, Schurig M, Böhme M, Steffens M, Plank-Kiegele B, et al. The phenotype of adverse drug effects: Do emergency visits due to adverse drug reactions look different in older people? Results from the ADRED study. Br J Clin Pharmacol. 2020;86(11):2144–54.
8. Naganathan V. Cardiovascular drugs in older people. Aust Prescr. 2013;36(6):190–4.
9. Lauterbach M. Clinical toxicology of beta-blocker overdose in adults. Basic Clin Pharmacol Toxicol. 2019;125(2):178–86.
10. Kusumoto Fred M, Schoenfeld Mark H, Barrett C, Edgerton James R, Ellenbogen Kenneth A, Gold Michael R, et al. 2018 ACC/AHA/HRS guideline on the evaluation and management of patients with bradycardia and cardiac conduction delay. J Am Coll Cardiol. 2019;74(7):e51–e156.
11. Morrison LJ, Long J, Vermeulen M, Schwartz B, Sawadsky B, Frank J, et al. A randomized controlled feasibility trial comparing safety and effectiveness of prehospital pacing versus conventional treatment: 'PrePACE'. Resuscitation. 2008;76(3):341–9.
12. Tortosa-Alted R, Reverte-Villarroya S, Martinez-Segura E, Lopez-Pablo C, Berenguer-Poblet M. Emergency handover of critical patients. A systematic review. Int Emerg Nurs. 2021;56:100997.
13. Iedema R, Ball C, Daly B, Young J, Green T, Middleton PM, et al. Design and trial of a new ambulance-to-emergency department handover protocol: 'IMIST-AMBO'. BMJ Qual Saf. 2012;21(8):627–33.
14. Gupta R, Arora VM. Merging the health system and education silos to better educate future physicians. JAMA. 2015;314(22):2349.
15. Burgess A, Van Diggele C, Roberts C, Mellis C. Teaching clinical handover with ISBAR. BMC Med Educ. 2020;20(S2):459.

Providing End-of-Life Care for an Older Adult in the Emergency Department

28

Target Learner Group: Emergency Medicine Trainees and Doctors

Alice Gray

Background

Emergency medicine (EM) physicians see and manage patients at end-of-life (EoL) frequently in the Emergency department (ED). However, EM training often lacks palliative care education and the application of palliative care in the acute setting. Goals of care conversations are common in many settings, but the ED requires a specific skill set where healthcare providers must be able to quickly establish a patient's level of care and communicate clearly and concisely with patients and their families. This session has been offered to senior residents training in emergency medicine as part of a geriatric EM curriculum to help build the skills required to have these often challenging conversations in a time-sensitive environment. It has also been offered to EM physicians as part of a local conference, as many staff lack formal training or practice in delivering palliative care in the acute setting.

This scenario was developed to train emergency physicians to recognize EoL trajectories and hold goals of care conversations in a time-sensitive, high-pressure environment. These conversations are challenging even when there is an established therapeutic relationship but even more challenging in the ED with time constraints and lack of familiarity with the patient. Furthermore, the emergency provider must effectively deliver EoL care and manage common symptoms, such as pain, shortness of breath, and airway secretions.

A. Gray (✉)
University Health Network, Toronto, ON, Canada
e-mail: alice.gray@uhn.ca

Key Session Information

Description of the scenario	A 78-year-old patient presents with worsening shortness of breath in the context of known advanced cancer. The patient is too ill to communicate their wishes and participants must have an expedited goals of care conversation with the family member at the bedside. They must also simultaneously manage the patient's pain, shortness of breath, and airway secretions
Setting	Simulated emergency department
Learning objectives	By the end of this session, learners will be able to: 1. Manage common EoL symptoms: pain, dyspnea, and airway secretions in the emergency room setting 2. Hold EoL conversation under time constraints in the ED
Adjunct materials	Mannequin to simulate the patient who is dying and show a video of a patient with abnormal breathing nearing the end of their life
Participants	Learners: • 3–4 learners, one taking the lead role to facilitate the discussion with the family member Faculty/SPs/others: • 2 facilitator(s) • 1 SP as family member undertaking the goals of care discussions
Age of SP	SP should appear to be the stated age of the role
Scenario length	50 min
Session schedule	15-min setup and pre-briefing 15-min for simulations 20-min debriefing
Room setup	• Hospital bed in the middle of the room with a patient (mannequin) • One chair for family member SP
Props	• IV tubing with fluids • IV medications (can have one syringe for all medications learners request) • Discharge summary from recent admission • Simple oxygen system with nasal prongs and face mask • Cardiorespiratory monitor to show HR, BP, RR, O_2, and temperature (can also be written on a board by hand as the scenario develops)
Wardrobe	Casual clothing for family member.
Moulage	Shaving cream is placed around the mouth of the mannequin to simulate secretions

C. M. Smith et al. (eds.), *Comprehensive Healthcare Simulation: Geriatric Simulation*, Comprehensive Healthcare Simulation,
https://doi.org/10.1007/978-3-031-65742-9_28

Instructions to Learners

You are seeing a 78-year-old patient in the ED presenting with shortness of breath, pain, and decreased level of consciousness.

Please assess and manage them the way you would manage a similar patient in the emergency department.

You can give IV medications by specifying the name, dose, and route of delivery. The patient's vitals will change according to the scenario.

Instructions to SP

You are Avery Diamond, the partner of the patient Riley Persaud, who has metastatic lung cancer. You are concerned about the quick deterioration of your partner. You are aware that their cancer is very advanced and active treatment is no longer an option. You are concerned about them and want them to be comfortable, but you won't offer any knowledge about disease trajectory unless specifically asked by participants. You need learners to use simple, non-medical language to describe the situation. If they are able to do this, you are calm and able to have a discussion with the participants. You are sad and emotional but not hysterical or agitated. If the participants try very aggressive measures (e.g., intubation) without confirming the goals of care, you may become agitated and annoyed.

History of Current Situation

What brings this person to a healthcare provider at the starting point of the scenario?

- Concerns for rapid deterioration at home.
- Your partner was diagnosed with lung cancer 2 years ago. They underwent chemotherapy, which was initially successful, but in the last year, they have not been responding to treatment, which was stopped 6 months ago. They were reasonably well until 2–3 months ago, when their health started to decline significantly.
- Your partner was recently admitted to the internal medicine ward, where fluid was removed from their lung (thoracentesis) to help with the worsening shortness of breath. Their pain medication was titrated by the palliative care team. They were discharged home with palliative care support at home along with daily personal support workers.

Current and Past Medical History

- Your partner's past medical history includes metastatic, end-stage lung cancer, hypertension, and coronary artery disease.
- Your own past medical history (if asked) includes diabetes, hypertension, and arthritis.

Social/Lifestyle Information

- Your partner lives at home with you. You do not have any children. Your partner is a retired teacher.

Person's Ideas, Concerns, and Expectations

- You expect that learners will treat your partner's symptoms of pain and shortness of breath, as well as address secretion management.
- You understand that your partner's condition is terminal but will not volunteer this information unless asked directly by learners.

Opening Line

I'm concerned that Riley isn't eating. They're only taking sips of water and tea for a few days.

Other Scripted Lines

They live with me, and other caregivers just started coming into the home now.

I think they're in pain. Their breathing is so noisy. They just make these grunting noises…they have not been really communicating much in the last couple of days.

They've been like this for the last 2 days. But it's been a rapid decline over the last 2 months.

Considerations for Working with Older Adult SPs

The SP in this scenario is the patient's partner. The patient is a mannequin. The older adult SP can be any gender and is >65 years old.

Before the Scenario

- Screen older adult SPs for comfort with being involved in such a difficult conversation and if similar recent EoL discussions involving their family members happened in real life, which might trigger raw emotions.
- Send the scenario to the older adult SP 1–2 weeks prior to training.
- Train 3–5 days prior to the session.
- Training should be no more than 2 h long with a break half-way through the session.
- Work with older adult SPs to generate a list of possible questions. Write them down so they can take them into the room for use (as much as an actual relative would do).
- Simplify the quantity of role details.

During the Scenario

- Ensure that chairs are accessible for older adult SPs.

After the Scenario

- Provide an opportunity for older adult SP to de-role.
- Provide an opportunity for them to give you feedback about the session for future iterations, if appropriate.

Lessons Learned

- Learners are generally very comfortable treating patients in a simulated environment but are less comfortable taking time to establish goals of care before rushing to treatment.
- The language used by many healthcare providers is complicated by medical jargon. Simulated practice is needed in order to use simpler and clear terminology. It was helpful to have an older adult SP who is not well versed in medical jargon to facilitate discussions and to give authentic feedback about the EoL and goals of care conversation.
- It was easier to break the scenario into two parts, the first part being symptom management before the older adult SP (partner) arrives. Once the older adult SP arrives, the team can have a conversation about the goals of care. This helps to focus the whole team on one task at a time.
- To simulate dyspneic, dying patients, a video can be used showing a patient in respiratory distress. This addresses some of the fidelity lost with simulation that is important for learners to recognize EoL clinical situation.

Resources

1. McEwan A, Silverberg JZ. Palliative care in the emergency department. Emerg Med Clin North Am. 2016;34(3):667–85.
2. Mierendorf SM, Gidvani M. Palliative care in the emergency department. Perm J. 2014;18(2):77–85.
3. Baile WF, Buckman R, Lenzi R, Glober G, Beale EA, Kudelka AP. SPIKES-A six-step protocol for delivering bad news: application to the patient with cancer. Oncologist. 2000;5(4):302–11.
4. VandeKieft GK. Breaking bad news. Am Fam Physician. 2001;64(12):1975–8.

Part VI

Applications: Older Adult Care—Advanced Conversations

Conversations About Driving Retirement with Older Adults

29

Target Learner Group: Fourth Year Medical Students in a 6-Year Program

Beate G. Brem and Daniel Bauer

Background

The scenario serves to train breaking bad news (BBN) following a six-step protocol based on the SPIKES model [1].

BBN is one of the four topics in the communication training for fourth year medical students at the University of Bern. The other three topics are taking a sexual history, informed consent, and motivational interviewing. In this communication training, eight students practice these four different challenging conversations in pairs.

In each scenario, one of the students actively communicates (simulating the physician) with the SP (in the patient's role), while the peer student observes. The maximum duration of this conversation is 15 min. Fifteen minutes is then scheduled for feedback immediately after each simulation. At the end of the simulation, the students step out of the room for a moment and are encouraged to exchange their thoughts on the simulation with each other as the SP de-roles and prepares their feedback using a feedback form (see Fig. 29.1.). The students return to the room and the SP moderates the feedback process which involves encouraging reflection and the integration of their perspective with the student's self-reflections.

The four sequences of simulation and feedback are followed by a debriefing session. The format of the debriefing session has been iteratively developed. While initially lecturers randomly observed some of the conversations and held a 15-min informal session with the eight learners afterwards, in 2019 a new format of debriefing was developed. The eight learners now review and annotate a video recording of their own conversations and of conversations of a peer student. They then meet 1–2 weeks later with a lecturer in a 90-min seminar to discuss their experiences based on the annotated video sequences. The Simulated Participants (SPs) are not involved in this session. This debriefing process is described in detail by Pless et al. [2].

After 4–6 weeks, students come back to the simulation center and practice conversations with the same underlying topics again, trying to integrate lessons learned during the first simulation and the debriefing.

In the first few years of this course, the same four scenarios (one for each topic) were used in two sessions separated by 4–6 weeks. The lecturers thought it to be advantageous for learners to improve their skills by engaging in the exact same case twice, with learning about these topics in between. The students, however, lamented a lack of opportunity to transfer their skills to different situations from those they encountered in the first session. To meet this need, a second set of four alternative scenarios for each topic was developed. A general practitioner on the steering committee suggested creating a scenario around driving cessation to supplement the original BBN scenario about communicating the relapse of cancer. The rationale was that this conversation was just as common as delivering a cancer diagnosis, especially with older adults, and could be just as devastating for patients. While not being allowed to drive is not immediately life-threatening, many patients may fear a significant loss of independence and self-determination. Additionally, an aspect of feeling judged and invalidated as "being not good enough any longer" can add to the stress of these conversations.

B. G. Brem (✉) · D. Bauer
Faculty of Medicine, Institute for Medical Education, University of Bern, Bern, Switzerland
e-mail: beate.brem@unibe.ch; daniel.bauer@unibe.ch

C. M. Smith et al. (eds.), *Comprehensive Healthcare Simulation: Geriatric Simulation*, Comprehensive Healthcare Simulation,
https://doi.org/10.1007/978-3-031-65742-9_29

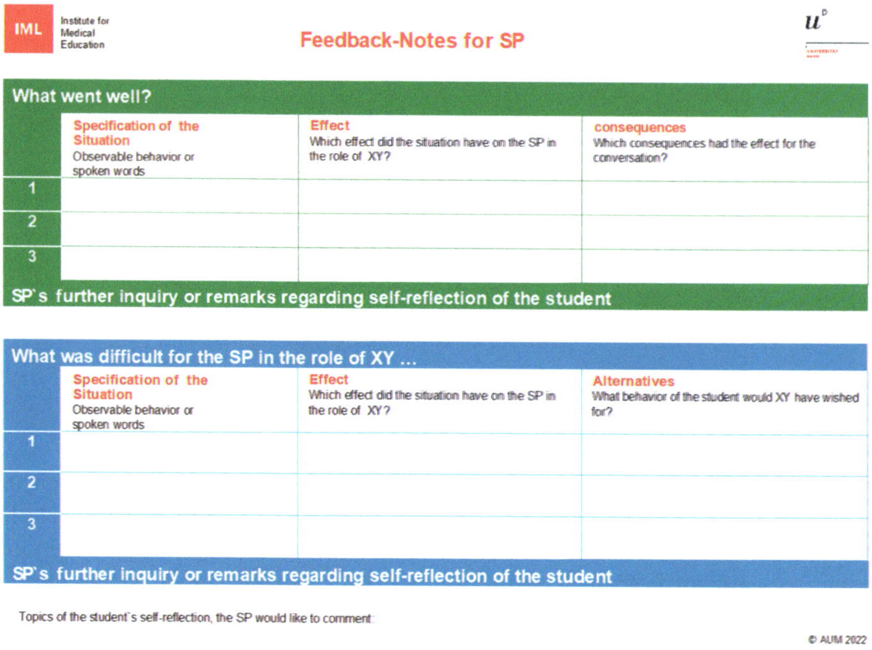
IML Institute for Medical Education

Feedback-Notes for SP

What went well?

	Specification of the Situation Observable behavior or spoken words	Effect Which effect did the situation have on the SP in the role of XY?	consequences Which consequences had the effect for the conversation?
1			
2			
3			

SP's further inquiry or remarks regarding self-reflection of the student

What was difficult for the SP in the role of XY ...

	Specification of the Situation Observable behavior or spoken words	Effect Which effect did the situation have on the SP in the role of XY?	Alternatives What behavior of the student would XY have wished for?
1			
2			
3			

SP's further inquiry or remarks regarding self-reflection of the student

Topics of the student's self-reflection, the SP would like to comment:

© AUM 2022

Fig. 29.1. Feedback-Notes for SP

Administrative Details

Description of the scenario	The 76-year-old patient has a left-sided residual hemiparesis of the arm and leg, and a homonymous hemianopsia to the left, following a stroke with hospitalization and rehabilitation. The patient is meeting the doctor for follow-up bloodwork. The doctor will also take the opportunity of today's visit to disclose the patient's (current) unfitness to drive.
Setting	Family doctor's office
Event format	Multi-station communication training, 15-min encounter, 15-min feedback (incl. feedback preparation)
Learning objectives	The simulation's learning objective is the ability to deliver bad news according to a six-step approach (modified SPIKES model [1]): 1. Setting up the conversation (cannot be practiced in this actual simulation, since the time for setup already passed, when the simulation starts) 2. Determining the previous knowledge of the patient while paying attention to the emotional content of the patient's answers to the inquiry 3. Asking if the patient is ready for a discussion 4. Sharing the information 5. Providing emotional support 6. Establishing a plan and follow-up
Preparation material for students	1. Minichiello TA, Ling D, Ucci DK. Breaking Bad News: A Practical Approach for the Hospitalist, J Hosp Med. 2007; 2: 415–421 2. Dias L, Chabner BA, Lynch TJ, Penson RT. Breaking Bad News: A Patient's Perspective. 2003 Oncologist 8: 587–596 3. Fallowfield L, Jenkins V. Communicating sad, bad and difficult news in medicine. 2004 Lancet 363: 312–319 4. DocCom (interactive learning resource for communication in healthcare) – Module 33: Giving Bad Newshttps://webcampus.med.drexel.edu/DocCom/db/readDocComDemo.aspx?m=33 (accessed June 11th, 2023) 5. ICAA's Guidelines for effective communication with older adults. Published June 2011 by the International Council on Active Aging. Available at: https://www.icaa.cc/business/whitepapers/communicationguidelines.pdf (accessed June 11th, 2023) 6. Backman WD, Levine SA, Wenger NK, Harold GJ. Shared decision-making for older adults with cardiovascular disease. 2020 Clin Cardiol 43(2): 196–204 7. DocCom (An Interactive Learning Resource for Communication in Healthcare) – Module 23: The Geriatric Interviewhttps://webcampus.med.drexel.edu/doccom/db/readDocCom.aspx?m=23#tree_node_name_730 (please note that in contrast to the module 33: Delivering Bad News, this module is only accessible with subscription to DocCom) 8. Chihuri S, Milelenz TJ, DiMaggio CJ, et al. Driving cessation and health outcomes in older adults. 2016 J Am Geriatr Soc 64(2): 332–341

Potential areas for feedback	• Establishment of a relationship according to steps 2 and 3 of the protocol before sharing the news • Information provided in a clear and factual way without preaching or moralizing, ensuring that the patient understands the risk of driving • Allowing sufficient time to be silent, talk, express concerns, and/or ask questions • Active listening • Identification of the cause of the patient's resentment regarding the information • Achieving patient's agreement by responding to their objections and suggesting possible solutions • Information about the physician's right to inform the authorities without appearing threatening
SP recruitment guideline	Age: should appear to be 76 years old Gender: any Other: no history of anxiety about aging, loss of physical abilities, or declining independence
Props	Walking cane
Wardrobe	SP can wear own clothes (appears neat but unobtrusive). SP uses a walking cane
Moulage	Not necessary
Room setup	Table and 2 chairs (student and SP); additional chair for observing peer
Adjunct materials	Piece of paper and pen for student's notes (optional); feedback form and pen for SP's notes

Instructions to Learners

Setting and task: You are simulating a family doctor, standing in for Dr. Werren, who is on vacation. You are about to see Jan Gerber, whom you have never met before. The patient is registered for an INR check today. The files reveal that the patient was discharged from a rehabilitation facility a few days ago, following a cerebrovascular incident. Because of a newly diagnosed normocardiac atrial fibrillation, the patient is now taking oral anticoagulation. As result of the stroke, Jan Gerber suffers from a residual left-sided hemiparesis and a homonymous hemianopsia also to the left. Apart from that, the medical history does not reveal anything remarkable.

Dr. Werren made a note in the file that you should inform the patient that they are no longer medically fit to drive. Moreover, the practice assistant points out to you that the patient almost hit another car in the parking lot when parking their car. After your introduction, your objective is to inform Jan Gerber that they are unsafe to drive.

You are expected to enter the consultation room/area where Jan Gerber is seated and start the conversation.

Instructions to SPs

History of Current Situation.

Your name is Jan Gerber. You are 76 years old. About 4½ weeks ago you had a stroke. Today you are going to see the doctor for a blood test. You have been told that your regular family physician is on vacation and you will be seeing another doctor.

You have been healthy all your life. You have never had a serious medical condition and almost think of yourself as "invincible." The stroke really surprised you as it came out of nowhere. Out of the blue, as you were sitting reading the paper in the morning, your left arm and leg were paralyzed. Fortunately, you were quick to realize what was happening and got your partner to notify the ambulance right away. You were taken to the emergency room. While in the emergency room, you noticed some strength returning to your arm and leg. After just 24 h, you were almost back to normal. Your 4-year-old granddaughter made a joke and called your stroke a "stroke of luck." You agree. It could have been much worse!

The doctors prescribed some new medications (you don't know the names):

- A pill to make your blood thinner
- A pill to manage your blood pressure
- A pill to manage your cholesterol

You spent 2 weeks in the hospital and another 2 weeks in a rehabilitation care facility and you came home a few days ago. You continue to have some weakness in your left arm and leg. You limp a bit when walking and sometimes stumble a bit, but you are using a cane for support. However, these symptoms don't really limit your daily activities, and in any case, it's quite handy that you are able to drive.

You recall that the doctors mentioned that your eyesight is limited on the left side, and this would be a problem for driving. True, you cannot see anything in the left side of your field of vision (e.g. objects lying around). You are not concerned, though, about how your limited vision may affect your driving. You consider yourself to be a very skilled and careful driver. You feel that if you just turn your head to the left more often and are very careful, everything will be ok. Since being discharged from the rehabilitation facility, you have been driving with no issue.

You were told to make this appointment with your family doctor to get your blood tested when you were discharged a few days ago. You expect that this appointment will be short. You are in a bit of a hurry as you must pick up your grandchildren.

Past Medical History

You have generally been in good health. You have never been in a hospital. (Note: For women, you were in the hospital for the birth of your two children.) When you were 34, you had an accident while skiing and dislocated your left shoulder, but this was handled through outpatient care and did not result in any residual issues.

Family History

Your father died at 73 from a heart attack; your mother died at age 80 from lung cancer. She had been quite a heavy smoker.

Social History

You are married and have two children. Your son lives near you and has two children (Nicole is 2 and Emma just turned 4). You look after your two grandchildren on Tuesdays and Thursdays and are available to drive them around on other days. You adore spending time with them. Your other child lives in another city, but she visits often, and you talk online frequently. Your partner has arthritis and occasional seizures.

You are retired. You previously worked as a real estate consultant. Being able to get around with the car is, and always was, crucial for your lifestyle. You and your partner live in a rural area and rely on being able to drive for daily activities, shopping, etc. You still travel to the theatre and concerts in town, about 20 km away. You and your partner pick up your two grandchildren twice a week to support your son and his wife. Public transportation is not an option. The public transport is limited in your area, the bus is on a 2-h schedule on weekdays, and it runs just three times on the weekends. Your partner is not allowed to drive, because of occasional epileptic seizures. You love where you live and can't imagine moving to an apartment in a crowded city. Just thinking about that makes you upset.

Opening Line

Let the learner initiate the conversation. Respond to their greeting. Then add:

> I'm here for a quick blood test, because of that pill I take that makes my blood thinner.

Affect, Nonverbal Communication, and Posture

You are relaxed at first as you are just anticipating a simple blood test. When the learner delivers bad news about driving, you become both sad and angry. This is reflected in your facial expression and body language (defensive posture).

As trained, follow the learner's cue. If the learner is empathetic, you may express sadness and loss to them. You may get upset. If the situation escalates to a point where a constructive conversation is not possible anymore, you may leave the room early. Otherwise you stay in the room till the learner ends the conversation (max. 15-min). The lines below are ideas of things you might say. Feel free to improvise your responses, based on the information provided in the SP role and the questions the learner asks you.

Other Things You Might Say

- After a few minutes, if the learner does not tell you that your license will be taken away, you can say things like:
  - *Is this going to take long? I have to drive over to pick up my grandchildren soon.*
  - *When can I expect the vision in my left eye to return to normal?*
- If the learner tells you that you are no longer able to drive, some things you might say include:
  - *Who do you think you are, a greenhorn like you, taking away my license?*
  - *But I've driven almost 50 years accident-free! I bet I'm a better driver than you!*
  - *Without a car there is no way I can manage my life!*
  - *Who will do the shopping then because my partner can't drive! I need to drive to a supermarket to get food.*
  - *How will I take care of my grandchildren?*

Considerations for Working with Older Adult SPs

As pointed out in the framework for working with older adult SPs [3], possible cognitive impairment and memory problems are a key consideration in working with older adult SPs. At the same time, communication training with scenarios focused on older adults is an important domain to keep working with aging SPs. In contrast to Objective Structured Clinical Examinations (OSCEs), in which standardization is crucial, communication training is often a lot more flexible regarding exact language used, and the scenarios allow for much more improvisation.

Having said this, it is important to keep in mind that memorizing critical moments during the conversation for feedback during debriefing is a key challenge in this format. Providing a list of potential areas for feedback can help guide the SPs' reflection after the scenario is completed. This list can be reviewed (and supplemented) during the SP training. Another template can be provided that allows the SPs to document and link a student's behavior during the simulated consultation to the emotional reaction and impact on the patient (see Fig. 29.1.).

Another consideration in older adult scenarios is that, for authenticity, these scenarios are simulated by older adult SPs, so they can draw on their own life experiences. As in other scenarios, special concerns with respect to ethical and psychological safety can arise from this practice. As Picketts et al. point out, it is not impossible or unsafe to implement this kind of simulation, but special care has to be taken in selecting the SPs, monitoring them during the simulation and debriefing them afterward [4].

Lessons Learned

- The scenario was developed as an example of BBN. Thus, the preparatory materials for the students were focused on BBN only (see preparation material for students, 1–4). The fact that communication with older adults requires additional considerations was missed by authors and lecturers in the initial version of the case.
- To successfully communicate in this scenario, students need instructions on communication with older adult patients as well as instructions on BBN. Thus, additional resources were added to the students' preparation material (see preparation material for students, 5–7).
- During the debriefing many students commented on the scenario as being "too easy" and "not being really about breaking bad news." Many of them did not realize the significance of the news for a patient in terms of losing autonomy and independence. They did not recognize the fear of aging and the emotions that arise from perceiving one's own body as not being able to perform tasks anymore that once could be taken for granted. Neither were they aware of the fact that not only declining health may lead to driving cessation but that also driving cessation, in turn, may result in adverse health outcomes. Considering the general age of the students and the fact that talking about aging and loss of physical capacities like driving can be a taboo topic in any context, lecturers need to make students aware of the importance of this conversation during preparation (see preparation material for students, 8).

Acknowledgement The authors would like to thank Andreas Born and Adrian Göldlin for their contributions in the development of the scenario.

Disclosure The authors operate "DocCom.Deutsch" the equivalent of "DocCom" at Drexel University in Philadelphia, PA, USA, in German language. "DocCom.Deutsch" was developed in cooperation with the team of "DocCom" at Drexel University.

References and Resources

1. Kaplan M. SPIKES: a framework for breaking bad news to patients with cancer. Clin J Oncol Nurs. 2010;14(4):514–6.
2. Pless AHR, Brem B, Woermann U, Schnabel KP. Using self and peer video annotations of simulated patient encounters in communication training to facilitate the reflection of communication skills: an implementation study. GMS J Med Educ. 2021;38(3):1–15.
3. Smith CM, Sokoloff LG, Alsaba N. Collaborative framework for working with older simulated participants (SP). BMJ Simul Technol Enhanc Learn. 2021;7(2):112–5.
4. Picketts L, Warren MD, Bohnert C. Diversity and inclusion in simulation: addressing ethical and psychological safety concerns when working with simulated participants. BMJ Simul Technol Enhanc Learn. 2021;7(6):590–9.

Goals of Care Discussions at End-of-Life with Families and Caregivers of Older Adults

30

Target Learner Group: Family Physicians

Kerry Knickle, Nancy McNaughton, and Anita Singh

Background

This innovative, experiential workshop was developed to help family physicians overcome identified barriers: (1) their ability to discuss and break bad news, (2) acknowledging suffering and impending death, and (3) talking to patients about suffering by allowing them the opportunity to engage in a difficult communication encounter with SPs in a supportive, facilitated environment [1].

Discussing goals of care with patients and families is an important aspect of caring for patients with life-limiting illnesses and is considered an essential component of high-quality care.

Scenario Overview

Max Goldstein is an 88-year-old gentleman living in a long-term care home who develops a sudden change in condition. The family doctor organizes a family meeting with his 75-year-old wife and 52-year-old son to discuss goals of care.

K. Knickle (✉)
Communication Matters: INESRA, Toronto, ON, Canada

N. McNaughton
Communication Matters: INESRA, Toronto, ON, Canada

Institute of Health Policy, Management and Evaluation, University of Toronto, Toronto, ON, Canada

The Wilson Centre for Research in Education, University of Toronto and University Health Network, Toronto, ON, Canada
e-mail: n.mcnaughton@utoronto.ca

A. Singh
University of Western Ontario, London, ON, Canada
e-mail: anita.singh@lhsc.on.ca

Key Session Information

Description of the scenario	A family meeting to discuss the goals of care for Max Goldstein, an 88-year-old man who lives in a long-term care home
Setting	Long-term care home's quiet family meeting room
Participants	Learners: family physicians in small groups SP: 2 SPs to play role of wife and son Faculty: facilitators
Age of SP	The SPs should appear to be the stated age of the role
Session schedule	Small group sessions are scheduled for approximately 45–55 min with 5 min to rotate between cases. This timeframe includes simulation (10–15 minutes) timeout discussions (5–10 minutes) followed by SP feedback immediately after the interaction (5–10 minutes) and facilitated discussion (15–20 minutes)
Facilitation	Each interaction is facilitated by an experienced palliative care physician and a facilitator experienced in communication and simulated participant pedagogy

Key Learner Information

Unique to this case is that Max is not present in the scenario. The encounter takes place between Max's wife, her son Peter, and the participant learner.

Max Goldstein is an 88-year-old Jewish holocaust survivor with metastatic lung cancer, diagnosed incidentally after an admission to hospital 6 months ago for pneumonia. He was not a candidate for chemotherapy or radiation due to his advanced emphysematous chronic obstructive lung disease and frail condition.

Mr. Goldstein was a heavy smoker for many years and has used bronchodilators for years to help his shortness of breath. He has had two previous episodes of pneumonia. At age 76, he required admission to a critical care unit and required ventilation through a tracheostomy for several weeks before he could be weaned off the ventilator. It took him months to recover. He said to his wife shortly after this hospital episode that he would never want to be intubated again, "no more tubes."

C. M. Smith et al. (eds.), *Comprehensive Healthcare Simulation: Geriatric Simulation*, Comprehensive Healthcare Simulation,
https://doi.org/10.1007/978-3-031-65742-9_30

At age 83, he began to get quite forgetful and was diagnosed with Alzheimer's. His condition deteriorated very quickly. He became totally disoriented except for remembering names of his wife Georgia and his son Peter. He had unsteadiness of gait and had frequent falls, one of which led to a fractured hip and hip replacement. He became quite agitated at night and began to wander.

His wife Georgia, and power of attorney for his personal care, had signed a Do Not Resuscitate (DNR) order when he was admitted.

Since his hospital discharge 6 months ago following his hip surgery, his condition has continued to deteriorate. He has been having more difficulty recognizing his family. He has been experiencing some pain in his back that seems to be controlled with morphine 5 mg q4h prn.

Three nights ago, Max developed a fever and increased chest congestion. You suspected aspiration pneumonia and started him on oral antibiotics. Today when you see him during your rounds, his condition has worsened. He has a decreased level of consciousness. He does not seem to be responding to the oral antibiotic. You give him oxygen 5 LPM by nasal prongs. He keeps pulling off his oxygen. You cannot provide any aggressive treatment including IV antibiotics in your facility.

Today you will be meeting with Georgia and Peter in the long-term care home's quiet family meeting room, to discuss Max's condition and goals of care.

Learning Objectives

- Communicate and discuss end-of-life decision-making that is sensitive to issues of culture and religion
- Communicate prognosis and its uncertainty
- Demonstrate empathy and caring using verbal and nonverbal language
- Demonstrate an approach to effectively communicate with angry and/or challenging patients and family members

Facilitation

The facilitator in each small group will support and guide a faltering participant to:

- Acknowledge the thoughts and perspective of both Georgia and Peter
- Engage and respond empathically in the goals of care discussion
- Set ground rules for the heightened conversation
- Explore the common ground Georgia and Peter share in their love for Max and anticipation of his death

SP Role Description

Georgia Goldstein

You are 75 years old. You and Max have been married for 52 years. Max came to Canada after surviving the holocaust. Most of his family died in concentration camps. He talks about this rarely, but he has shared with his son how important the will to survive was at that time in his life and how he learned to never give up. Your son Peter has never forgotten those talks.

Max was a bus driver with the local public transit company for many years, and he retired at age 63 to pursue his carpentry and furniture building hobbies and his work as a volunteer driver for cancer patients. You did not work outside the home. Your only son Peter, age 52, lives in Barrie, 1 h from your home. Peter is married and has three children, ages 19, 17, and 16. Peter has tried to visit you and Max every month and speaks to you frequently on the phone.

You come to visit your husband today and find him very ill. He is agitated and less responsive than usual. The doctor wants to meet with you to discuss what is happening with your husband and the treatment options. You call Peter, who takes time off work to come to the meeting.

You realize how much your husband has changed. He is far from the man you married. You are aware that when he was well, he made it clear to you that he would not wish to go on in this condition. You also know he did not want aggressive treatment. You do not want to transfer him to hospital but want him to be comfortable and allowed to die in peace. Your son wants aggressive treatment. You don't know how to talk to Peter regarding your wishes for your husband. You feel if you do not agree to do further treatment, your son will never forgive you when Max dies. You have not told Peter yet that you have signed a DNR order.

Peter Goldstein

You are 52 years old. You live in a small town, an hour from your parents' home. You are married and have three children, ages 19, 17, and 16. You try to visit your parents every month and speak to your mother frequently on the phone.

You want aggressive treatment for your father. You remember that your dad talked to you about how his will to survive saved his life and that you should never give up. You feel the medical system has given up on him just because he is old. You haven't really thought about the issue of quality of life. You just think your dad's life should be prolonged for as long as the medical system can intervene.

During the scenario, Peter and Georgia are at extreme odds about Max's care. Peter is furious to discover the DNR order, feeling betrayed and helpless. He lashes out at Georgia and the physician, whose challenge is to listen, allows Peter to vent and express his anger. Georgia is fearful and anxious about Peter's reaction and needs support to share her thoughts and explain her position clearly.

Training Considerations

SPs are trained and oriented to the overarching objectives of the day so that they are familiar with the workshop goals, the case objectives, and any associated challenges. This ensures that the facilitators and SPs can support learning integration over the course of the day. It also provides important contextual information for the SPs about the cues or prompts they may provide and contributions they make.

It is critical that the training contains a logistics review of the pre-brief, the length of time in role, the number of portrayals, and the nature of feedback to be provided. See Table 30.1.

Revisiting the SP's comfort level with the original role expectations and the associated stamina requirements is a critical element. We have found that all SPs (including our older demographic) appreciate this attention.

When recruiting the SPs, the SP should appear the age of the role.

Debriefing

After the simulation, learners are asked to share their experience, followed by feedback provided by the SP who will also contribute to the large group debrief led by the facilitators. At the end of the day, all SPs meet with the large group to participate in a reflective discussion about what went well and what

Table 30.1 Logistics for the full-day workshop that includes the scenario with the Goldstein family

The day is designed as a formative experience. Participants are divided into small groups with an opportunity to both engage in interactions and observe their colleagues in practice. Each simulation is punctuated with time-outs and facilitated discussion over the course of the day. Smaller group sessions are scheduled for approximately 45–55 min with 5 min to rotate. This includes simulation (10–15 min) and time-out discussions (5–10 min) directly followed by SP feedback detailing the impact and effect that the participant's words and actions have during the encounter (5–10 min in length) and facilitated discussion (15–20 min). Each interaction is facilitated by an experienced palliative care physician and a facilitator experienced in communication and simulated participant pedagogy		
7:30–8:30	Registration, continental breakfast	An informal opportunity for participants to register, meet, and chat prior to session start
8:30–9:30	Pre-brief Large group orientation, communication skills review and discussion	Welcome and introductions • Orientation to simulation with Q and A opportunity • A short didactic introduction to challenging palliative care conversations and the associated challenges • A review of beneficial communication skills and techniques
9:30–11:15	Williams family conference (one portrayal each)	• A large group introduction to conducting a volatile family meeting on home premises • A participant volunteers to have the conversation with a facilitator present to support participants and highlight common challenges
11:15–11:30	Refreshment break	
11:30–12:30	Group splits into two smaller groups (pain management)	• The pain management scenario runs simultaneously in two rooms. (one portrayal each)
12:30–1:30	Lunch	
1:30–2:30	Group splits into four small groups: 2 scenarios—Robert Skinner/Max Goldstein	• 2 groups will encounter Robert Skinner • 2 groups will encounter Max Goldstein's family (two portrayals per scenario)
2:30–2:45	Refreshment break	
2:45–3:45	Return to four groups: Max Goldstein/Robert Skinner	• Each group will now rotate and encounter the role they have not yet seen
3:45–5:00	The whole group reconvenes in the boardroom with the SPs for wrap-up and evaluations	• A facilitated large group debrief and discussion • Overarching feedback from the SPs • An opportunity for Q and A • Lessons learned, uptake going forward • 10 min for evaluation

empathic skills and techniques they appreciated in their encounter with the participant. The participants share their experience and detail how they might integrate and apply what they have learned into their future professional practice.

Post-session

SPs are invited to follow up with the trainer and/or facilitators, or to request a further debrief if needed. Similarly, the trainer or SP facilitator may wish to follow up if they sense that the SP needs to talk about their experience. Follow up serves as a wellness check as well as a quality improvement opportunity for revisions to the scenario or the SPs' performance.

Considerations for Working with Older Adult SPs

The training for a case such as this involves initial storytelling with reflective opportunities for deep empathic understanding about how Max's life experience shaped both his own ideas and values and impacted the family's perspective. Although this approach is not particular to an older demographic per se, it allows all SPs latitude to appreciate emotional details prior to reading through the case.

An SP with more years of life experience can often bring a rich emotional depth to training. Their thoughts and ideas greatly contribute to the discussion regarding rationale for heightened or more moderate affect levels during portrayal. Anecdotally the older SP may have greater confidence to ask for what they need with less concern related to judgment, esteem, or embarrassment.

To preserve both the realism of this case for the learner and to avoid suspension of disbelief, it is critical to preserve Georgia's demographic for an authentic simulation experience. This brings credibility to the circumstance of the case and affords the participant greater ability to engage without distraction (i.e., SPs portraying Georgia and Peter appearing much younger than the case descriptors) [2].

Thoughtful consideration for physical and psychological safety of the SP portraying Georgia is also critical. Regard for the possibility that the older SP's own lived experience may be too close to the circumstances of the case, perhaps resulting in triggering memories, and vicarious suffering is an essential responsibility when recruiting and discussing roles with all SPs, paying particular attention to vulnerable cohorts [3].

Lessons Learned

This scenario is designed as a formative learning experience. No one sits down following these complex conversations about end-of-life care without achieving some measure of success. The SPs involved in this day walk away feeling valued for the contribution they have made for professionals caring for people like themselves.

Participants indicate in session evaluations that they benefit from both observing their peers in interactions and engaging in the simulation experience.

The weighted life experience of the older SP and their feedback are of enormous import to participants both as observers and participants. We benefit from the enormous privilege of engaging with older adult SPs who are experienced and confident portraying complex emotional affect and leveraging important experiential opportunities for the learner through simulation-based education.

References

1. Ambuel B, Mazzone MF. Breaking bad news and discussing death. Prim Care. 2001;28(2):249–66.
2. Knickle K, Weir K, McNaughton N. Authoring and othering: examining bias in scenario design. Int J Healthcare Simul. 2021;1(1):45–8.
3. Smith CM, Sokoloff LG, Alsaba N. Collaborative framework for working with older simulated participants (SP). BMJ Simul Technol Enhanc Learn. 2020;7(2):112–5.

Social Determinants of Health: Diabetes Management in Older Adults

31

Target Learner Group: Pre-licensure Baccalaureate Nursing Students

Nick Miehl, Calvin Miller, Emma Vick, and Jesika S. Gavilanes

Background

The Interprofessional Care Access Network (I-CAN) brings interprofessional teams of learners together to address complex healthcare needs of vulnerable and disadvantaged individuals, families, and populations [1]. The program focuses on care coordination in the community setting which often includes home visitation. Similarly, the Oregon Veteran Affairs Nursing Academic Partnership (VANAP) program seeks to train learners and expand the workforce of nurses trained to provide high-quality veteran-centric care across multiple and diverse care settings [2]. For learners beginning their clinical experiences in these programs, this scenario provides a formative, introductory experience to meeting with clients in the home setting, where resources and roles differ from other areas of practice, such as a hospital or clinic setting.

Learners prepare for the scenario by reviewing the client's chart from the clinic and reading faculty-selected articles and clinical documentation resources in advance of the simulation. On the day of the simulation, groups of 8–12 learners come together for a 15-min faculty-led pre-simulation briefing. Following the pre-briefing, two learners, in the role of nurses in the I-CAN program, take part in the 15-min scenario, interacting with simulated patients/participants (SPs) portraying John and Carol. The remaining learners observe the interaction via streaming video from a debrief room or classroom. A faculty-led debrief occurs after each encounter. SPs may provide feedback to learners directly or indirectly through faculty or SP trainers. After each simulation-based learning experience, learners are asked to submit feedback using a QR code linked to the Simulation Effectiveness Tool – Modified (SET-M) (see Table 31.1).

This scenario is used each term as new learner groups prepare for their clinical experiences in the I-CAN program. Learners have noted in their feedback how impactful it is to work with SPs in this context, including "Real patient actors contributed to a productive learning experience for me"; "I think using real actors made the simulation one of the most valuable ones I've ever done"; "Excellent and very helpful as we prepare for I-CAN experiences"; and "Helpful to learn that home health visits can go a different direction than expected and helping the spouse can be the priority in getting to the underlying issues that patient is facing."

N. Miehl · C. Miller · E. Vick (✉) · J. S. Gavilanes
Oregon Health and Science University, Portland, OR, USA
e-mail: miehl@ohsu.edu; millcal@ohsu.edu; vickem@ohsu.edu; gavilane@ohsu.edu

C. M. Smith et al. (eds.), *Comprehensive Healthcare Simulation: Geriatric Simulation*, Comprehensive Healthcare Simulation,
https://doi.org/10.1007/978-3-031-65742-9_31

Table 31.1 Description of the Simulation Effectiveness Tool—Modified (SET-M)

SET-M domains	Description
• Pre-briefing • Learning • Confidence • Debriefing	• The SET-M is a 19-item tool designed to evaluate the learner's perception of the efficacy of simulation-based learning experiences across four domains • The SET-M has a high degree of overall reliability ($\alpha = 0.936$) • Examples of the statements include "I am more confident communicating with my patient" and "Debriefing provided opportunities to self-reflect on my performance during simulation" • Data from the SET-M are reviewed quarterly for educational effectiveness, facilitator effectiveness, and process improvement opportunities

Note: Data for description of the Simulation Effectiveness Tool – Modified (SET-M) from [3] and Leighton, K, Ravert, P., Mudra, V., & Macintosh, C. (2018). Simulation Effectiveness Tool - Modified. Retrieved from https://sites.google.com/view/evaluatinghealthcaresimulation/set-m

Key Session Information

Description of the scenario	Carol Frazier (61 years old) has been referred for home nursing services by the social worker at the health clinic where she receives care. I-CAN learners are visiting Carol and her husband, Jack, for continued care coordination. This is the third in-home visit for Carol and Jack.
Setting	Carol and Jack's residence
Learning objectives	By the end of this simulation-based learning experience, learners will be able to: 1. Demonstrate therapeutic relationship application and rapport building with the family unit 2. Recognize personal feelings and bias 3. Adjust priorities and practice client-centered care within the community setting
Adjunct materials	• Client chart, with clinic notes • Relevant clinically related articles, including the Four Habits Model [4] and diabetes management in low-income populations • Documentation resources for I-CAN charting and SOAP notes • Observer questions for debriefing
Participants	Learners: • 8–12 learners per session • 2 learners interact with Carol and Jack, while the remainder observe. The learners all come back together for debriefing after the case Faculty/staff/SP: • One clinical faculty and one simulation faculty • One simulation operations specialist • Two SPs portraying Carol and Jack
Age of SP	SP should appear to be the stated age of the role
Scenario length	15-min
Session schedule	60 min: • 15-min pre-briefing • 15-min scenario • 30-min debriefing with faculty (can include SPs)
Room setup	Plain and sparse 1-bedroom apartment, tidy and clean (living room area only), screen off any other areas
Props	• Prescription medications on the table • Glucometer and insulin syringes • Empty test strip bottle • Lancets
Wardrobe for SPs	Modest, comfortable dress

Instructions to Learners

All the intake forms have been completed. Carol and Jack have identified the following goals.

- Carol wants to help support the family financially (feels stressed and unempowered), and she wants to be supportive of Jack
- Jack wants to find a job, stop drinking for good, and find ways to provide for his family's needs
- The previous nursing team suggested the next steps including continuing relationship building; investigating Carol's understanding of her diabetes and hypertension (HTN); and following up steps regarding employment status for Jack

Instructions to SPs

History of the Current Situation

Carol is a 61-year-old woman who lives with her husband Jack, 63, in a one-bedroom apartment. Carol has type I diabetes (insulin-dependent diabetes) and has recently had high blood glucose readings. The family is struggling to make ends meet and is unable to afford Carol's medications and supplies. Carol was referred to home health nursing by her clinic social worker; the nurse team made three visits to Carol, with Jack present each time. Jack is a veteran. Their daughter, Priscilla, moved away from home at age 16 and has not been in contact with her parents for over 20 years.

Current and Past Medical History

Type 1 diabetes, hypertension (high blood pressure), and hyperlipidemia (high cholesterol) medications:

- Lantus insulin multidose vial (clear) (insulin that works all day and she takes every morning)
- Regular insulin multidose vial (clear) (insulin she takes if blood sugar is high before eating a meal)

- Lisinopril, 10 m.g. po daily (medication for high blood pressure)
- Lipitor, 10 m.g. po daily (medication for high cholesterol)

Person's Ideas, Concerns, and Expectations

Carol: Carol understands that she needs to take her insulin to keep her blood glucose in a controlled range. She's not supposed to eat high-carbohydrate foods. She's been stressed, is not really paying attention to her diet, and feels helpless and hopeless. She is worried about finances. This worry impacts her buying the right kinds of foods based on her income. They are eating more processed foods, frozen dinners, and fast foods. She doesn't feel like cooking and doesn't feel like they can afford to buy fresh food. Carol is not checking her sugars; she ran out of strips a couple of weeks ago. She has been taking her insulin (she reduced her dose from 15 units to 10 units) and is feeling fine but doesn't know her sugar levels. Carol feels unempowered and wants to be supportive of the family. She's looking for a job too. Carol is demure. She frequently looks to her husband for guidance during the interview but answers questions when directed toward her. Otherwise, she is quiet.

Jack: Jack is more verbal and tends to dominate the interview. He may answer questions for Carol. Jack seems nervous and his left leg shakes. He has been unemployed for 6 months and his unemployment will run out soon. He was previously employed as a custodian at the local school for the past 5 years until there were layoffs due to budget cuts. Jack is depressed since losing his job. "After 5 years, they canned me. I had great relationships with the kids. Now look where we are…." Jack is interested in finding a job.

Jack interrupts Carol (e.g. she says "I don't really feel like cooking" and Jack says "You do just fine, it's not a problem…"). He's worried about Carol and feels bad that she doesn't have enough financial support for food and the management of her diabetes. Jack is depressed and has a history of alcoholism. Jack says he has been so worried and busy looking for work that he is skipping his AA meetings and is concerned about a possible relapse.

Opening Line

Carol: "Hi, come in. Please sit down; be comfortable."
Jack: "Hi, come on in."

Special Instructions for Portraying This Scenario

Carol and Jack dynamic:

- Carol seems sad, hopeless, and helpless
- Jack looks visibly anxious and talks over Carol a lot

Types of questions learners might ask:

- How low are you on your medications? How have you been feeling?
- Can you tell me what you know about your diagnosis of diabetes?
- What are your goals for our visit today?
- Do you have insurance coverage? Do you have a primary care provider?
- Tell us about your job search. What are the biggest barriers?
- What is your access to food like? Tell us about your typical diet.
- What do you use for transportation?

Ending the scenario: The scenario ends with Jack needing to go for a job interview and asking the nurses to leave so that he can use the computer downstairs for his interview.

Considerations for Working with Older Adult SPs

Before the Scenario

Asking the SPs involved in the case the way they prefer to communicate if there are follow-up questions after training and prior to the event date.

During the Scenario

Often earbuds are used for providing cues to SPs when they are performing in a simulation theatre. Making sure to test out the technology prior is important and especially when working with SPs who may have hearing issues. This tends to be more common with older adults but is certainly not true with all older adult SPs.

After the Scenario

Debriefing with everyone involved to see what went well and what areas can be improved for the future is an important practice to incorporate, as well as exploring considerations for the integration of SPs and feedback into the debriefing with learners and faculty.

General Considerations

Many SPs are hired as contract employees and may or may not have health insurance in connection to their role at a given facility. Therefore, it is important to consider the health and well-being of all SPs regarding physical and psychological safety. With COVID there was an increase in concern for older adult SPs due to age being a consideration for an increase of potential COVID complications.

- During COVID, operational safety guidelines and documents were created by many simulation programs that looked closely at multiple considerations. Some of the safety adaptations integrated during COVID are considerations that will remain under non-COVID operations.
- Some older adult SPs are at higher risk for in-person simulations due to potential comorbidities and their overall health considerations. This is an important consideration when SPs sign up for cases.
- Not all SPs have health insurance, and it is important for SPs to know what the case parameters are up front so that they can decide as to whether to participate and can be included as a consideration in recruiting for roles.
- Making sure older adults can see, hear, and feel comfortable with new technologies is important. This is true for all adults not specifically older adults but rather depends on people's level of experience and comfort.
- Explore with human resources and additional local avenues, such as retirement homes, for recruitment to an SP program if there is a need for additional older adult SPs on the team. This is also a consideration if directed and deliberate recruitment is needed for additional demographics within an SP program.
- Train on bias within cases and for teams to make sure not to perpetuate bias based on expectations or stereotypical social norms of various ages. In this case, having older adult SPs play older patient roles can lessen ageist stereotypes.

Lessons Learned

- The scenario is effective as a telehealth scenario with modifications.
- Occasionally, learners will want to separate Jack and Carol to speak with each individual but are not certain if they can in simulation. For observers, it can be hard to clearly distinguish the audio between the two simultaneous conversations. A pre-simulation orientation, including the logistics of the event, can help alleviate the learners' uncertainties. The separate conversations can be debriefed and explored further after the simulation.
- For SP pair dynamics, having individuals that know each other and can work well together is ideal.
- Having older adults in the roles versus younger people playing the part of an older adult is beneficial for authenticity and realism.
- Consider training remotely to reduce or minimize risk of people coming for in-person training when not necessary. This also saves reimbursement for parking and travel time.
- For remote training, it is important to make sure all SPs have the technology needed to be set up for success. Having technical checks prior to training and telehealth implementations is important for all participants to ensure a successful event.
- Safety considerations for physical and psychological safety are important for all SPs. Given the nature of the content of this case, it is important for the older adult SPs to understand what the case involves at the onset when signing up to participate [5].

References and Resources

1. Interprofessional Care Access Network (I-CAN) | OHSU [Internet]. [cited 2022 Nov 30]. Available from: https://www.ohsu.edu/school-of-nursing/interprofessional-care-access-network-i-can
2. VA Scholar Program | OHSU [Internet]. [cited 2022 Dec 6]. Available from: https://www.ohsu.edu/school-of-nursing/va-scholar-program
3. Leighton K, Ravert P, Mudra V, Macintosh C. Updating the simulation effectiveness tool: item modifications and reevaluation of psychometric properties. Nurs Educ Perspect. 2015;36(5):317–23.
4. Lundeby T, Gulbrandsen P, Finset A. The Expanded Four Habits Model—a teachable consultation model for encounters with patients in emotional distress. Patient Educ Couns. 2015;98(5):598–603.
5. Smith CM, Sokoloff LG, Alsaba N. Collaborative framework for working with older simulated participants (SP). BMJ Simul Technol Enhanc Learn. 2020;7(2):112–5.

Counselling Family Members About an Older Adult's Test Results and Treatment Plan

32

Target Learner Group: Master's Level Speech-Language Pathology Students

Lisa Guttman Sokoloff, Cathy M. Smith, and Regina Jokel

Background

For the most part, SLP students have limited practice sharing information with clients/families during their training. They frequently request more practice regarding counselling. Although there are accounts of Simulated Participants (SPs) working with SLP students [1–4], there is nothing specific to counselling.

For this session, learners worked in small groups (up to 12 learners); two SLP students collaborated to counsel family members, while the rest of the learner group actively observed and took notes. Students prefer smaller groups so they have more opportunity to actively participate. However, any configuration can be chosen.

This was a formative session; the assessment of student performance was informal by design as these students had limited experience with simulation. Students were debriefed, completed a final evaluation, and had the opportunity to reflect on their experience in their final course portfolio.

Immediately after the session, the SPs were debriefed in another room by the simulation educator who had trained them. They were asked to complete a written reflection that included opportunities to provide feedback about their experiences with the students and evaluate the interaction. This feedback was collated and forwarded to the session organizer by the SP educator and was also used to improve future processes. SPs did not provide direct oral feedback to the learners as, in our program, there have been very few opportunities for them to provide oral feedback. In other contexts where oral feedback is regularly trained and practiced, SPs could do so for this simulation.

While this scenario can stand alone, it was designed to take place toward the end of a 1-day integrated learning experience consisting of several components. Typically, this day includes didactic presentations about aging, facilitated small group work where the students review assessment findings from the client and develop a treatment plan, an in-person meeting with a patient and their family member, and the simulation. If run as a stand-alone exercise, students should be provided with assessment findings and a treatment plan by whoever is running the scenario.

This session has been run for several years, with overwhelmingly positive feedback from students. Students noted how useful and realistic it was working with the SPs and that the simulation "tied everything together." Comments included "I enjoyed the simulation because it was like what we would see in real life"; "The SPs were an amazing experience and the closest I've come to real world counselling experience"; and "Working with SPs was a great way to practice clinical counselling in a safe setting."

Key Session Information

Description of the scenario	Family member(s) of 77-year-old Janice Peters is (are) attending a meeting with SLP students to receive results of Janice's communication and swallowing testing and discuss treatment planning and next steps
Setting	Private outpatient clinic room in a memory disorders clinic

L. G. Sokoloff (✉)
Faculty of Applied Health and Community Studies, Sheridan College, Brampton, ON, Canada

Department of Speech Pathology, Temerty Faculty of Medicine, University of Toronto, Toronto, ON, Canada
e-mail: lisa.sokoloff@sheridancollege.ca

C. M. Smith
Baycrest Academy for Research and Education, Baycrest Centre for Geriatric Care, Toronto, ON, Canada
e-mail: CSmith4@baycrest.org

R. Jokel
Rotman Research Institute, Baycrest, Toronto, ON, Canada

Department of Speech Pathology, Temerty School of Medicine, University of Toronto, Toronto, ON, Canada
e-mail: rjokel@research.baycrest.org

C. M. Smith et al. (eds.), *Comprehensive Healthcare Simulation: Geriatric Simulation*, Comprehensive Healthcare Simulation,
https://doi.org/10.1007/978-3-031-65742-9_32

Learning objectives	By the end of this session, learners will be able to: 1. Share information about assessment findings and treatment plans with family members 2. Respond to questions and concerns from family members with appropriate information 3. Demonstrate supportive counselling techniques
Adjunct materials	• De-identified SLP report containing medical diagnosis, findings from the speech, language and swallowing assessments and a treatment plan for students (for this scenario the material was related to communication and swallowing; however, any diagnostic and assessment materials could be used, depending on the topic and/or profession of learners) • Other material might include a video of a client the case is based on for student and SP review, written language samples, etc. (review organization privacy policy to ensure confidentiality)
Participants	Learners: • 2 SLP students who lead the meeting • Remaining students in small group observe Faculty/SPs/others: • Facilitator(s) • 1 or 2 SPs portraying Janice's sibling and/or partner
Age of SP	SP should appear to be close to 77 years old
Scenario length	15 min
Session schedule	90 min total: • 30 min—briefing for learners; dry run/final briefing for SPs • 30 min—running of scenario, travel time to get to and from simulation rooms • 30 min—debrief of learners; separate debrief of SPs
Room setup	• Chairs at the front of the room; enough chairs for the SPs and the 2 students • Student observers sit in a semicircle facing the SPs and student interviewers
Props	• Students may carry notes/pen, laptop, tablet, etc. • Samples of patient's test results including swallowing X-rays as appropriate (e.g., in case students want to show to family) • SPs may carry questions and/or bring paper and pen to take notes during the session

Instructions to Learners

You have completed communication and swallowing assessments with Janice Peters and are now meeting with her family in an outpatient clinic room at a memory disorders clinic to share the findings. During her assessment, the client has requested that you refer to her as Janice. Janice is not here because she becomes upset about her situation and did not want to come to this meeting. She asked her family members to attend in her place. She gave consent for you to share this information with them.

In particular, you will:

- Discuss the results of Janice's speech, language, and swallowing assessment
- Discuss a treatment plan for Janice
- Respond to questions about what Janice's family can expect in the future

At any time you can call a "time-out" to reflect and/or discuss the scenario and next steps with the other learners.

Instructions to SPs

You are portraying the partner or sibling (any gender) of Janice (who is 77 years old). You are close in age to Janice.

Today, you are meeting with Speech-Language Pathology students in an outpatient clinic room at a memory disorders clinic. Janice has a progressive brain disease and over the last few days, she has had a thorough assessment at this clinic.

You are here today:

- To discuss the results of Janice's speech, language, and swallowing assessment
- To discuss a treatment plan for Janice
- To find out about what you can expect in the future

Janice is not here because she becomes upset about her situation and did not want to come to this meeting. She asked you to attend in her place. She gave consent for information to be shared with you.

History of Janice's Situation

(Information About Janice that You May Be Asked).

Two Years Ago

- Janice started to experience weakness and drag her right foot.
- She had tests and was diagnosed with a "progressive brain disease." You can't remember the name of it.
- The doctor said that it would get worse over time, affecting other things such as her ability to communicate.

Over the Last 12 Months

- Janice has started to have problems communicating, e.g., she has a hard time getting her words out and expressing what she wants to say. She will say things like "I know what I want to say but I can't get it out!"
- She has become increasingly impatient, frustrated, and withdrawn, e.g., she does not like to participate in conversations or social gatherings.
- Her family doctor referred her to a neurologist for testing at this memory disorders clinic.

Social/Lifestyle Information

- You were all born and raised in Toronto.
- Janice and her spouse have two children with whom they are close.

- If the SPs are Janice's spouse or siblings, you are retired. If the SPs are Janice's children, you are still working and raising your own families.

Past Medical History

- Janice's other medical conditions include a heart murmur and high cholesterol—both diagnosed several years ago and under control with medication.
- She tried a drug for her memory but had to stop it a while ago because it upset her stomach.

Your Ideas, Concerns, and Expectations

- It upsets you to see Janice this way.
- It's challenging and sometimes frustrating for you because you don't always know what Janice wants.
- You are concerned about what will happen to her in the future.
- You will do anything to help her.
- You are eager for any information.

Opening Line

Thank you for taking time to talk to me/us about my wife/mother/sister.

Special Instructions to SPs Portraying This Scenario

- You are wearing casual clothing.
- Students will be in small groups of 12; 2 students will present the treatment plan to you; 10 students and 2 facilitators will observe.
- The interview will last 15 min.
- If you are a pair of SPs, you will take turns asking questions. The order will be determined in training.
- If the student asks about something that you are not sure of, say "No" or "I don't know" or "I can get that information for you."
- If the student gets stuck and the facilitator calls a *time-out*, go into neutral. Do not engage in the conversation or make eye contact with the students. Pick up the interview where you left off when *time-in* is called again.
- Ask questions that flow from the student's behaviors. Do not drive the interview forward with questions if the student gets stuck. Quietly wait until they get on track again.
- You carry your list of questions and a pen if you wish to write down anything the learners might say. During the meeting, feel free to write any additional questions down or take notes.
- You may ask any relevant questions that come to mind. Feel free to use your own words. Here are some examples of questions that you might ask:

Related to the Diagnosis

- What are the test results?
- Ask for clarification if the student expresses something in a way that you don't understand, such as:
  - What does that word mean?
  - Could you explain that to me more clearly?
  - I don't have a medical background, so I'm not sure what that means.

Related to the Treatment Plan

- What is the follow-up?
- When will her treatment start?
- How will it help her?
- How many times a week will she have it?
- Where do I bring her?
- How long will she have this treatment?

Related to the Future

- Do I change anything about how I communicate with her?
- How do I help her?
- Is it better to have different people giving care or better for her to have a single caregiver?
- Who can I call if I am having problems?
- What happens if I can't cope anymore?

Considerations for Working with Older Adult SPs

Before the Scenario

- Screen SPs for comfort with subject matter and memory ability.
- Send the SP the scenario just prior to training.
- Train less than 1 week prior to the session.
- Training should be no more than 2 hours long with a break halfway through the session.
- Work with SPs to generate a list of possible questions. Write them down so they can take them into the room for use (as much as an actual relative would do).
- Simplify the quantity of role details.

During the Scenario

- Ensure that room is free of fall hazards and chairs are comfortable and accessible for SPs.
- Ensure facilitators face SPs when calling a time-in or time-out so SPs with hearing loss are clear when the simulation starts and stops.
- Ensure lighting is bright enough so SPs can read their notes.

After the Scenario

- Provide an opportunity for the SP to de-role.
- Provide an opportunity for them to give feedback to you about the session for future iterations of the session if appropriate.

Lessons Learned

- SP life experience being a caregiver of a family member with dementia helped to increase comfort with the simulation for both students and SPs.
- Modifications to the scenario design (e.g., allow for SPs to participate in pairs, simplify information presented, provide written questions) helped SPs feel more confident and allowed more experienced SPs to provide peer support.
- Incorporating SP feedback into training processes (e.g., they asked to see the video of the patient and this step was added in subsequent years) may have deepened the SPs' empathy and understanding of the patient and enhanced the authenticity of their role portrayal.
- Creating a written briefing guide for facilitators related to specific modifications for working with older adult SPs helped ensure a safe and effective session for all.
- This is good introductory session for students who are new to simulation and for novice SPs because of the low stakes and ability to partner/observe with other students/SPs.

References and Resources

1. Hewat S, Penman A, Davidson B, Baldac S, Howells S, Walters J, Purcell A, Cardell E, McCabe P, Caird E, Ward E. A framework to support the development of quality simulation-based learning programmes in speech–language pathology. Int J Lang Commun Disord. 2020;55(2):287–300.
2. Howells S, Cardell EA, Waite MC, Bialocerkowski A, Tuttle N. A simulation-based learning experience in augmentative and alternative communication using telepractice: speech pathology students' confidence and perceptions. Adv Simul. 2019;4(1):1–1.
3. Syder D. The use of simulated clients to develop the clinical skills of speech and language therapy students. Eur J Disord Commun. 1996;31(2):181–92.
4. Zraick RI. Standardized patients in communication sciences and disorders: past, present and future directions. Teach Learn Commun Sci Disord. 2020;4(3):4.

An Older Adult with a Malignant Melanoma: A Sequential Simulation

33

Target Learner Group: Plastic and Reconstructive Surgery Trainees

Marc Seifman and Debra Nestel

Key Session Information

Box 33.1 Key session information

Description of the scenario	A 70-year-old man presents at a specialist clinic with a skin lesion for management
Setting	Outpatient department
Learning objectives	After this simulation, trainees will be able to: 1. Identify key elements in a pathology report for malignant melanoma that guides management *(medical expertise)* 2. Outline priorities in the management of a patient with an upper limb malignant melanoma *(clinical decision-making and judgement)* 3. Demonstrate empathic communication with an older adult patient relative to the initial assessment, post-procedure care, diagnosis and treatment options *(communication)*
Adjunct materials	Competency statements Framework for patient-centred communication and for difficult conversations Referral letter Pathology report
Participants	Plastic and reconstructive surgeons in training
Age of SP	SP should appear to be the stated age of the role
Scenario length	Two scenarios—10 and 15 min
Session schedule	70 min for trainees
Scenario room setup	A consultation room with video capture facility—2 chairs, desk, pen and blank paper, cups, water bottle/jug, tissue box, hand sanitizer
Briefing/debriefing room setup	A meeting room—4 chairs for briefing and debriefing
Props	Malignant melanoma skin transfer
Wardrobe	SP dresses for a scheduled visit to see a doctor; shirt that enables easy access to right hand; recommend bringing a separate garment for the second scene
Others	• SP to have fair complexion • Given the very high number of older adults who have treatable skin lesions, SPs could identify with this patient role

Supplementary Information The online version contains supplementary material available at https://doi.org/10.1007/978-3-031-65742-9_33.

M. Seifman
Plastic, Reconstructive and Hand Surgery Unit, Peninsula Health, Frankston, VIC, Australia

Plastic, Reconstructive and Hand Surgery Unit, Eastern Health, Box Hill, VIC, Australia

D. Nestel (✉)
School of Clinical Sciences, Faculty of Medicine, Nursing & Health Sciences, Monash University, Clayton, VIC, Australia

Department of Surgery (Austin Precinct), University of Melbourne, Parkville, VIC, Australia
e-mail: debra.nestel@monash.edu

C. M. Smith et al. (eds.), *Comprehensive Healthcare Simulation: Geriatric Simulation*, Comprehensive Healthcare Simulation,
https://doi.org/10.1007/978-3-031-65742-9_33

Background

Melanoma is a subtype of skin cancer that is relatively common in Australia and is considered within the purview of plastic and reconstructive surgeons. A detailed understanding of the pathological aspects of the disease is therefore necessary for all plastic and reconstructive surgeons. Despite its incidence in the population, the ramifications of a diagnosis of melanoma can be devastating for patients. Accordingly, an appreciation of the factors influencing decision-making, as well as the communication to the patient, is critical.

It is expected that a plastic and reconstructive surgery trainee achieve a level of competence relating to an appreciation of these features, the formulation of a management plan and the discussion of these with a patient, within the early phase (first 2 years) of their training [1].

The aim of this sequential simulation is to enable a surgical trainee to combine their skills in the competencies of *medical expertise*, *clinical decision-making and judgement* and *communication* [2] in the context of a diagnosis of malignant melanoma and to compress elements of the arc of care to a single simulation session. A patient will move through several phases in their healthcare experience:

1. Initial assessment with GP or dermatologist and initial biopsy
2. Initial referral to specialist care
3. Formal excision and post-procedure care
4. Discussion of diagnosis and treatment options
5. Longer-term care

In this scenario, we focus on phases 2 and 4, but it would be possible to address other phases as required.

Trainee Preparation

Before attending the session, trainees are recommended to review:

1. The Calgary-Cambridge Observation Guide on patient-centred communication [3]
2. The SPIKES model for breaking bad news [4]
3. RACS Surgical Competence and Performance [2]

The scenario takes place in a consultation room. It is designed as a formative activity. Faculty may include plastic and reconstructive surgeons, general surgeons, general practitioners, nursing staff, or clinical educators all of whom have experience in facilitating simulations. Prior to the session, the faculty are sent the scenario document and the SP is sent relevant sections. SPs have been trained to portray the patient role prior to attending the session (see below). Immediately prior to the trainee arriving, there will be verbal briefings for faculty and SPs conducted by the faculty lead. The session lead is hereafter referred to as the facilitator. Approximate timings for the simulation activity are outlined in Box 33.2. The total duration of this simulation involving the trainee will be 70 min.

Box 33.2 Timings for the simulation session

Minutes		Who is involved?	Where?
0–10	Faculty lead briefs SP	Faculty lead and SP	Outpatient clinic meeting room
10–20	Faculty lead briefs session faculty (facilitator) including introduction to SP; SP has simulated melanoma (mole) applied to right hand	Faculty lead, facilitator and SP	Outpatient clinic meeting room
20–35	Trainee arrives and is briefed on the overall session and specifically scene 1: initial referral to specialist care	Facilitator and trainee	Outpatient clinic meeting room
35–45	Scene 1	Trainee and SP	Consultation room
45–55	Debriefing scene 1	Facilitator, trainee and SP	Outpatient clinic meeting room
55–60	Briefing for scene 2: discussion of diagnosis and treatment options SP has a bandage placed over mole	Facilitator and trainee Facilitator and SP	Outpatient clinic meeting room Consultation room
60–75	Scene 2	Trainee and SP	Consultation room
75–90	Debriefing scene 2 and the overall session	Facilitator, trainee and SP	Outpatient clinic meeting room
90–115	Faculty lead (if available) debriefs with facilitator and SP; otherwise facilitator debriefs with SP Removal of bandage and silicone mole	Faculty lead, facilitator and SP	Outpatient clinic meeting room

Briefing for Trainee

After a welcome and introductions, orient the trainee to the simulated environment, the structure of the session and the task. Briefly explore their experience of working with SPs. Invite discussion of the preparatory information, the learning objectives and the trainee's experience of the topic. Establish any specific goals the trainee has and invite questions. Pay attention to the psychological safety of the trainee. Remind the trainee that this is a formative assessment and that the video recording is for observation purposes. Offer start and finishing cues. Start with the specific briefing for scene 1.

Trainee Task Briefing for Scene 1: Initial Referral to Specialist Care
This is your initial meeting with the patient, Mr. John Smith, at the specialist skin clinic about the mole on his right hand. You have about 10 min to assess Mr. Smith and make recommendations as to what will happen next. Here's the referral letter addressed to the consultant (Dr Louis Henry) with whom you are working (Appendix 1).

Debriefing for Scene 1

While the PEARLS framework for debriefing will be used as a guide, [5] the facilitator is expected to be experienced in debriefing and may use variations. The SP is included in the facilitator-led debriefing and must be given an opportunity to share their experience of the trainee. As a sequential simulation, this will enable further flexibility with the framework leading into scene 2.

Trainee Task Briefing for Scene 2: Discussion of Diagnosis and Treatment Options
You have received the pathology report and are meeting Mr. Smith in a follow-up appointment where you will explain the results and propose a treatment plan (Appendix 2).

Debriefing for Scene 2 and the Overall Session

Again, the PEARLS framework will be used flexibly. Return to the learning objectives and any specific goals that the trainee raised during the briefing. Provide further opportunities for the SP to share their experience of the trainee.

Session Evaluation

At the end of the session, trainees complete a brief evaluation form that also facilitates their reflection on the session (Appendix 3).

The SP completes a rating form about their role and their experience of the session (Appendix 4).

The facilitator completes an evaluation form (Appendix 5).

Before leaving the session, the faculty lead, facilitator and SP meet briefly to discuss how the session went, what worked and what might be improved.

Faculty Considerations for Working with Older Adult SPs

Before the Session

- In recruiting the SP, consider someone with fair skin, likely 65–75 years—they need to look believable as 70 years (pathology report is age specific).
- Provide the written information in user-friendly presentation (e.g. larger font size to support visual changes with aging, hard copy to support any memory changes).
- Check SP's emotional comfort with playing this role.
- Provide training for role portrayal in advance of the session, on a different day to avoid fatigue and to give the SP a chance to think more about the role.
- During briefing, agree on a "safe word" so that they can stop the simulation at any time.
- Rehearse applying the silicone mole before the session (possible source: https://www.mentone-educational.com.au/simulation/clinical-skills-and-patient-care/wound-care/malignant-melanoma-small).
- Adjust any details of the SP role that make it easier for the SP to remember information while staying true to the educational goals.

During the Session

- Observe for the safe word during scenes and respond if used.
- Observe for any unexpected emotional response from the SP and pause the scene if necessary.
- Check in for psychological safety between scenes. The first debriefing may have surfaced something that needs to be addressed.

After the Session

- Ensure that the SP has de-roled—engage them in a conversation about what they might be doing after the session or some other conversation that is grounding.
- Remind the SP about encouraging everyone to have regular skin checks with their GP.

Box 33.3 Information for the SP

The simulation session will take approximately 2 h and will take place in the outpatient department.
The learners will be surgeons in training.
There will be a faculty lead and one other faculty member. You will meet the faculty on arrival and the trainees soon after.
There is a schedule that states what is happening, where, when and who is involved (Box 33.2).
You will be invited to participate in the debriefings after the simulations to share your experiences of the simulation.
The faculty member will ask you questions about your experience.
Dress as you would if you were going to see a doctor; wear a top that allows for easy access to your right hand/arm. You should bring a different top for the second simulation.
There will be two scenes in the simulation:

- The first scene is your initial meeting with a surgeon at the specialist skin clinic. It will last ~10 min, and the surgeon will ask you questions about why you've come to the clinic and will look at the melanoma we have placed on your right hand.
- The second scene is a follow-up meeting with a surgeon to explain the results of your test, diagnosis and treatment plan.

The patient's characteristics including overall demeanour and behaviour
You are **Mr. John Smith and aged 70**.
You are feeling a little nervous about your consultation although relieved to have an appointment. You've been worried about the mole on your right hand for a while now. You've had it for years but it's changed recently—it has become itchy and has grown slightly, becoming darker as well.
You're cooperative and able to answer questions that you've been asked. You're a bit light on the detail you give just because you're not that comfortable talking about yourself. If the trainee shows empathy to you and also asks you to say a bit more, you will start to offer more information. In scene 1, you'll have a small silicone mole on your right hand. In scene 2, you'll have a bandage over the mole.
The patient's questions
You do not have to state these questions verbatim and there's not a set time in the consultation to state these things. Remember that the surgeon is learning to explain complex information to patients and to have these difficult conversations. If you keep this in mind, then you'll probably find moments in the consultation to ask these or similar questions.
Scene 1
"Do you think it's serious?"
"How do you know if it's one of the dangerous skin cancers?"
"When will you be able to tell me if it's one of the dangerous ones?"
Scene 2
You're feeling nervous about the test result. If asked, you can confirm this.
After you've been told the diagnosis, **"Can you say that again. I didn't quite get that."** You're probably a bit stunned by the first message. While you've been thinking about it, now it's become a reality. You're not really processing information well.
"What does this mean?"
"Will I get through it?"
"What are my chances?"
The patient's ideas about the problem, their concerns and expectations
Ideas: You are aware that you are at risk for skin cancer given your fair complexion. You remember many hours spent outdoors without any sun protection across your lifetime—especially playing cricket and gardening. While you take care now with sun protection, it was not something that was really spoken about when you were younger. You've had the mole for years but it's changed and you're a bit concerned. You don't know anyone with "dangerous skin cancer" but you hear about it in the news.
Concerns: You are concerned that you may have one of the **"dangerous skin cancers"**. You're mainly nervous about how **"serious"** it might be. On a more immediate note, you're also concerned about your skin healing. It seems to take longer to heal now than when you were younger. You've heard your friends talk about skin grafts that sound "pretty awful".
Expectations: You will have the mole removed and tested to see if it is a dangerous cancer. At minimum, you'll probably have another appointment to have some stitches out and find out if it's cancer. You haven't really thought much beyond that.
The patient's history of the problem
You went to your general practitioner (GP) because the mole started to itch and change colour. The GP has referred you to the specialist skin clinic. You've had the mole for at least 10 years.
The patient's past medical history
You have some heart issues that if you're probed, you can call it by its name (ischaemic heart disease).
You also have high blood pressure.
You also have high cholesterol.
And you have type 2 diabetes (for about 10 years now but you manage it well through your diet).
If asked about medication, then you can pull out a piece of paper that you've prepared that states the names of the drugs that you take. We'll have this available for you at the session.
Here's the list of drugs—apixaban, atenolol, rosuvastatin and irbesartan.

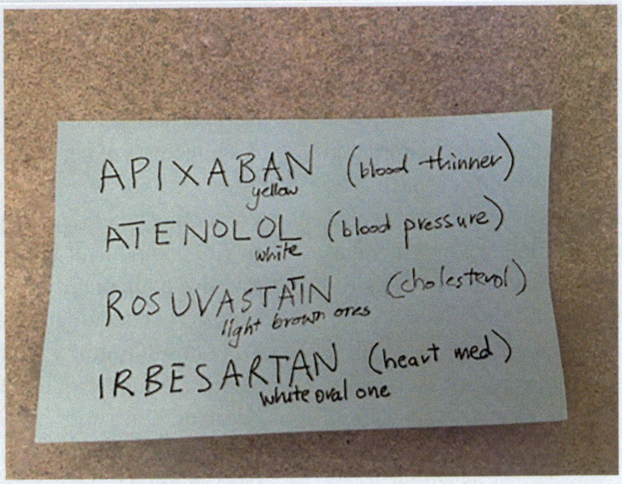

The patient's family medical history
Your father died of melanoma 20 years ago.
The patient's social information (work, lifestyle, habits)
- You're retired now.
- You're married and have two adult children who live in the city. You're making the most of this visit to spend a night with them in town.
- Your wife has come to the city with you. She dropped you at the hospital and she'll pick you up. She doesn't want to come in. She doesn't like hospitals.
- You were a teacher at a country high school for almost all your working life. You can decide on your subject area. You were also really involved in your local cricket club.
- You have a busy retirement with participation in many activities in your town.

Considerations in playing this role
- Please wear clothes that you think John would wear coming to the hospital—probably smart casual clothes. You might have a hat in your hand. Please bring a second shirt/jacket for scene 2 to help imagine that a couple of weeks have passed.
- You will be provided with a written list of medications so you do not need to memorize them.
- Since this simulation has a couple of scenes, it is important to try to remember what has happened in each of the scenes because they are intended to be linked.

Resources

Appendix 1: Referral Letter.
Appendix 2: Histopathology Report.
Appendix 3: Trainee Evaluation Form.
Appendix 4: SP Evaluation Form.
Appendix 5: Facilitator Evaluation Form.

Appendix 1: Referral Letter

Western Medical Centre

04/05/2021
Dr. Louis Henry
Peninsula Health
2 Hastings Road, FRANKSTON VIC 3199

Dear Louis
Re: MR JOHN SMITH
157 Sommerton Road, Westhall VIC 3759
DOB: 01/03/1955
Medicare number: 309487771
Telephone number: 0469386273

Would you kindly see JOHN SMITH for management of his newly diagnosed Malignant Melanoma of his right arm. I would appreciate you seeing him to organise a full clearance.

John has a significant past medical history of ischaemic heart disease, hypertension, hyperlipidaemia, Type 2 diabetes mellitus; and is maintained on Apixaban, Atenolol, Rosuvastatin and Irbesartan. There are no known allergies. John lives at home with his wife, is a non-smoker and is retired. John has a family history of melanoma, with his father having died from melanoma 20 years ago.

John presented for a routine skin check where I noticed a pigmented lesion on his right arm. He is unsure of how long it has been present for.

On examination, there was a 12 mm irregularly bordered and irregularly pigmented lesion on his right mid arm. The lesion was mobile. There was no axillary lymphadenopathy.

I performed an excisional biopsy of the lesion which has returned with a malignant melanoma. I have attached the histopathology report for your information.

Thank you for your opinion and management,

Kind regards,

Dr Vera Blain

Provider No. 0438965K

Appendix 2: Histopathology Report

SMITH, John

157 Sommerton Road, Westhall VIC 3759 **Phone:** 0469386273		
Birthdate: 01/03/1955	**Sex:** M	**Medicare number:** 309487771
Your Reference: Lab Reference: 21-394876-HIS-0		
Laboratory: HistAnat.		
Addressee: Dr. Vera Blain	**Referred by:** Dr. Vera Blain	
Name of Test: HISTOLOGY		
Requested: 02/05/2021	**Collected:** 02/05/2021	**Reported:** 04/05/2021

Histology

Clinical Notes

Partial excision. Bx right mid arm pigmented lesion? MM

Macroscopic Description

Specimen: Right mid arm. A skin ellipse 24 × 14 × 6 mm with an off centre ill-defined brown patch 14x12mm. TS-2A spp/adb (sb/jg)

Microscopic Description

Synoptic report – malignant melanoma

Site: Right mid arm

Thickness (Breslow): 1.10 mm

Level (Clark): 3

Architectural type: Superficial spreading with naevoid features

Predominant cell type: Epithelioid

In-situ component: Present

Invasive component Present

Mitoses per square mm: 1

Tumour infiltrating lymphocytes: Absent

Microsatellites: Not identified

Perineural invasion: Not identified

Lymphovascular invasion: Not identified

Ulceration: Absent

Regression: Absent

Associated naevus: Possible background naevus

Margins:

In-situ: Extends to involve a transverse margin in consecutive sections

Invasive: Extends to involve a transverse margin and is 3 mm to deep margin

Preferred block for molecular testing: B

Conclusion

Right mid arm lesion

Level 3 malignant melanoma, 1.1 mm thick, superficial spreading type with naevoid features, extending to a transverse margin.

Appendix 3: Trainee Evaluation Form

Thanks for participating in the session. Please take a few minutes to complete the evaluation form so we can improve the quality of the session.

To what extent did the session help you to meet the learning objectives?

Identify key elements in a pathology report for malignant melanoma that guides management *(Medical expertise)*	Not at all helpful 1	2	Partially helpful 3	4	Completely helpful 5
Outline priorities in the management of a patient with an upper limb malignant melanoma *(Clinical Decision Making and Judgement)*	Not at all helpful 1	2	Partially helpful 3	4	Completely helpful 5
Demonstrate empathic communication with an older adult patient relative to the initial assessment, post-procedure care, diagnosis and treatment options *(Communication)*	Not at all helpful 1	2	Partially helpful 3	4	Completely helpful 5

Please rate the following parts of the session:

The learning objectives were relevant to me	Not at all relevant 1	2	Partially relevant 3	4	Completely relevant 5
Overall, the preparation information sent before the today's session was helpful in preparing me	Not at all helpful 1	2	Partially helpful 3	4	Completely helpful 5
Overall, the briefing information immediately before the session was helpful in preparing me for the task	Not at all helpful 1	2	Partially helpful 3	4	Completely helpful 5
Overall, the simulation design was helpful in addressing the learning objectives	Not at all helpful 1	2	Partially helpful 3	4	Completely helpful 5
Overall, the debriefing was helpful in supporting my learning	Not at all helpful 1	2	Partially helpful 3	4	Completely helpful 5

What was the best thing about the session?

How can we improve in the session?

Please give any other specific feedback that you'd like us to know about any aspect of the session. (e.g., level of challenge for you, the simulated patient feedback, the time allocations, the facilitator's debriefing etc.)

List three learning points that you will take from the session.

1.
2.
3.

Please return the form before you leave.

Thank you for participating.

Appendix 4: Simulated Patient Evaluation Form

Thanks for participating in the session. Please take a few minutes to complete the evaluation form so we can improve the quality of learning activities. *[This is a generic SP evaluation form – Nestel D, Simulated Patient Evaluation Form, in Nestel D, Smith C, Harlim J. Module 2, https://learn.healthysimulation.com/course/spn-m2-creating-standardized-patient-roles]*

1. What do you think worked well in the session?
2. What did not work well in the session?
3. What role did you play today?
4. Did you need any further information during the briefing at today's session? Yes/No

   If yes, please outline.
5. Do you think the role had 'coherence'? *[That is, did the character, health issue, setting and learning objectives "hold" together?]* Yes/No

   If no, please outline.
6. What aspects of the role were challenging to play?
7. Did the learners have any unexpected challenges in the simulation? Yes/No

   If yes, please outline.
8. Is there any advice you would give to someone else playing this role?
9. Are there any other considerations in playing the role?

Please return the form before you leave.

As always, thank you for your contribution to healthcare simulation practice.

Appendix 5: Faculty Evaluation Form

Thanks for participating in the session. Please take a few minutes to complete the evaluation form so we can improve the quality of learning activities.

To what extent do you think the trainees met the learning objectives?

Identify key elements in a pathology report for malignant melanoma that guides management *(Medical expertise)*	Not at all met 1	2	Partially met 3	4	Completely met 5
Outline priorities in the management of a patient with an upper limb malignant melanoma *(Clinical Decision Making and Judgement)*	Not at all met 1	2	Partially met 3	4	Completely met 5
Demonstrate empathic communication with an older adult patient relative to the initial assessment, post-procedure care, diagnosis and treatment options *(Communication)*	Not at all met 1	2	Partially met 3	4	Completely met 5

Please rate the following parts of the session:

Overall, the communication before today's session was helpful in preparing you for your role	Not at all helpful 1	2	Partially helpful 3	4	Completely helpful 5
The relevance of the learning objectives to the trainees	Not at all relevant 1	2	Partially relevant 3	4	Completely relevant 5
Overall, the briefing for the trainee was helpful in preparing them for the task	Not at all helpful 1	2	Partially helpful 3	4	Completely helpful 5
Overall, the briefing for the simulated patient was helpful in preparing them for their role and for their feedback	Not at all helpful 1	2	Partially helpful 3	4	Completely helpful 5
Overall, the simulation design was helpful for this trainee in addressing the learning objectives	Not at all helpful 1	2	Partially helpful 3	4	Completely helpful 5
Overall, the debriefing was helpful in supporting the trainee's learning	Not at all helpful 1	2	Partially helpful 3	4	Completely helpful 5

Did you implement the session as outlined in the scenario document? Yes/No.

If no, what changes did you make, why and what was the outcome?

What was the best thing about the session?

How can we improve in the session?

Please give any other specific feedback that you'd like us to know about any aspect of the session. (e.g., level of challenge for you, the simulated patient role portrayal, the simulated patient feedback, the time allocations, the debriefing etc.)

Please return the form before you leave.

Thank you for your contribution.

References

1. Australian Society of Plastic Surgeons. Plastic and Reconstructive Surgery: Curriculum 2019. St. Leonards; 2019.
2. Royal Australasian College of Surgeons. Surgical Competence and Performance East Melbourne: Royal Australasian College of Surgeons; 2020 [Third]. Available from: https://www.surgeons.org/-/media/Project/RACS/surgeons-org/files/Louise-Pfrunder/Surgical-Competence-and-Performance-Framework_V16.pdf?rev=120ec964eb9e4c26a1f266eba17eaf79&hash=BA49820B4620667CA9F007C72856E346.
3. Silverman J, Kurtz S, Draper J. Defining what to teach and learn: an overview of the communication skills curriculum. Skills for communicating with patients. Oxford: Radcliffe Medical Press; 2013. p. 7–34.
4. Baile WF, Buckman R, Lenzi R, Glober G, Beale EA, Kudelka AP. SPIKES-A six-step protocol for delivering bad news: application to the patient with cancer. Oncologist. 2000;5(4):302–11.
5. Eppich W, Cheng A. Promoting excellence and reflective learning in simulation (PEARLS): development and rationale for a blended approach to health care simulation debriefing. Simul Healthc. 2015;10(2):106–15.

Telehealth Opportunities and Challenges: Recognizing Abuse of an Older Adult During a Telehealth Consultation

34

Target Learner Group: Third Year Medical Students

Melih Elcin

Background

"Communicating with Vulnerable Groups" is an elective course in the third year of a 6-year medical school. The students (max. 20) enrol in the 14-week course, experiencing 6 cases of patients from various vulnerable groups. The weekly topics include domestic violence (young housewife married with three children, a middle-aged divorced woman staying with her parents, an elderly woman living with her brother's family), elder abuse (three variations: neglect, psychological/verbal, and physical), patients with disabilities (hearing loss, visually impaired, patient in wheelchair), LGBTIQA+ patients, patients from underserved groups, and patients with a language barrier. Students have two sessions for each topic: one for encounters with SPs and one for debriefing in the larger student group.

Telehealth is an emerging modality in health sciences' curricula that had not been implemented in our program prior to the introduction of this scenario. Care of older patients and hypertension management had been studied recently, so telehealth was added to the elder abuse cases to present a challenging situation in delivering healthcare service for medical students [1–5]. This session, and the scenario, are the only opportunity for the students to experience and discuss telehealth in our medical school.

This education session is based on individual performances in communicating with and counselling older patients. The students have encounters with older adult SPs via online communication tools [6–8]. SPs do not formally provide verbal feedback to the students because of time constraints, but they are encouraged to share what they feel about the encounter with students if there is time at the end of the session. The students are debriefed as a small group activity and have the opportunity to discuss telehealth, communication with older patients, and alternately hypertension management and elder abuse, or both in some instances. As the students are in their preclinical years, they may have difficulty managing this situation. The debriefing sessions also serve as a type of formative assessment for the students, allowing them to gain insight into what they did more and less effectively.

The students have provided positive feedback on this particular session of the elective course as the use of telehealth is unique. The context of elder abuse in the scenario is often unexpected for most of the students, as culturally, in Turkey, older people living with younger generations in a family are regarded as a "gift of life" and are perceived to be well respected within the family. Health professionals do not usually think of or imagine a case of abuse in a regular patient interview, and are hesitant to ask a question to an older patient about abuse. However, this perception is also changing, and despite many cases of elder abuse not being reported, a number of them are, and this is becoming a recognized issue in the population [9]. This aspect of the scenario provides perhaps the most powerful educational experience to the students.

Key Session Information

Description of the scenario	A 68-year-old female patient, Canan Kara, is calling via an online platform to request an intervention to control her blood pressure
Setting	Telehealth service of a private hospital
Learning objectives	By the end of two sessions, learners will be able to: 1. Take the history of the patient suffering from uncontrolled blood pressure while using her medication regularly 2. Ask questions about recent lifestyle changes 3. Diagnose the possibility of elder abuse 4. Manage the case

M. Elcin (✉)
Department of Medical Education and Informatics, Hacettepe University Faculty of Medicine, Ankara, Turkey
e-mail: melcin@hacettepe.edu.tr

C. M. Smith et al. (eds.), *Comprehensive Healthcare Simulation: Geriatric Simulation*, Comprehensive Healthcare Simulation,
https://doi.org/10.1007/978-3-031-65742-9_34

Participants	Third year medical students 3 SPs portraying three patients (with variations in types of abuse) 1 faculty member to facilitate the debriefing session
Age range of SP	SP should appear to be the stated age of the role
Scenario length	10–15 min
Session schedule	10–15 min for each encounter in the first session 50 min for debriefing as a group in the second session
Room setup	SPs join the encounters from their own houses, sitting in the living room or kitchen via computers or mobile phones Students join the sessions from the simulation center via computers in outpatient clinic rooms

Instructions to Learners

You are the primary care physician on duty for the telehealth service of a private hospital today. Patients call the service and request intervention for a new complaint or any changes in their ongoing treatment processes. Your responsibility is to learn about the current complaint and take a brief history focusing on the complaint. You can manage the case on your own or refer the patient to another department.

Instructions to SPs

You are portraying a 68-year-old patient, Canan Kara. You were diagnosed with hypertension 10 years ago. You have been using amlodipine 5 mg daily so far to control your blood pressure. You have never had a problem controlling your blood pressure before. However, you have been having difficulties controlling your blood pressure for the last 4–6 months. You have a wrist blood pressure monitor. You take your blood pressure if you have a headache. You are having headaches a few times a week. You have recently measured high values such as 160/95 mmHg and 170/100 mmHg.

Today, you are calling the telehealth service of a private hospital to get suggestions for controlling your blood pressure. Your expectation is a change in the dose of your medication, or a change in your medication.

History of Current Situation

Part I: Common for Three Options

You are a retired primary school teacher. You were living in Sinop. Your husband, Celal, died 5 years ago. You have a son, Arif. He is married to Ayşe. They have a 13-year-old daughter, Sinem, and a 10-year-old son, Mehmet.

You were living alone in your house in Sinop. You had an active social life with your friends. You liked walking at the park next to your house every morning. You met with your friends two times a week at a coffee shop and enjoyed your time.

You were diagnosed with hypertension 10 years ago and have been using amlodipine, 5 mg daily since then. You do not have any additional medical conditions. You do not smoke, drink alcohol, and use any other substances.

Your son, Arif, told you that you were getting older and might have new health issues. He told you to sell your house and move into their house. Experiencing the pandemic alone made you accept his suggestion. You moved to Ankara 2 years ago.

You have your own room in the house, and you are happy to be with them. You do not have to clean the house, go shopping, or cook any more. You do not have any friends in Ankara, and their house is in a commercial district with no park around.

You have been experiencing headaches for the last 6 months. You take your medication regularly. However, you recently measured high blood values such as 160/95 or 170/100. Arif and Ayşe both work long hours outside the home. They are very busy, and do not have the time to take you to a clinic.

If the physician does not ask any questions about your daily routine, lifestyle changes, or your feelings and thoughts about your new life with your son's family, the interview will go on as a medical case. You will not mention anything about your family/social life.

Part II: Option 1 (Neglect)

If the physician asks any questions about your daily routine, lifestyle changes, or your feelings and thoughts about your new life with your son's family, you are expected to express or say any of the following (one at a time), in your own words:

- You feel upset and exhausted.
- You wish you had never moved here.
- You have a room in the house, but not in their life.
- You do not have a social life or friends here.
- You cannot go outside; you just read and watch TV.
- Arif and Ayşe come home very late, generally just say hello, but no more.
- Sinem and Mehmet come from school earlier but go directly to their room; there is no interaction.
- You cannot cook your own meals, and they add too much salt and prefer fried food.

You think all your loneliness, new style of diet, and lack of activity have impacted your blood pressure. You cannot talk to Arif about these things as you do not want to become a problem for him. You do not think you have any power, even the chance to change your life. You are trying to adapt to your new situation, and it is not so easy. You are open to any kind of medication, but nothing more (e.g. psychologist, family interview, social worker) as you are concerned what your family will think.

Part II: Option 2 (Psychological/Verbal Abuse)

If the physician asks any questions about your daily routine, lifestyle changes, or your feelings and thoughts about your new life with your son's family, you are expected to express or say any of the following things (one at a time), in your own words:

- You feel upset and exhausted.
- You wish you had never moved here.
- You do not have a social life or friends here.
- You cannot go outside; you just read and watch TV.
- You cannot cook your own meals, and they add too much salt and prefer fried food.
- You have a room in the house, but not in their life.
- You feel yourself alone, isolated, and desperate.

You stop talking at that moment and wait for 10–15 s as if you want to say something more but cannot talk. You are about to cry but you will not. Wait till the physician asks what happened; then begin to talk very slowly, sharing comments (one by one) in your words:

- Arif and Ayşe come home very late, and generally do not talk to you too much.
- Arif and Ayşe have guests at the weekend, and they do not let you stay with them. They want you to stay in your room.
- When Sinem and Mehmet are home, they want to watch TV or play games on TV. If you are watching TV at that moment, they tell you that you watch all day long, and it is now their turn. They want you to leave the room.
- When they come home with their friends, they also want you to go to your room.
- They sometimes go out for dinner as a family, but they want you to stay home.
- You feel that they are waiting for the day you will die—that you are a problem for them that they cannot get rid of. You should not have been here.
- You cannot manage this situation in your mind and heart.
- You think you need professional help.

You should give the impression that it is difficult for you to share all these things; these are your family secrets, very private and confidential and hard to share with a third party. You may come closer to the screen, use a lower voice tone, check your environment from time to time, etc. If the physician does not ask what happened, just wait for another 10–15 s, and then ask what their suggestions are for controlling your blood pressure.

You are expecting some suggestions from the physician such as psychological support (e.g. referring you to a psychologist or a psychiatrist) or a medication to relieve your feelings, support you in handling the situation, and clear your mind from bad thoughts and feelings. Any suggestion related to engaging your son and his family is unacceptable. This includes inviting them to negotiate your feelings or their behavior toward you; any appointments as a family with a professional to discuss the situation; and any legal professional support.

Part II: Option 3 (Physical Abuse)

If the physician asks you directly whether your life has changed so far, or whether you think your health issues are because of your new lifestyle, you tell them (one by one) in your own words, things like:

- You feel upset and exhausted
- You wish you had never moved here
- You do not have social life or friends here
- You cannot go outside; you just read and watch TV
- You cannot cook your own meals, and they add too much salt and prefer fried food
- You have a room in the house, but not in their life
- You feel that they are waiting for the day you will die

You stop talking at that moment and wait for 10–15 s as if you want to say something more but cannot talk. Wait till the physician asks what happened or if you are okay. You begin sobbing. When the physician asks whether you want to share what happened, you begin to tell them in your own words (one by one) what has been happening while you are still sobbing:

- While Ayşe and you are in the kitchen or when you meet each other at the door of a room, she pushes you but pretends it is an accident.
- Once, she pulled your arm very roughly (she said she was trying to help you), and you had pain in your arm for 2 weeks. In another instance, you had a large bruise on your shoulder.
- You sometimes think that you are exaggerating. However, this is all happening.
- You cannot talk to your son about it.
- You fear the situation may become more chaotic.

If they do not ask you to share what happened, just wait for another 10–15 s, and ask what their suggestions are for controlling your blood pressure.

You are expecting real help and an intervention from the physician (e.g. a referral to a psychologist, an appointment with a social worker). The physician may tell you that they suspect physical abuse and they must report this situation. If this happens you are both fearful and grateful.

Considerations for Working with Older Adult SPs

Before the Scenario

- Assess the SP's comfort with technology when working online (e.g. through a separate rehearsal with the online platform, comfort level with the type of device used, support from family members).
- Send the SP the scenario 1 week prior to training.
- Meet with the SP in the morning of the session and review the case.
- Work with the SP to generate a list of possible questions they may use or answers to possible questions.

During the Scenario

- Ensure the SP can comfortably portray the character, particularly in options 2 and 3.

After the Scenario

- Provide an opportunity for the SP to de-role.
- Provide an opportunity for SPs to debrief (schedule time after a session, provide phone numbers of trainers for additional support, create an online group where they can share their general experiences with other SPs).
- Ask the SP to provide feedback about what worked in the interaction or where there might be gaps in the information provided.

Lessons Learned

- There is the potential that this type of situation is close to the SP's own experience, so careful screening is required.
- It is important to provide the SPs with techniques to de-role and debrief as they can become psychologically triggered and experience strong feelings similar to what the patient experiences in this scenario.
- Older adult SPs may forget components of the scenario while portraying the elevated feelings/emotions.
- Experiencing the interaction via screen as opposed to being in person may lessen the SP's ability to portray a strong affect.
- SP feedback to students may improve the students' performance in such intense cases.

References and Resources

1. Şahin E, Yavuz Veizi BG, Naharci MI. Telemedicine interventions for older adults: a systematic review. J Telemed Telecare. 2024;30(2):305–19.
2. Bashshur RL, Shannon GW, Smith BR, Alverson DC, Antoniotti N, Barsan WG, Bashshur N, Brown EM, Coye MJ, Doarn CR, Ferguson S, Grigsby J, Krupinski EA, Kvedar JC, Linkous J, Merrell RC, Nesbitt T, Poropatich R, Rheuban KS, Sanders JH, Watson AR, Weinstein RS, Yellowlees P. The empirical foundations of telemedicine interventions for chronic disease management. Telemed J E Health. 2014;20(9):769–800.
3. Omboni S, McManus RJ, Bosworth HB, Chappell LC, Green BB, Kario K, Logan AG, Magid DJ, Mckinstry B, Margolis KL, Parati G, Wakefield BJ. Evidence and recommendations on the use of telemedicine for the management of arterial hypertension: an international expert position paper. Hypertension. 2020;76(5):1368–83.
4. Hoover RM, Polson M. Detecting elder abuse and neglect: assessment and intervention. Am Fam Physician. 2014;89(6):453–60.
5. Rosen T, Stern ME, Elman A, Mulcare MR. Identifying and initiating intervention for elder abuse and neglect in the emergency department. Clin Geriatr Med. 2018;34(3):435–51.
6. Smith CM, Sokoloff LG, Alsaba N. Collaborative framework for working with older simulated participants (SP). BMJ Simul Technol Enhanc Learn. 2020;7(2):112–5.
7. Harendza S, Gärtner J, Zelesniack E, Prediger S. Evaluation of a telemedicine-based training for final-year medical students including simulated patient consultations, documentation, and case presentation. GMS J Med Educ. 2020;37(7):Doc94.
8. Maynard K, Knickerbocker J. A telemedicine standardized patient experience: enhancing the virtual classroom and preparing for alternative modalities of care. Nurs Educ Perspect. 2023;44(3):181–2.
9. Gok Metin Z, Karadas C, Balci C, Cankurtaran M. The perceived caregiver burden among Turkish family caregivers providing care for frail older adults. J Transcult Nurs. 2019;30(3):222–30.

Part VII

Future Directions and Possibilities

Looking to the Future of Older Adults as Simulated Participants

35

Nemat Alsaba, Debra Nestel, Cathy M. Smith, and Lisa Guttman Sokoloff

Overview

This book was designed as a resource for anyone working with older adult SPs and/or simulation related to the care of older adults. We purposefully focused on integration of evidence-informed SP methodology practices, relevant clinical evidence of aging, and evidence-based care related to the care of older adults. In this chapter we focus on challenges and opportunities in (1) changes in the epidemiology of the older adult population, (2) increased focus on interprofessional and team-based clinical practice, (3) advances in technology-enhanced educational practices, and (4) shifting societal and educational values.

N. Alsaba (✉)
Faculty of Health Sciences and Medicine, Bond University, Gold Coast, QLD, Australia

Department of Emergency Medicine, Gold Coast Hospital and Health Service, Gold Coast, QLD, Australia
e-mail: nalsaba@bond.edu.au

D. Nestel
School of Clinical Sciences, Faculty of Medicine, Nursing & Health Sciences, Monash University, Clayton, VIC, Australia

Department of Surgery (Austin Precinct), University of Melbourne, Parkville, VIC, Australia
e-mail: debra.nestel@monash.edu

C. M. Smith
Baycrest Academy for Research and Education, Baycrest Centre for Geriatric Care, Toronto, ON, Canada
e-mail: CSmith4@baycrest.org

L. G. Sokoloff
Faculty of Applied Health and Community Studies, Sheridan College, Brampton, ON, Canada

Department of Speech Pathology, Temerty Faculty of Medicine, University of Toronto, Toronto, ON, Canada
e-mail: lisa.sokoloff@sheridancollege.ca

Key Messages

- In preparation for the exponential growth of the older adult population, it is essential to support health professions' educators, simulationists, and clinicians involved in the care of older adults. Older adult simulated participants (SPs) may provide some of this support.
- We anticipate future challenges and opportunities that may impact SP methodology when working with older adults including (1) changes in the epidemiology of the older adult population, (2) increased focus on interprofessional and team-based clinical practice, (3) advances in technology-enhanced educational practices, and (4) shifting societal and educational values.

Introduction

Throughout this book, we have offered guidance to design, run, maintain, and evaluate simulations for the care of older adults. The book offers tools, tips, and wisdom from experts. We have also shared scenarios developed by colleagues who work with older adult SPs. The trajectory of SP methodology targeting the care of older adults will likely be shaped by diverse factors. This chapter presents future challenges and opportunities that may impact SP methodology with older adults. These include:

1. Changes in the epidemiology of the older adult population.
2. Increased focus on interprofessional and team-based clinical practice.
3. Advances in technology-enhanced educational practices.
4. Shifting societal and educational values.

C. M. Smith et al. (eds.), *Comprehensive Healthcare Simulation: Geriatric Simulation*, Comprehensive Healthcare Simulation,
https://doi.org/10.1007/978-3-031-65742-9_35

Changes in the Epidemiology of the Older Adult Population

While the World Health Organization (WHO) defines an older adult as any person who is 60 years and older, [1] this definition is based only on age and does not consider other factors, such as physical or cognitive abilities. As everyone ages differently, older adults will present with tremendous variation in cognitive, physical, and sensory abilities that cover a broad spectrum of aging, health status, and level of frailty. Therefore, the perception of the term "older adult" will likely change.

Globally, older adults are living longer [2, 3]. Further, the effective management of chronic conditions and acute injuries has contributed to a cohort of older adults living well with chronic medical conditions and physical disability [4].

The scenarios in Parts 4–6 of this book reflect current common health and social issues affecting older adults (e.g., falls, delirium, dementia, elder abuse) [2, 5, 6]. As we get better at recognizing and managing these issues, and new conditions arise, priorities and focus will shift.

The COVID-19 pandemic disrupted every aspect of our lives, affecting society, health, well-being, economy, and education. Although we do not yet know the full impact of the COVID-19 pandemic on the older adult population, it clearly negatively impacted older adults' health, psychosocial status, and well-being [7, 8] resulting in a rise in social isolation, loneliness, long COVID syndrome, [9] and mental health issues. Although ageism and age discrimination have always been present in society, these were highlighted during the COVID-19 pandemic [10, 11]. Furthermore, since the beginning of the COVID-19 pandemic there has been a rise in depression, sleep disturbance, and physical deterioration in many older adults along with a reduction in quality of life, social connectedness and difficulty accessing services [7–9]. These changes will impact the future epidemiology of the older adult population.

The predicted epidemiology of the older adult population in the next decade will likely feature increased mental health issues, depression, loneliness, drug and alcohol-related dependency and illness, and long COVID syndrome. This epidemiology has implications that will affect the choice of simulation topics, the design and delivery of future simulations, and the roles that older adult SPs may be asked to portray.

Increased Focus on Interprofessional and Team-Based Clinical Practice

The multidimensional and complex medical and pyschosocial aspects of aging and frailty make it essential to ensure interprofessional care for older adults, their families, and caregivers to achieve the intended healthcare outcomes [12, 13].

To facilitate interprofessional and team-based clinical practice, we believe it is important to embed interprofessional simulations for the care of older adults into curricula for healthcare students and trainees. The challenges with any interprofessional education activity are well documented and often revolve around logistics such as staffing and scheduling [14] and rarely about the idea and concept of interprofessional education. In this book, we share two interprofessional scenarios (Chaps. 21 and 27).

Further, as we have emphasized throughout the book, inviting all relevant parties, including older adult SPs, to engage in the simulation from the conception phase is important in designing an authentic, collaborative interprofessional simulation that reflects the "real world."

We anticipate more interprofessional and team-based practices with more fruitful collaborations across care systems, including community, paramedical, prehospital, emergency, postoperative, acute, and rehabilitation care.

Advances in Technology-Enhanced Educational Practices

Technological opportunities will shape future simulation practices and impact research. For example, the use of wearable and eye-tracking devices can aid in generating varied forms of data for simulation research [15] which can positively impact the field. Since the rise and improved accessibility of generative AI (e.g., ChatGPT), [16] simulationists have been considering the implications for simulation-based education (SBE). Some have used AI to write learning objectives and generate debriefing outlines [16]. However, the intersection of AI, simulation, and the care of older adults is complex [17]. Some of these complexities are attributed to the challenges AI engineers face with regard to understanding the intricate nature of aging [17]. An example of the challenges with AI and the care of older adults that might impact simulation is the implicit bias in perpetuating gender and racial prejudices in healthcare data [17]. This issue reflects the existing societal biases, such as ageism, and can unfortunately lead to widening the gap of inequity and neglecting the needs, values, and preferences of older adults [17, 18]. All of these factors can impact the use of AI in the care of older adults, including using AI in simulation. AI is here to stay, so we need to use it responsibly, knowing the opportunities and risks. AI in SBE may be used to reduce workload in some tasks, such as generating drafts of learning objectives and debriefing outlines. This may ultimately help simulationists focus on other tasks that AI currently cannot achieve, such as debriefing. In the future, the simulation community should determine how best to leverage this new technology in simulation research and practice, including simulation for the care of older adults.

The book shares an example of simulation innovation and advanced technology (Chap. 13), such as virtual reality (VR), to de-escalate responsive behaviors for caregivers of persons with dementia.

Irrespective of the technological advances, we are confident that the need for human-based interactions, such as those we experience in older adult SBE, will not be replaced. Instead, they will be supported by AI and other emerging technologies.

Shifting Societal and Educational Values

Health disparities for persons of diverse socioeconomic, ethnic, racial, gender, and sexual backgrounds exist. Such disparities can result in bias, racism, and stereotyping, leading to poor health outcomes and compromising patient safety [19]. The same health disparities and their outcomes exist when providing care for a diverse older adult population [20]. Our scoping review [21] highlighted the need for more diversity in older adult SP characters and scenario context regarding culture, ethnicity, and social determinants of health. It also highlighted the lack of diversity in older adult SP recruitment. Addressing this gap requires a cultural shift and intentional efforts to explicitly showcase and embed diversity in healthcare training, education, and curricula [19].

The future offers simulationists the opportunity to design scenarios that includes diversity in both the contexts represented and in the recruitment of older adult SPs who portray the people in these contexts. Picketts et al. [22] noted that while educators have an ethical obligation to promote diversity and inclusion, we also have a responsibility to mitigate harm to SPs to ensure their psychological safety. Simulationists may consider using Purdy et al.'s conversational tool (SIM-EDI), [23] which prompts simulation teams to regularly reflect on equity, diversity, and inclusion (EDI) in their simulation program, allowing for ongoing awareness and growth.

Conclusion

We have positioned this book as a resource for educators interested in using simulation for the care of older adults. Our focus has been on working with older adults as SPs. Again, we remind readers that older adult SPs can portray roles such as parents, grandparents, siblings, caregivers, partners, and friends, which may open new opportunities for them. In Chap. 2, we noted that in some programs older adult SPs are recognized as members of the education team and co-creators of simulations and participate in research [21].

We hope the book prompts conversations with and about older adult SPs in all facets of SP methodology—education, training, and research.

References

1. Ageing [Internet]. Who.int. [cited 2024 Feb 1]. Available from: https://www.who.int/health-topics/ageing
2. Crimmins EM. Lifespan and healthspan: past, present, and promise. The Gerontologist. 2015;55(6):901–11.
3. Storey A. Living longer - Office for National Statistics [Internet]. Gov.uk. Office for National Statistics; 2018 [cited 2024 Feb 1]. Available from: https://www.ons.gov.uk/peoplepopulationandcommunity/birthsdeathsandmarriages/ageing/articles/livinglongerhowourpopulationischangingandwhyitmatters/2018-08-13
4. Molton IR, Yorkston KM. Growing older with a physical disability: a special application of the successful aging paradigm. J Gerontol B Psychol Sci Soc Sci. 2017;72(2):290–9.
5. Carpenter CR, Heard K, Wilber S, Ginde AA, Stiffler K, Gerson LW, Wenger NS, Miller DK, Society for Academic Emergency Medicine (SAEM) Geriatric Task Force. Research priorities for high-quality geriatric emergency care: medication management, screening, and prevention and functional assessment. Acad Emerg Med. 2011;18(6):644–54.
6. Hwang U, Carpenter C, Dresden S, Dussetschleger J, Gifford A, Hoang L, Leggett J, Nowroozpoor A, Taylor Z, Shah M. The Geriatric Emergency Care Applied Research (GEAR) network approach: a protocol to advance stakeholder consensus and research priorities in geriatrics and dementia care in the emergency department. BMJ Open. 2022;12(4):e060974.
7. Lebrasseur A, Fortin-Bédard N, Lettre J, Raymond E, Bussières EL, Lapierre N, Faieta J, Vincent C, Duchesne L, Ouellet MC, Gagnon E. Impact of the COVID-19 pandemic on older adults: rapid review. JMIR Aging. 2021;4(2):e26474.
8. Martins Van Jaarsveld G. The effects of COVID-19 among the elderly population: a case for closing the digital divide. Front Psychiatr. 2020;11:1211.
9. Mansell V, Dykgraaf SH, Kidd M, Goodyear-Smith F. Long COVID and older people. Lancet Healthy Longev. 2022;3(12):e849–54.
10. Barrett AE, Michael C, Padavic I. Calculated ageism: generational sacrifice as a response to the COVID-19 pandemic. J Gerontol Ser B. 2021;76(4):e201–5. https://doi.org/10.1093/geronb/gbaa132.
11. Silva MF, da Silva DSM, de Bacurau AGM, Francisco PMSB, de Assumpção D, Neri AL, Borim FSA. Ageism against older adults in the context of the COVID-19 pandemic: an integrative review. Rev Saúde Pública [Internet]. 2021;55:4. https://doi.org/10.11606/s1518-8787.2021055003082. [cited 2024 Feb. 18]
12. Brown DK, Graor CH, Chiu SH, Kidd L, Grand JA. The effect of a geriatric simulation-enhanced interprofessional education on health profession students. Clin Simul Nurs. 2021;61:33–41.
13. Balogun SA, Rose K, Thomas S, Owen J, Brashers V. Innovative interprofessional geriatric education for medical and nursing students: focus on transitions in care. QJM. 2015;108(6):465–71.
14. Fox L, Onders R, Hermansen-Kobulnicky CJ, Nguyen TN, Myran L, Linn B, Hornecker J. Teaching interprofessional teamwork skills to health professional students: a scoping review. J Interprof Care. 2018;32(2):127–35.
15. Eppich W, Reedy G. Advancing healthcare simulation research: innovations in theory, methodology, and method. Adv Simul. 2022;7(1):23.
16. Rodgers D, Ahmed RA, Misra A. Artificial intelligence in healthcare simulation: hype or hope. Int J Healthcare Simul. 2023; https://doi.org/10.54531/nzqf1198. Published online 2023

17. Abadir P, Chellappa R. Artificial intelligence in geriatrics: riding the inevitable tide of promise, challenges, and considerations. J Gerontol Ser A Biol Sci Med Sci. 2024;79(2):glad279.
18. Neves BB, Petersen A, Vered M, Carter A, Omori M. Artificial intelligence in long-term care: technological promise, aging anxieties, and sociotechnical ageism. J Appl Gerontol. 2023;42(6):1274–82.
19. Ibrahim S, Lok J, Mitchell M, Stoiljkovic B, Tarulli N, Hubley P. Equity, diversity and inclusion in clinical simulation healthcare education and training: an integrative review. Int J Healthcare Simul. 2023;10(null):1–4.
20. Providing care to a diverse older adult population [Internet]. National Institute on Aging. [cited 2024 Feb 2]. Available from: https://www.nia.nih.gov/health/health-care-professionals-information/providing-care-diverse-older-adult-population
21. Smith CM, Alsaba N, Nestel D, Sokoloff LG. Older adults as simulated participants: a scoping review. Int J Healthcare Simul. 2023;12:1–10.
22. Picketts L, Warren MD, Bohnert C. Diversity and inclusion in simulation: addressing ethical and psychological safety concerns when working with simulated participants. BMJ Simul Technol Enhanc Learn. 2021;7(6):590.
23. Purdy E, Symon B, Marks RE, Speirs C, Brazil V. Exploring equity, diversity, and inclusion in a simulation program using the SIM-EDI tool: the impact of a reflexive tool for simulation educators. Adv Simul. 2023;8(1):11.

Correction to: A Systematic Approach to Designing Scenarios Involving Older Adult Simulated Participants

Linda Ní Chianáin, Suzanne Gough, and Debra Nestel

Correction to: Chapter 3 in: C. M. Smith et al. (eds.), *Comprehensive Healthcare Simulation: Geriatric Simulation*, Comprehensive Healthcare Simulation, https://doi.org/10.1007/978-3-031-65742-9_3

The chapter was inadvertently published with the incorrect surname of the author. It has been updated as "Linda Ní Chianáin" in this corrected version.

In current print version:
Linda Ní Chianiáin
Updated author name to be included:
Linda Ní Chianáin

The updated version of this chapter can be found at https://doi.org/10.1007/978-3-031-65742-9_3

C. M. Smith et al. (eds.), *Comprehensive Healthcare Simulation: Geriatric Simulation*, Comprehensive Healthcare Simulation,
https://doi.org/10.1007/978-3-031-65742-9_36

Index

C. Smith et al. (eds.), *Comprehensive Healthcare Simulation: Geriatric Simulation*, Comprehensive Healthcare Simulation,
https://doi.org/10.1007/978-3-031-65742-9

9783031657412